RD

THE
COMPLETE
BOOK OF
WOMEN'S
HEALTH

GAIL CHAPMAN HONGLADAROM
RUTH McCORKLE
NANCY FUGATE WOODS

A SPECTRUM BOOK

Prentice-Hall, Inc., Englewood Cliffs, New Jersey 07632

Library of Congress Cataloging in Publication Data

Main entry under title:

The Complete book of women's health.

    "A Spectrum Book."
    1. Women—Health and hygiene.   2. Women—Diseases.
3. Women's health services.   I. Hongladarom, Gail.
II. McCorkle, Ruth.   III. Woods, Nancy Fugate.
RA778.C728   610'.88042   AACR2   81-17941

ISBN 0-13-158634-3 {PBK}

ISBN 0-13-158642-4

Editorial/production supervision by Cyndy Lyle Rymer
Interior design by Don Chanfrau
Medical illustrations by Dr. Charles D. Wood
Cover design by Jeanette Jacobs
Manufacturing buyer: Cathie Lenard

Chapter Twelve, *Women and Alcohol,* was excerpted with minor changes from
Estes, Nada J., Smith-Dijulio, Kathleen, and Heinemann, M. Edith: Nursing
diagnosis of the alcoholic person, St. Louis, 1980, The C.V. Mosby Co.

Prentice-Hall International, Inc., *London*
Prentice-Hall of Australia Pty. Limited, *Sydney*
Prentice-Hall of Canada, Ltd., *Toronto*
Prentice-Hall of India Private Limited, *New Delhi*
Prentice-Hall of Japan, Inc., *Tokyo*
Prentice-hall of Southeast Asia Pte. Ltd., *Singapore*
Whitehall Books Limited, *Wellington, New Zealand*

list of contributors

editors

Gail Chapman Hongladarom,
R.N., Ph.D.
Fred Hutchinson Cancer
Research Center
Seattle, Washington

Ruth McCorkle, R.N., Ph.D.
University of Washington
Seattle, Washington

Nancy Fugate Woods, R.N.,
Ph.D.
University of Washington
Seattle, Washington

contributors

Jeanne Quint Benoliel, R.N.,
D.N.Sc.
University of Washington
Seattle, Washington

Ann Birnbaum, Ph.D.,
M.P.H.
Former Director
Washington State Cervical
Cancer Screening Project

Jeanne Brooks-Gunn, Ph.D.
Educational Testing Service
Princeton, New Jersey

Laura S. Brown, Ph.D.
University of Washington
Seattle, Washington

Marie Annette Brown, R.N.,
Ph.C.
University of Washington
Seattle, Washington

Carole Browner, Ph.D.
Wayne State University
Detroit, Michigan

iii

Ann Wolbert Burgess, R.N.,
  D.N.Sc.
Boston University
Boston, Massachusetts

Nada Estes, R.N., M.S.
University of Washington
Seattle, Washington

Barbara Germino, R.N.,
  Ph.C.
University of Washington
Seattle, Washington

Marcia Gruis Killien, R.N.,
  Ph.C.
University of Washington
Seattle, Washington

T. Hongladarom, M.D.
Virginia Mason Medical
  Center
Seattle, Washington

Lydia Kotchek, R.N., Ph.D.
University of Washington
Seattle, Washington

Sharon Krumm, R.N.,
  M.S.N.
Ellis Fischel State Cancer
  Hospital
Columbia, Missouri

Louise Kruse, R.N., M.A.
University of Iowa
Iowa City, Iowa

Helen I. Marieskind, Dr. P.H.
Editor, Women and Health
Seattle, Washington

Bonnie Metzger, Ph.D.
University of Michigan, Ann
  Arbor; and Pennsylvania
  State University

Nancy Milio, Ph.D.
The University of North
  Carolina
Chapel Hill, North Carolina

Pamela Holsclaw Mitchell,
  R.N., M.S.
University of Washington
Seattle, Washington

Donna Moniz, R.N., M.N.
University of Washington
Seattle, Washington

Catherine M. Norris, R.N.,
  ED.D.
University of Minnesota
Minneapolis, Minnesota

Linda Peters, R.N., M.N.
University of Washington
Elliott Bay Health Associates
Seattle, Washington

Jean Reese, R.N., M.N.
University of Iowa
Iowa City, Iowa

Diane N. Ruble, Ph.D.
University of Toronto
Toronto, Ontario, Canada

Joan Shaver, R.N., Ph.D.
University of Washington
Seattle, Washington

Sherry Shamansky, R.N., Dr.
  P.H.
Yale University
New Haven, Connecticut

Barbara Sommer, Ph.D.
University of California at
  Davis
Davis, California

Karen VanDusen, M.S.P.H.
University of Washington
Seattle, Washington

contents

V

preface

In the past few years women have become increasingly involved in their own life situations and have sought opportunities to be active participants in national, state, and community activities. Most importantly, they have sought the opportunity of taking responsibility for themselves. To be full participants in the broad range of activities now available to women, their health has become of primary importance to them. In fact, women who have taken charge of many aspects of their own lives—their finances, their family relationships, their educational aspirations, and their careers—have recently chosen to become knowledgeable about their greatest personal resources, their bodies and their health. They want to know how and why their bodies act and react in certain ways and how to assess and manage many of their unique health situations and problems.

Traditionally, women have been rather passive recipients of health information and treatment, but the women's movement and the consumer movement have changed both the system and women to be more interactive partners. The health care system frequently blames its clients for their lack of "self-control," "willpower," and "compliance with treatment regimens." However, unless a woman believes that she is a full partner in the management of her health situations, and has been given all the necessary information in order to choose among the options that should be presented, she cannot exercise "self-control" or "willpower." So, it is not surprising that women have been poorly characterized by the health care system. For all too long, when women listed their symptoms and concerns when they entered the system, they were discounted and treated with tranquilizers, sugar-coated pills, and sugar-coated talk.

Rapid change has occurred in health care as a result of economic, legal, and humanistic pressures. Women are now more frequently believed, without having to rigorously prove that their symptoms are real and worthy of care and attention. However, the better informed women are about how to present themselves and interpret their health situations and concerns, the better able they are to be participants in their health care maintenance and management.

For too many years, information about women's health has focused—as has society— on a woman's reproductive system. This book presents for the first time an introduction to the broad range of health situations, concerns, and problems that most women face during their lifetimes. It is written for many people: women wanting to learn about the uniqueness of their health and how to manage or seek care for related problems; women who are beginning careers in the health professions; students in women's studies programs; and for men who are interested in learning more about the health of women.

Throughout history, women have managed and coordinated complex situations. Frequently they did so without knowing how great their accomplishments were. Today women have to, and are taking the opportunity to, manage their own health situations. For women just beginning in this new area, this book will provide the information they need for that adventure into themselves.

Gail Chapman Hongladarom

To my "family of orientation," my roots: *Ruby Gwendolyn Ironside*, my mother, and *Leslie Kenneth Douglas Chapman*, my father;
To my "family of procreation"; *Ty Hongladarom*, my husband, *John Grawn Hongladarom*, my son, and *Nuan Gail Hongladarom*, my daughter;
To my "fictive family": *Thelma Mary Melder*, and *Max McDonough Allison*, *Mark Melder Allison*, and *Mary McDonough Allison*.

Gail Chapman Hongladarom

To *Dr. Helen S. Grayum*, a friend, teacher, and scholar.

Ruth McCorkle

To my foremothers: *Mary Magdalene, Anna Laura, and Elizabeth Magdalene;*
To my sisters: *Susan Mary, Elisabeth Jane, and Patricia Jean;* and
To my daughter: *Erin Elizabeth.*

Nancy Fugate Woods

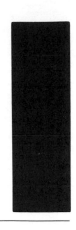

AN INTRODUCTION
TO WOMEN'S HEALTH

GAIL HONGLADAROM, R.N., Ph.D.

wellness for women

Women are the majority users of health care, and women also comprise the majority of workers in the health care system. We will be discussing the reasons behind both facts throughout this book. As consumers of health care, women are the primary users of the system for themselves and for their family members. The health needs of women require a comprehensive approach from early health education in elementary schools to women's health clinics, which provide appropriate services for women in the middle years and beyond. This comprehensive approach must not forget the needs of thousands of women who are the majority of the occupants in nursing homes. These women especially need and deserve good health care, not substandard warehousing.

Approximately 75 percent of health workers are women, yet women are under-represented at all levels of decision-making in the health care system. They face special and unique barriers to becoming leaders in the health industry. These psychological, social, and organizational barriers, which a woman teacher of management discussed in her book, *Making It In Management*, are very pertinent to women who must be able to manage their own health as well as to women health workers who want to move up the health career ladder. Perhaps, when we overcome these barriers, especially our lack of acceptance as women, and also come to like ourselves as women, we will have made a great step toward an increased state of wellness. When more women know about, understand, accept, and protect their bodies and the attendant functions as part of their total womanhood, we will be much more able to be full participants in decisions about our health care. Knowledge and information about our bodies—how they work, how and why they break down, how they can be protected, and, when needed, how they can be treated, is what all women need in order to bring their health choices and decisions into operation.

our health situations

In spite of the fact that women and the female role appear to be under lifelong surveillance by the health and medical system, women generally have not had the opportunity to learn how to manage their own health situations and concerns. The situations that bring most women into contact with the health care system are related to the female reproductive system. When women seek care, it most frequently involves menstruation, fertility control, abortion, pregnancy, or the menopause. The system of medical specialities has contributed to health care for women from two types of practitioners. Women may visit the obstetrician/gynecologist on a regular, continuing basis throughout their life-spans for health needs related to the reproductive system. They take other health problems to general practitioners or internists. Men tend to have one central care provider, and they go to medical subspecialists such as a heart specialist only when needed; even this is usually coordinated through the primary care provider. This division of care for women makes it all the more vital that they be informed about their treatment. If and when medicines are prescribed, women must know what they are so they can inform their other care providers and can avoid treatments that may not work well when combined with other treatments or medicines.

Health situations related to menstruation, fertility control, abortion, pregnancy, and the menopause have put women into a situation of being "done to" rather than encouraging us to be self-reliant, good managers of our health. Traditionally, the young girl with cramps is taken to the physician, and she has things "done to" her, such as pills, prescriptions for rest, or perhaps tests and other procedures. She could be taught how to manage this situation in a way that is much more conducive to her self-esteem as a developing woman, as well as in a way that contributes to her thinking of herself as "normal" rather than "sick."

The words *fertility control* should raise the question of "controlled by whom?" The answer should be "women," or is this, again, another health area in which women are "done to" rather than given information and encouraged to manage their reproductive functions? Women health care providers, women writers, and all women should adopt the words *reproductive management* rather than birth control, fertility control, or population control. Most women manage complex situations: a home, a career, a business, a transportation network, and/or a family in the broadest definition of that word. It is, therefore, sheer nonsense for them to turn over their very selves to have them "done to" rather than manage this part of living. Women manage for themselves, and frequently for one or two other persons, payment of bills, gas tank fill-ups, immunization visits, dental checkups, food, nutrition, warmth, and shelter needs. Why, then, do we abdicate managing ourselves?

Are we full participants in managing our pregnancies? Some women are taking charge of this aspect of their lives, but this is a very recent change, and, as yet, it involves far from the majority of women. Without sufficient valid information, women are not able to manage this special part of womanhood. Some later chapters will give women information to help them decide whether they, in fact, do want to become full partners with other care providers in the management of their own pregnancies.

As the life-spans of women increase, perhaps there is no phase we spend more time in than the "change of life," or the menopause. Many women are afraid of that time in their lives because they do not have the information that would allow them to manage the health concerns that occur during the years after age 45; women have long assumed that these health situations are related to meno-pause, but this may not be so. Although health classes on sex education and childbirth are frequently part of continuing education programs, rarely do we find classes to inform women about the facts of the menopause and how we can help ourselves manage the body's response to this health situation. A chapter later in this book talks specifically about these years to familiarize the reader with the self-assessment and self-management of conditions and concerns associated with the meno-pause. The term "self-management" is used many times in this woman's health book, and it must be emphasized that self-management does *not* mean that we diagnose and treat all our own health concerns and conditions. Self-management includes relating to a variety of health professionals—dieticians, nurses, physical therapists, physicians, and psychologists—to name just a few. The key idea is that the timing, degree of involvement, and inter-action with other health professionals in our health care are decisions that women can make when accurately and adequately informed.

health conditions and femaleness

Are some health conditions associated with being female? Women are fatter, sadder, more fragile, and more prone to suicide than men. Is this true? Or is that first sentence just another put-down of women? A significant chronic health problem of women in the United States is obesity. Being obese is nothing else but being fat. In spite of the cultural value put on thinness, 40 percent of women are classified as overweight. Whether this is because we are women, and whether this is related to physiology, or because culturally and socially women share a lot of other factors that lead to obesity are discussed in detail in a later chapter. It is, however, very important that we have information on the causes, effects, and management of being overweight. Being obese is uncomfortable and unhealthy, and whether it is unattractive depends on your personal views. The discomfort and the disease of excess fat should not be ignored by women in spite of those who promote the "fat lady's okay" kind of thinking.

Women can be depressed because they are too fat, and they can overeat and become fat because they are depressed. Depression is another health situation more common among women than men. Health studies show that women are more likely than men to be diagnosed as depressed. Admission data to state and county hospitals show that women are admitted more for depression than are men. In community mental health clinics, more women than men are treated for depression, and it is the formerly married female, now family head, who is most likely to be a depressed woman. This woman is very likely experiencing a large number of factors that definitely would contribute to depression. Whether the reported higher numbers for depressed women are real or whether they reflect additional instances of how women are categorized by a system and how we ourselves are taught by society to talk about our predicaments will be discovered only when sound investigations are conducted. Women investigators can bring a feminine perspective to these studies, and, in this way, the information gathered, as well as the findings, may be more likely to be free from the bias that has long been evident among male mental health specialists.

In 1974, Avery Weissman published the findings of an extensive survey of suicide attempts in the years 1960-1971. His study showed that those who attempted suicide were predominantly women in the 20-to-30 decade of life. The tragedy of women living in such social or physical pain that to end their lives becomes their only relief should be a number-one priority of the women's health movement as well as of the nation's mental health system. The causes—physical, social, economic, mental, and spiritual—must be investigated, and, here again, women researchers have much to contribute in addition to their scientific competency. Women who are not able to help solve this mental health puzzle through research can work with community and federal agencies and lobby for funds for women's mental health. Wellness in women is something we all can work toward whether it be as a health professional, an active community worker, or as a prod to the mental health system. Women who work or volunteer in support groups for women are another significant resource as we try to resolve the painful situations that lead to depression and suicide in women. Information about these support groups and other unique features of the women's health network are found later in this book in chapter 25 by Dr. Laura Brown and chapter 28 by Dr. Helen Marieskind.

do women break more easily than men?

If the question that introduces this section is asking about the brittleness of women's bones, which leads to many hip and wrist fractures, the answer is "yes." This is not because women are clumsy or skeletal weaklings, but because a bone condition known as osteoporosis (osteo = bone, porous = spongelike) is found more frequently in women than in men. Few women have probably even heard the word, let alone know that they are more likely to encounter the health condition, and, perhaps even more important, few know the preventive steps they can take and the treatments that are available. To maintain the strength of the body, we need access to information about osteoporosis; perhaps we even could benefit from learning "how to fall" to prevent the hip and wrist fractures that can result when brittle bones hit hard surfaces that cannot absorb the impact. (In chapter 21, this health condition is discussed in greater depth.) Awareness of this potential problem and information about preventive and protective measures can lead to increased wellness in women.

women's health—is it changing?

Women's health, like other complex systems, changes according to the things that happen to the system, as well as in relation to the basic strength of the system and the care and maintenance it receives.

The basic health of women can be strengthened by better care for female infants in the days before their birth and good infant care following birth. Many available programs assure the best health start possible, and these are discussed in chapter 16. Changes in the environment in which women live, work, and relax affect our health. New chemicals enter our environment much faster than they can be studied for their long-term effects. We must arm ourselves with this information and avoid exposure to chemicals when their potential risk is known. In addition, when we seek health care, we must be certain that we inform the nurse or physician who is taking the health history about the jobs we have had and the places we have worked that might provide clues to possible unhealthy exposure. If we have a hobby or leisure activity that brings us into contact with special substances that might be damaging, it is also important that we give such information to health professionals.

There are changes needed in the care and maintenance we give ourselves. More women must know about personal needs; nutritional needs and the need to reduce the stresses in our lives; the necessary exercise programs and "time away from it all," or leisure; and the all-important health care. Few women know all these things, which is why chapters in this book give you information about all of these topics—and many more that are vital for your wellness. Women's associations such as the YWCA have many classes on "how to care for and maintain your body." More women should attend them to help spread the information and increase our level of wellness.

Women's habits are changing and some, such as participation in volleyball, basketball, or soccer, are especially beneficial to health. The alarming increase in young female smokers, however, is not beneficial and will not let those women live longer, fuller lives. Lung cancer was once something men got; now, however, the cigarette ad that says "you've come a long way, baby" really means women have just about caught up with men—as far as getting lung cancer, anyway! Some people wonder if women will also have more heart attacks and other circulatory problems because we have begun to enter the "man's world" as far as stress goes. We need more information over longer periods to find this out. Cardiovascular problems may be more related to smoking habits than to the stress that the few women who have achieved middle or upper management positions now exhibit. Trends or patterns in the changes in

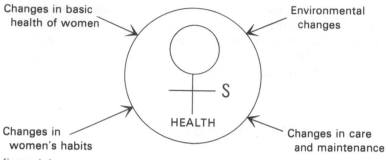

figure 1-1
shows the factors that lead to changes in women's health status.

our "health picture" and our health problems are looked at closely in the next chapter. As you read, think of yourself and how your health habits or activities have changed, or, perhaps, should change so that there can be more wellness in your life.

women seeking wellness

Many women believe that they and their health concerns receive different care and treatment from health professionals and the system than do men with similar concerns. Women very often report that they feel under pressure to prove that their symptoms or problems are "real." In fact, women may delay seeking care because they fear being told "you're neurotic; it's all in your head; get a hobby; do volunteer work; there's nothing the matter with you; it's your imagination." No one likes to have their credibility doubted, so women have developed ways of coping with these "put-downs." Often, to protect their self-esteem, they say:

"I know it's probably nothing."
"It's probably just nerves."
"My husband says it's stress."
"My boss says it's my age."

In this way, women play the game of using "anticipatory put-downs" of themselves to seem more credible or to jump the gun on the health professional who is liable to arrive at a similar, if not the same conclusion. Because confirmation of our self-esteem has traditionally come from others, we often anticipate what people's reactions to us are likely to be and adopt their assessment partly as our own. Women should not have to prove themselves as ill or as having "real" symptoms before a physician or nurse will listen to them thoughtfully and respectfully. We do not help ourselves as consumers of health care by using the kinds of excuses already mentioned, or by saying "I'm not as young as I used to be, I guess." A straightforward statement, such as "I want to find out why I have pain in my joints" or "I am not sleeping well and can't concentrate, and I want your opinion about these problems," is a useful approach when we seek care or consultation.

Most of our information about how women are treated as health care consumers in comparison to men has, until recently, come from casual comments, conversation, and anecdotes. But two studies (Armitage, Schneiderman, & Bass, 1979; Nathanson, 1975) did look at how we are treated in a more scientific way. In Karen Armitage's study, in the *Journal of the American Medical Association*, she reported her review of the records of men and women who were having male physicians investigate the following kinds of health problems; headache, backache, dizziness, chest pain, and tiredness. She concluded that male physicians took the problems of men more seriously. When a person goes to a physician with a health problem, for instance, a cough that lingers on for months, and the physician requests blood studies, a chest X-ray, a breathing capacity study, and a tuberculin test, that whole group of tests and studies is often referred to as a "workup." To discover if women's problems were treated differently from men's, Armitage, a physician herself, looked at the kinds and amounts of things requested in the workups of men and women who sought help for the same problem. She found that men received a more extensive workup for each of the five health problems, and it was even more extensive when men, rather than women, complained of low back pain and headache. Numerous ex-planations for these differences were considered and discarded other than the explanation that male physicians tend to take illness more seriously in men than in women. Women who know this are better prepared when they enter the system, and they should request a thorough workup if they believe their health concern has not been fully investigated.

Women do use the health care system more frequently than men, and this relates to visits concerned with pregnancy. Papanicolaou smears (Pap smears), and breast examinations. Women also live longer than men, and some people have suggested that perhaps women pay more and better attention to their health, seek health care more frequently, and thus live longer. Women report more physical and mental illness than men and utilize more hospital days than men do. This may be related to women's acceptance of the need to seek health assistance, whereas many men are taught to believe that they should "tough it out" on their own and only seek assistance when problems become extreme. Women may seek health care earlier than men and discover conditions and problems at an earlier stage, and therefore have more success in solving or managing their health problems—thus living longer lives.

arranging health care for others

In many cultures and for many centuries, women have arranged, managed, and provided health care for others. Women in the twentieth century have been responsible for the overall health maintenance and health management of their aging parents, husbands, children, life partners, and friends, as well as for themselves. Because they have a great deal of experience and a variety of contacts with the health care system, many women have become skilled navigators in this still relatively uncharted network. In our very mobile society, women have to use such skills each time they and their families move to a new place. Each health department, clinic, and hospital is different, which means that the woman who is trying to arrange health care must learn new ways to deal with or get around the rules and regulations.

In addition to managing health care for so many, women watch over what they and their families eat to make sure they are well nourished and that each person for whom they are responsible gets enough physical exercise.

Women frequently do all of these things *and* manage their own health, and they often carry on all these activities even when they are not feeling well or in the best of health themselves. Many women have been and still are the guardians of health for many people, and a number grow so accustomed to this role in the family that they continue the same functions outside by choosing nursing as a career.

women as health care providers

When some health problem occurs within a family unit, it is generally a woman in the family who cares for the sick or arranges for health care. Even when a woman is employed outside the home, she is expected to provide or arrange the health care. A man in the family unit rarely shares this responsibility and, if asked to, the usual response is, "*I* have to go to work, but *you* can take the time off." A woman's work is not yet considered of equal importance even though Department of Labor statements constantly remind us that most women work because it is economically necessary, not for self-fulfillment. It is very possible that the number of "sick days" working women request is not totally related to their own health situations, but because they must take some time off to provide or arrange for the health care of other family members. This use of women's sick time, however, is counted by government agencies in the overall total of women's "disability days" and may contribute to the conclusion that women are not generally as well as men.

Many women have had some structured preparation for the health care role through Red Cross home nursing courses. As recently as the 1960s, these kinds of courses were offered and, in some instances, required

through the physical education departments of many high schools. Young men in high school were rarely, if ever, a part of high school home nursing courses.

The play of little girls begins to socialize them toward providing care much earlier than the high school nursing courses. Little girls often receive "nurse's kits" for gifts, complete with white hats and thermometers; little boys receive "doctor's bags" with a stethoscope to drape around the neck and play doctor. Little girls are encouraged to develop nurturing, caring, serving ways very early in their lives, so it is not surprising that the nursing profession is at least 98 percent female. Men who do enter a health profession such as nursing usually rise more quickly to managerial positions than do women. Those positions are more frequently associated with the power and authority that women very much need to experience.

Health work is women's work in a real-life sense. Over 85 percent of all health service and hospital workers are women. Apparently little girls learn their lessons well and, through their low wage-earner jobs, they assist the health industry elite—physicians and administrators—to collect large incomes. Even though women work in great numbers in the health industry, they are usually clustered at the bottom of the hierarchy or decision-making ladder. The large numbers of women workers in the industry have little power or authority.

Women are still, today, the handmaidens of physicians in the health setting, whether it be as professional nurses, practical nurses, nurses' aides, or office assistants. This is not healthy for women—physically, mentally, socially, or professionally. The full participation of women professionals as respected and valued members of the health care team is the far healthier situation. Promoting and assisting wellness for people and providing care for patients and their families should receive society's respect and appropriate financial rewards from the health care industry. To achieve the goal of wellness for women, much more information must be available to all women about our specific health situations and our role as consumers, arrangers, and managers of health care. Finally, because so many working women are clustered in the health industry services, we should be aware of the ways in which the industry uses women

and decide whether this contributes to our goal of wellness. If it does not—surely the case—women should take action, now.

Armitage, K J., Schneiderman, L., & Bass, R. Response of physicians to medical complaints in men and women. *Journal of the American Medical Association* (May 18, 1979, *241 (20)*, 2186–2187.

Corea, G. *The hidden malpractice: How American medicine treats women as patients and professionals.* New York: Morrow, 1977.

Fenn, M. *Making it in management: A behavioral approach for women executives.* Englewood Cliffs, N.J.: Prentice-Hall, Inc., 1977.

Nathanson, C. A. Illness and the feminine role: A theoretical review. *Social Science and Medicine*, 1975, *9*, 55–62.

Proceedings of the international conference on women in health, June 16–18, 1975. Washington, D.C., DHEW Publication (HRA) 76–51.

Women and their health: research implications for a new era. Proceedings of a conference, San Francisco, Calif., Ed. Virginia Olesen, DHEW Publication No. (HRA) 77–3138.

Women's Health Issues. A report prepared for Wisconsin physicians on recommendations emanating from the Women's Health Issues Conference, Madison, Wisconsin, April 23, 1979. *Journal of the American Medical Women's Association* (June 1980), *35, 6,* 152–160.

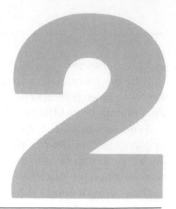

NANCY FUGATE WOODS, R.N., Ph.D.

women and their health risks—the paradox

One of the most fascinating observations recorded since the earliest investigations into incidence of disease is the paradoxical relationship between morbidity (illness) and mortality (death) rates for women and men. Although mortality rates for most causes of death are lower for wome ian for men, and women in the Western world live longer than men, women report more physical and mental illness and use health services at higher rates than men do.

mortality rates for women and men

The death rate for women of all ages in the developed countries is appreciably lower than for men. There has been a steady rise in the

Parts of this chapter appear in: Nancy Fugate Woods, "Women as Patients," in *Health Care for Women: A Nursing Perspective*, eds. Catherine Fogel and Nancy Fugate Woods. St. Louis: Mosby, 1981. Permission to reprint parts of this chapter granted by C.V. Mosby Co.

ratio of male to female mortality from 1930 to 1960 for each age group, indicating that the reduction in death rates was more rapid for females than males. Further, females held the highest ratio over males at ages 45 to 64 years and the lowest at ages 65 and over.

Relationships between mortality rates for

women and men in the United States parallel the patterns in other developed countries. Although more male than female infants are born alive, death rates for males exceed those for females at all ages. The female advantage in life expectancy has increased dramatically since 1900, and male life expectancy is now only 89.9 percent of that for females.

disparity in female-male death rates

The greater overall male death rate is attributed to a serious disadvantage for males reflected in most causes of death. An international comparison of death causes is limited by the differences in vital statistics for each of the countries as well as the social and economic habits of the population. Variations in death certificates come from the health habits of the people, the stage of illness at which health care was sought, the system of health care, training of health personnel, and the legal structure. To complicate matters, the countries may be using different versions of the International Classification of Disease. Also, the use of crude death rates (rather than age-adjusted rates) may be misleading due to the aging of the population. With these limitations in mind, we can examine some international comparisons of how the sexes fare. Excessive increases in mortality rates among males 40 to 69 years of age in 16 Western countries from 1930–1963 have been attributed to cardiovascular disease, cancer, and, to a smaller extent, bronchitis. Amount of smoking is a strong factor in the mortality change from these three diseases. Slight increases in female mortality rates for women 40 to 69 years may reflect a decline in mortality for women during the earlier childbearing years; since more women survive childbirth, more live to ages 40 to 69.

The age-adjusted death rates for selected causes of death in the United States for 1974 are shown in Table 2.1. It can be seen that the rates for every cause except diabetes mellitus show an excess of male deaths. And, if we restrict the comparison to white males and females, white males demonstrate an excess of mortality due to diabetes.

Although deaths from major cardiovascular-renal diseases have declined for men since 1940 and for women since 1920, the rate of decline has been greater for women. However, if we consider crude death rates rather than age-adjusted rates, we find a dramatic increase in cardiovascular disease for both sexes since 1915. Age-adjusted death rates for arteriosclerotic heart disease have also declined since 1950, although women retain their advantage.

Before 1950, women had higher mortality rates from cancer than men, but since then, cancer death rates have increased for men, with little change occurring for women since 1960. Lung cancer rates show a totally different trend: age-adjusted death rates from lung cancer have risen for both men and women, and the sex ratios have narrowed considerably since 1960 due to a higher relative rate of increase among females. The differences in death rates between the sexes for other disorders of the respiratory system (bronchitis, emphysema, and asthma) have also been narrowing since 1965.

The difference between sexes for death due to cirrhosis of the liver has been increasing slowly, and male incidence of suicide has increased from 1970 to 1973, even though the overall rates have declined slightly for both sexes since 1960. Death rates from homicide have increased for both sexes since 1960, but males continue to experience an excess of deaths from motor vehicle and other injuries.

Death rates from the infectious diseases of influenza and pneumonia have been fairly

table 2.1

age-adjusted death rates for selected causes, by color and sex: United States, 1974

Based on age-specific death rates per 100,000 population in specified group. Computed by the direct method, using as the standard population the age distribution of the total population of the United States as enumerated in 1940. Numbers after causes of death are category numbers of the Eighth Revision International Classification of Diseases, adapted 1965.

CAUSE OF DEATH		TOTAL			WHITE			ALL OTHER		
		BOTH SEXES	MALE	FEMALE	BOTH SEXES	MALE	FEMALE	BOTH SEXES	MALE	FEMALE
All causes		666.2	877.8	492.9	635.4	843.0	466.4	901.3	1,149.1	693.1
Major Cardiovascular Diseases	390–448	310.8	413.7	228.1	302.9	409.1	217.8	374.8	449.1	313.5
Diseases of Heart	390–398, 402, 404, 410–429	232.7	323.6	159.2	228.8	322.8	152.8	262.8	325.8	210.8
Hypertension	400, 401, 403	2.1	2.6	1.7	1.7	2.2	1.4	5.6	6.5	5.0
Cerebrovascular Diseases	430–438	59.9	66.5	54.9	56.4	63.0	51.4	90.9	98.3	84.7
Arteriosclerosis	440	7.6	8.6	6.9	7.6	8.7	6.9	7.3	8.2	6.6
Malignant neoplasms, including neoplasms of lymphatic and hematopoietic tissues	140–209	131.8	162.3	109.2	129.0	150.3	107.6	156.6	199.0	122.4
Accidents	E800–E949	46.0	69.4	23.8	44.3	66.6	22.9	58.5	92.3	29.0
Motor vehicle accidents	E810–E823	21.8	33.2	10.9	21.7	32.8	11.0	23.2	37.5	10.8
All other accidents	E800–807, E825–E949	24.2	36.2	12.8	22.6	33.8	12.0	35.3	54.8	18.2
Influenza and pneumonia	470–474, 480–486	16.9	22.6	12.8	15.7	21.0	12.0	25.4	35.1	17.5
Cirrhosis of liver	571	14.8	20.7	9.7	13.4	19.0	8.6	25.0	34.0	17.4
Diabetes mellitus	250	12.5	12.2	12.7	11.4	11.5	11.2	23.4	18.8	27.1
Suicide	E950–E959	12.2	12.2	6.7	12.8	19.0	7.1	7.2	11.7	3.3
Homicide	E960–E978	10.8	17.3	4.6	6.0	9.3	2.9	44.5	77.9	15.5
Bronchitis, emphysema, and asthma	490–493	9.2	15.9	4.3	9.4	16.4	4.4	6.5	10.4	3.2
Tuberculosis, all forms	010–019	1.3	2.1	0.7	0.9	1.5	0.5	4.6	7.2	2.5

From: Vital Statistics of the US 1974
Volume 11—Mortality. Part A 1978

stable since 1950, although the sex differential continues to increase. The sex differential for diabetes mellitus is of special interest because women have traditionally had higher rates than men. There is now, however, a trend toward a more equal rate. Johnson (1977) points out that if this trend continues, one of the rare examples of male mortality advantage will disappear.

morbidity rates for men and women

Mortality data provide only one index of ill health in a population. In developed countries, ill health frequently results from significant but nonfatal conditions, such as mental illness or orthopedic and sensory impairments. To paraphrase Cole (1974), here is the definition used in conjunction with the National Health Interview Survey: morbidity is a departure from physical or mental well-being as a result of disease or injury, which has an impact on the individual's life inasmuch as she or he is aware of the departure from health and how it restricts or disables the person in some way.

Estimates from a recent National Health Interview Survey show that in the United States women continue to report more illness than men and also use health services at higher rates. The following estimates are based on data from the Health Interview Survey of a stratified random sample of households drawn from the civilian, noninstitutionalized population of the United States, which measures several factors that affect morbidity and use of health services.

ACUTE CONDITIONS. Illnesses and injuries that last less than three months and involve one or more days of restricted activity or medical attention are called acute. The annual incidence of acute conditions is estimated by including only those conditions that began during the two weeks prior to interview. Table 2.2 shows that the incidence of acute conditions for females exceeded that for males in nearly every condition. In the category that includes fractures, dislocations, sprains, open wounds and lacerations, and other injuries, incidence for males was higher. The other exceptions to the higher rates for females were for common childhood diseases, diseases of the skin, diseases of the ear and the musculoskeletal system. The female rates were higher for infective and parasitic diseases, respiratory conditions, digestive system problems, and all other acute conditions. This higher rate for females appears less consistent during the earlier part of the life cycle than at later ages.

DISABILITY. Days of disability refer to a temporary or long-term reduction of an individual's activity due to either acute or chronic conditions. Four types of disability days are reported in the survey: restricted-activity days, bed-disability days, work-loss days, and school-loss days. A restricted activity day is one on which an individual reduces her or his normal activity for the entire day due to an illness or injury. By definition, bed-disability days are spent all or most of the day in bed; these are counted as days of restricted activity. Each day lost from work or school is also counted as a day of restricted activity.

Women report proportionately more days of restricted activity than men, with an average of 21.1 days of disability per year in comparison with 16.3 days for men. Women also report more bed-disability days per person per

table 2.2

number of acute conditions per 100 persons per year, by age, sex, and condition group: United States, 1978

Data are based on household interviews of the civilian noninstitutionalized population.

SEX AND CONDITION GROUP	ALL AGES	UNDER 6 YEARS	6–16 YEARS	17–44 YEARS	45 YEARS & OVER
	NUMBER OF ACUTE CONDITIONS PER 100 PERSONS PER YEAR				
BOTH SEXES					
All Acute Conditions	218.2	387.6	272.9	224.5	129.1
Infective and Parasitic Diseases	24.7	64.5	36.9	22.3	9.4
Respiratory Conditions	115.8	206.6	152.8	116.6	66.7
Upper Respiratory Conditions	59.1	133.9	80.2	55.9	29.8
Influenza	50.3	56.0	66.5	55.5	31.9
Other Respiratory Conditions	6.3	16.7	6.1	5.3	5.0
Digestive System Conditions	10.7	14.0	13.3	11.2	7.4
Injuries	33.1	33.5	39.6	36.4	24.5
All Other Acute Conditions	33.9	69.0	30.3	37.9	21.1
MALE					
All Acute Conditions	207.1	403.5	261.6	202.7	114.4
Infective and Parasitic Diseases	22.8	72.1	34.0	17.2	7.7
Respiratory Conditions	109.7	215.1	140.5	107.7	58.3
Upper Respiratory Conditions	55.3	134.5	70.1	51.0	26.6

year than men, with an average of 8.2 days versus 6.0 days for men. Women report 5.7 work-loss days per person per year compared with the 4.9 days for men. Female children have a greater number of school-loss days (5.2 per child per year); male children are absent 4.4 days per child per year. The trend for both sexes appears to increase with age, although the pattern of more restricted activity for females seems to be established before adulthood. Although the data in Table 2.3 are for 1978, the patterns for the sexes have been the same in previous years.

CHRONIC CONDITIONS. A chronic condition refers to long-term reduction in activity, such as being unable to carry on usual activity or being restricted in the amount and kind of activity. During 1978, males exceeded females in limitation of activity due to chronic conditions for every age group (Givens, 1979). Of those who experienced limited activity due to a chronic condition, 18 percent of males attributed it to heart conditions, 10.1 percent to arthritis and rheumatism, and 7.2 percent to impairments of the lower extremities and hips; 19.6 percent of the females attributed their

table 2.2 (cont.)

SEX AND CONDITION GROUP	ALL AGES	UNDER 6 YEARS	6–16 YEARS	17–44 YEARS	45 YEARS & OVER
	NUMBER OF ACUTE CONDITIONS PER 100 PERSONS PER YEAR				
MALE(cont.)					
Influenza	48.3	63.3	63.3	52.3	27.5
Other Respiratory Conditions	6.1	17.3	7.0	4.4	4.2
Digestive System Conditions	10.1	10.7	14.0	10.6	6.5
Injuries	38.4	35.8	48.8	44.0	24.1
All Other Acute Conditions	26.1	69.7	24.4	23.2	17.7
FEMALE					
All Acute Conditions	228.5	370.8	284.6	244.9	141.4
Infective and Parasitic Diseases	26.5	56.6	40.0	27.1	10.7
Respiratory Conditions	121.5	197.6	165.5	125.0	73.7
Upper Respiratory Conditions	62.7	133.2	90.7	60.5	32.5
Influenza	52.2	48.4	69.8	58.4	35.6
Other Respiratory Conditions	6.6	16.0	5.1	6.1	5.6
Digestive System Conditions	11.3	17.5	12.7	11.9	8.2
Injuries	28.1	31.0	30.1	29.2	24.9
All Other Acute Conditions	41.2	68.2	36.4	51.7	23.8

NOTES: EXCLUDED FROM THESE STATISTICS ARE ALL CONDITIONS INVOLVING NEITHER RESTRICTED ACTIVITY NOR MEDICAL ATTENTION.
From Givens 1979

limitations to arthritis and rheumatism, 14.5 percent to heart conditions, and 8.9 percent to hypertension.

UTILIZATION OF HEALTH SERVICES. Information for utilization of health services obtained by the Health Survey concerns the hospitalization experiences in each household during the year preceding the interview. There were 16.3 hospital discharges per 100 persons per year for females, and 11.8 for males. Close inspection of the data shows that the excess of female hospitalizations occurred during the child-bearing years. Although females were hospitalized at greater rates than males, the length of stay was shorter for females than males (7.3 vs. 8.7 days). Females were also more likely to make dental visits than males. On the average, women in the survey for 1976 reported 1.7 dental visits per year as compared with 1.6 for males (Black, 1977).

During 1978, young adult females made more physician visits than did males. However, males under 17 years of age or over 65

table 2.3

death rates per 100,000 population for ten leading causes of death for each age group in the female population: all women, whites and nonwhites

RANK	UNDER 1 YEAR	1–4 YEARS	5–14 YEARS
1	Mortality in early infancy—820.2, 699.3, 1420.7	Accidents—23.4, 21.1, 35.0	Accidents—11.4, 10.9, 14.2
2	Congenital Anomalies—262.9, 262.4, 265.0	Congenital Anomalies—8.8, 8.6, 9.7	Malignant Neoplasms including Lymphatic and Hematopoietic—4.5, 4.6, 4.0
3	Symptoms and Ill-Defined Conditions—129.8, 93.8, 308.5	All Other Diseases—7.4, 7.2, 8.6	All Other Diseases—3.8, 3.8, 3.7
4	Influenza and Pneumonia—78.4, 60.0, 169.9	Malignant Neoplasms including Lymphatic and Hematopoietic—5.4, 5.9, 3.2	Congenital Anomalies—2.1, 2.2, 2.0
5	All Other—53.8, 46.3, 91.1	Influenza and Pneumonia—4.5, 3.5, 9.3	Major Cardiovascular Diseases—1.6, 1.4, 2.3
6	Accidents—42.9, 36.5, 74.8	Major Cardiovascular Diseases—2.8, 2.5, 4.5	Influenza and Pneumonia—1.2, 1.2, 1.5
7	Septicemia—26.2, 20.9, 52.0	Symptoms and Ill-Defined Conditions—2.5, 2.0, 5.2	Homicide—0.8, 0.6., 2.0
8	Major Cardiovascular Diseases—25.8, 19.1, 58.9	Homicide—2.0, 1.4, 5.4	Symptoms and Ill-Defined Conditions—0.6, 0.5, 1.1
9	All Other Forms of Heart Disease—18.3, 13.1, 43.9	All Other Forms of Heart Disease—1.7, 1.4, 3.2	All Other Forms of Heart Disease—0.6, 0.6, 0.8
10	Meningitis—17.1, 12.5, 39.8	Meningitis—1.5, 1.1, 3.2	Cerebrovascular Disease—0.6, 0.6, 0.6

RANK	15–24 YEARS	25–34 YEARS	35–44 YEARS
1	Accidents—23.9, 24.5, 20.3	Accidents—17.2, 16.0, 24.9	Malignant Neoplasms including Lymphatic and Hematopoietic—60.9, 57.9, 80.1
2	Homicide—6.3, 3.8, 20.5	Malignant Neoplasms including Lymphatic and Hematopoietic—15.5, 15.0, 19.1	Major Cardiovascular Diseases—42.7, 32.8, 107.3
3	All Other Diseases—6.2, 5.2, 12.1	All Other Diseases—11.0, 8.6, 26.4	All Other Diseases—21.7, 17.1, 51.4
4	Malignant Neoplasms including Lymphatic and Hematopoietic—5.4, 5.3, 6.1	Major Cardiovascular Diseases—10.7, 8.0, 27.9	Accidents—17.8, 16.4, 26.9
5	Suicide—4.6, 4.8, 3.9	Suicide—8.4, 8.7, 6.3	Cirrhosis of Liver—13.1, 9.8, 34.3

table 2.3 (cont.)

RANK	15–24 YEARS	25–34 YEARS	35–44 YEARS
6	Major Cardiovascular Diseases—3.7, 3.2, 7.2	Homicide—7.5, 4.3, 27.9	Suicide—11.1, 12.1, 4.5
7	Symptoms and Ill-Defined Diseases—2.5, 2.0, 5.1	Symptoms and Ill-Defined Diseases—3.5, 2.4, 10.0	Homicide—6.5, 3.9, 23.1
8	Influenza and Pneumonia—1.5, 1.3, 2.1	Cirrhosis of the Liver—3.0, 1.7, 11.6	Symptoms and Ill-Defined Diseases—6.3, 4.5, 18.1
9	Congenital Anomalies—1.5, 1.5, 1.4	Influenza and Pneumonia—2.1, 1.7, 4.5	Influenza and Pneumonia—4.4, 3.5, 10.4
10	Other External Causes—1.2, 1.0, 2.7	Other External Causes—1.8, 1.5, 3.5	Diabetes Mellitus—3.8, 2.8, 10.6

RANK	45–54 YEARS	55–64 YEARS	65–74 YEARS
1	Malignant Neoplasms including Lymphatic and Hematopoietic—177.5, 172.4, 218.3	Major Cardiovascular Diseases—416.1, 372.2, 824.8	Major Cardiovascular Diseases—1296.0, 1224.7, 2005.9
2	Major Cardiovascular Diseases—135.5, 112.1, 322.7	Malignant Neoplasms including Hematopoietic and Lymphatic—361.4, 354.5, 425.2	Malignant Neoplasms including Lymphatic and Hematopoietic—566.4, 560.0, 629.9
3	All Other Diseases—41.0, 36.1, 80.6	All Other Diseases—77.0, 72.5, 118.4	All Other Diseases—152.5, 147.2, 205.4
4	Cirrhosis of the Liver—25.8, 22.9, 48.7	Cirrhosis of the Liver—32.5, 31.4, 42.2	Diabetes Mellitus—85.0, 74.5, 189.4
5	Accidents—21.8, 20.6, 31.8	Diabetes Mellitus—31.4, 25.5, 86.1	Accidents—45.6, 44.6, 55.2
6	Suicide—13.0, 14.1, 4.0	Accidents—28.5, 27.3, 39.4	Influenza and Pneumonia—44.8, 42.3, 69.9
7	Diabetes Mellitus—11.1, 8.3, 33.7	Influenza and Pneumonia—16.9, 15.8, 27.2	Bronchitis, Emphysema, and Asthma—26.6, 28.1, 12.6
8	Influenza and Pneumonia—8.9, 7.8, 17.6	Bronchitis, Emphysema, and Asthma—14.4, 15.1, 8.4	Cirrhosis of the Liver—26.1, 26.4, 22.2
9	Symptoms and Ill-Defined Diseases—8.6, 6.6, 24.5	Symptoms and Ill-Defined Diseases—14.2, 10.8, 45.9	Symptoms and Ill-Defined Diseases—25.4, 19.5, 85.0
10	Bronchitis, Emphysema and Asthma—5.0, 5.0, 4.6	Suicide—10.3, 11.0 3.4	Nephritis and Nephrosis—11.4, 8.8, 37.4

table 2.3 (cont.)

RANK	75–84 YEARS	85 YEARS AND OLDER
1	Major Cardiovascular Diseases–4297.7, 4322.9, 3982.9	Major Cardiovascular Diseases—11691.8, 12070.7, 7515.5
2	Malignant Neoplasms—902.0, 911.7, 780.3	Malignant Neoplasms—1133.9, 1164.8, 792.8
3	All Other Diseases—317.5, 317.6, 316.4	Influenza and Pneumonia—701.7, 730.3, 386.6
4	Influenza and Pneumonia—192.5, 195.1, 159.5	All Other Diseases—596.7, 614.4, 402.1
5	Diabetes Mellitus—180.4, 175.0, 247.8	Accidents—330.9, 342.9, 197.9
6	Accidents—119.5, 121.7, 91.3	Diabetes Mellitus—252.1, 254.7, 223.7
7	Symptoms and Ill-Defined Diseases—54.9, 46.4, 160.2	Symptoms and Ill-Defined Diseases—178.3, 155.2, 433.0
8	Bronchitis, Emphysema, and Asthma—39.6, 41.4, 17.4	Hernia and Intestinal Obstruction—70.8, 74.2, 34.0
9	Hernia and Intestinal Obstruction—31.0, 31.6, 23.7	Infections of the Kidney—62.7, 64.2, 46.4
10	Infection of the Kidney—28.3, 28.1, 39.8	Bronchitis, Emphysema, and Asthma—48.9, 51.7, 17.5

made more physician visits than females.

PREVENTIVE CARE. Data from the Health Interview Survey for 1973 indicated that women tend to have some procedure associated with preventive care performed more often than men. More women respondents (89.6 percent) reported eye examinations for visual correction; more females (56.7 percent) than males (50.1 percent) had glaucoma tests; there were no sex differences for chest X-rays, but more men (64.6 percent) than women (56.8 percent) had electrocardiograms.

Three-fourths of the female sample had a Pap smear and a breast examination, with the frequency greatest in the 25 to 44 age group for whites. On the average, women had about 11 prenatal visits per pregnancy. The frequency of women seeking preventive services increases with their socioeconomic status.

The National Center for Health Statistics initiated the National Ambulatory Medical Survey in the United States. This survey is based on a continuing national probability sample and is unique in that it incorporates the need for seeking care as expressed in the client's own words. One limitation of the survey is its inclusion of only patient-physician in-office meetings, neglecting meetings with primary care professionals such as nurses and meetings outside the physician's office. In brief, patterns of primary care show 3.7 visits per person for women, a rate 50 percent higher than that for males.

the paradox explored

What are some of the explanations for the paradox between sex differences in mortality versus morbidity and the use of health services? If women have a lower general death rate and lower general incidence of illness, why do they use health care services more than men do? Crucial *biological differences* between males and females may influence mortality and morbidity in early parts of the life cycle. However, their influence becomes less clear for older age groups where other factors come into play. Hormonal influences may also have a protective effect for females, but experts agree that the sharp increase in sex differences in mortality during the twentieth century cannot be explained solely by biological factors. Perhaps it involves differences in exposure to nonbiological factors. Even if marked differences in biological processes could account for the changes in sex mortality differentials in this century, sociocultural factors must also be looked at in trying to explain the seeming biological advantage for females and their apparently unfavorable incidence of illness.

Although *social stress* has been suggested to account for both greater male mortality rates and greater female morbidity, this explanation has problems. First, there is controversy about what causes stress in women's and men's lives. Who can say which role is most stressful? Second, there is no well-refined theory to account for the mechanisms by which sex differences influence health. Is there a mechanism that causes males to die from exposure to social stress, but causes fe-

males to report symptoms and use health services because of it? Are there combinations of types of exposure and mechanisms of response that are more prevalent among women versus men?

Changing health technologies may have had some influence on sex differences in mortality, morbidity, and use of health services, although these have not been carefully documented. Reduction in maternal mortality rates would have to be counterbalanced by reviewing illness incidence for females resulting from thrombophlebitis and cerebrovascular accidents (strokes) associated with birth control pills. This might provide one example of how a decrease in death is accompanied by an increase in illness, caused by changing health technologies.

Life-style differences are one of the most popular explanations of the paradox. The way most men and women live their lives and the norms that regulate those differences probably expose each sex to different kinds of risks. Environmental and occupational hazards may account for higher death rates for men and greater incidence of injuries and injury-linked disability. Furthermore, men are taught by society to engage in high-risk behavior to a greater extent than women. Some modal female-male personality differences, such as aggressiveness among males, may also predispose men to both increased high-risk behavior and mortality rates. Our culture generally restrains men from acknowledging illness, altering their activities to accommodate illness, or seeking health services (all translated as weakness). Women, on the other hand, are encouraged to be more responsive to perceived illness and to avoid exposure to high risks. Perhaps women report more illness than men because it is culturally more acceptable for them to do so. Women may be more able than men to add illness to their other responsibilities because of the more flexible nature of their roles. Thus, the attitudes and activities ascribed to women are more self-protective than those ascribed to men.

A final explanation for the paradox may lie in how the behaviors and attitudes of health practitioners vary with respect to women and men as patients. It is likely that the sex differences in both illness and use of services are influenced by the one who gives health aid as well as the one who seeks it. Thus, sex role expectations held by the health practitioner are likely to affect the definition and treatment of complaints presented by women and men. For example, assumptions that women's complaints are psychosomatic may result in artificially inflated rates of psychological morbidity. Many health practitioners seem to be inclined to equate "male" with "normal." For example, the greater use of health services by women is sometimes labeled "excessive" rather than reflecting what may be merely appropriate use.

In summary, it would seem that the most credible explanation for the paradoxical relationship between higher mortality rates for males and higher morbidity and utilization rates for females probably lies in the life-styles that are generally characteristic of men and women.

special risks for women

A comparison of sex differences in the cause of death, morbidity, and use of health services suggests some important guides for the study of women's health. It is also important, however, to carefully consider the causes of death and illness affecting women and to compare some of the differences that exist between groups of women.

The four leading causes of death for both white and black women are: heart diseases, malignant neoplasms (cancers), cerebrovascular diseases, and injuries. However, there are some important differences. Diabetes mellitus is a more common cause of death for black women than for white women. Certain causes of death, such as influenza and pneumonia, in early infancy account for a greater proportion of nonwhite deaths. White women die more as a result of suicide; black women are more likely to die from homicide. Nephritis and nephrosis are among the 10 major causes of death for black women, but this is not the case for whites. For a more detailed inspection of the leading causes of death for females of all ages, see the data from the Vital and Health Statistics for the United States, which show causes of death for various age and racial groups. By carefully analyzing causes of death, health professionals as well as consumers can note the preventive measures that seem most applicable to each group.

An inspection of the major causes of death in Table 2.3 suggests many measures that might reduce mortality for females of all ages. Although some of the causes of death in early infancy and congenital anomalies remain unknown, early prenatal care can help women identify certain practices that may lead to health problems in their infants, for example, smoking and use of alcohol and drugs during pregnancy. Other causes of infant death are linked to infectious diseases. While exposure to an infectious agent is necessary for these diseases to occur, the immune system of the infant influences whether he or she will actually contract the disease. Breastfeeding is an important influence on an infant's immune status. Injuries are a major cause of death in infants. Mortality due to motor vehicle injuries can be reduced by use of car seats and seat belts, judicious use of alcohol and drugs, and driver education. Other causes of infant deaths include poisoning, drownings, and other non-motor-vehicle accidents such as falls. Careful child care and other preventive measures could reduce mortality in these areas.

For female children ages 1 to 4 years, injuries are the major cause of death. Motor vehicle injuries are responsible for nearly one-third of these; other causes include poisonings and drownings. Reducing the possibility of drowning accidents by teaching water safety and the use of poison deterrents such as special child-proof bottles, locks on cabinets, and decals that discourage children from swallowing poisons are recommended.

In addition to congenital anomalies and infectious diseases during the ages of 1 to 4 years, malignancies, especially the leukemias, appear as major threats to health. Major cardiovascular diseases account for many deaths in this age group—cerebrovascular disease, pericarditis, endocarditis, cardiomyopathies, pulmonary heart diseases, and ill-defined heart diseases. Homicide is a major cause of death. An end to violence in the society could eradicate it.

For females 5 to 14 years, injuries remain the leading cause of death, and motor vehicle injuries account for nearly half of this number. Malignant neoplasms (cancers) are sec-ond, with the leukemias accounting for most deaths. Congenital anomalies and cardiovascular disease threaten this group. Some of the cardiovascular disease deaths in this age band are attributed to acute rheumatic heart disease. Culturing sore throats for beta hemolytic streptococcal infections, followed by appropriate antibiotic therapy, could prevent some of these childhood deaths. Influenza and pneumonia are major threats in this group.

During the transition to the young adult years (15 to 24), females are at their greatest risk from injuries and homicide. The automobile is responsible for the majority of deaths, which could be prevented with seat belts and the judicious use of alcohol and drugs. In the young adult female, malignancies, especially the leukemias and the lymphomas, contribute heavily to deaths.

Suicide becomes a major cause of death for this 15 to 24 group, over major cardiovascular diseases, influenza and pneumonia, and other causes. Early identification and treatment of depression could prevent at least some of these deaths. Cerebrovascular diseases account for many deaths. Smoking, untreated high blood pressure, elevated blood cholesterol level, or uncontrolled diabetes all place women at greater risk for cerebrovascular disease. Appropriate use of antibiotics can reduce risk of death from chronic rheumatic heart disease, and reduction in smoking and alcohol use can lessen the risk of death from pneumonia.

Motor vehicle injuries remain the leading cause of death for women aged 25 to 34. Malignant neoplasms emerge as the second major cause; cancer of the breast, uterus, brain, and nervous system, leukemia, and Hodgkin's Disease account for most of the deaths. A more detailed discussion of risk factors for cancer of the breast, cervix, and uterus is found in chapter 22, chapter 26, and chapter 27. The major cardiovascular diseases also claim the lives of many woman during this period, with active rheumatic fever and chronic rheumatic heart disease, ischemic heart disease, acute myocardial infarction, and cerebrovascular disease being responsible for most of the deaths. Factors that increase the risk of the major cardiovascular diseases include untreated elevated blood pressure and cholesterol, uncontrolled diabetes, smoking, and untreated rheumatic fever. Sedentary lifestyles and obesity are also implicated in cardiovascular disease. Suicide and homicide continue as major causes of death, with cirrhosis of the liver emerging as an important cause for this age group. Alcohol abuse is the primary factor associated with cirrhosis. Influenza and pneumonia remain major causes of death, with alcohol use, smoking, and previous lung diseases such as bacterial pneumonia and emphysema increasing the mortality risk for women 25 to 34.

The major causes of death for women 35 to 44 are similar to those in the previous age group. Cancer of the breast, lung, uterus, ovary, colon, and rectum are major causes. In addition, the leukemias and the lymphatic and hematopoietic neoplasms are also major causes of death. Regular breast self-examination can aid in the early detection of breast cancer, and regular Pap smears aid the early detection of cervical cancer. Cardiovascular diseases are the second major cause of death for this group, with injuries, cirrhosis of the liver, suicide, homicide, influenza, and pneumonia included in the 10 major causes of death for women 35 to 44. Obesity, a serious health problem for women, has been implicated in adult onset diabetes, and diabetes mellitus emerges as major cause of death for this age group.

For women 45 to 54 years of age, cancer is the major cause of death, followed by cardiovascular diseases, cirrhosis of the liver, injuries, suicide, diabetes mellitus, influenza and pneumonia, and the other respiratory diseases—bronchitis, emphysema, and asthma. The cardiovascular diseases that affect women in this age group are the ischemic heart diseases and cerebrovascular diseases.

Women who are between 55 and 64 years of age are threatened primarily by heart disease and cancer. These disease groups persist as the two major causes of death throughout a woman's remaining life-span, including the 65 to 74 period. Diabetes mellitus and injuries remain important causes of death, along with influenza and pneumonia, bronchitis, emphysema, and asthma, and cirrhosis of the liver. The kidney diseases, nephritis and nephrosis, emerge as a major cause of death in this age group. Causes of death for women 75 to 84 and older include cardiovascular diseases and cancer. In these age groups, the major cardiovascular deaths are attributable to ischemic heart disease, hypertension, and the cerebrovascular diseases, especially cerebral thrombosis and hemorrhage and arteriosclerosis. The most common cancers affecting women over 75 are colon, rectum, breast, lung, pancreas, and uterus.

This review suggests a number of areas in which women can take preventive actions. First, to protect their children, women can seek early prenatal and infant health care, as well as avoiding smoking and using alcohol and drugs during pregnancy. Injuries and deaths can be reduced or prevented through general safety measures, defensive driving, and not driving under the influence of drugs and/or alcohol, and using seat belts and certified safe car seats for children. There is some evidence to suggest that breast feeding can bolster the infant's immunities to infectious agents. Violence can be reduced, as can suicide by early identification of depression and prompt initiation of therapy.

Collaboration with a health professional may improve women's life chances, but many of the most important contributions to our health are those that we, ourselves, control. In addition, women can try to bring about the social changes necessary to insure that all women have access to health care, adequate nutrition, and opportunities for living in an environment that enables them to seek and maintain optimum health.

the future health of women

The future health of women will depend on many variables, including changing health technologies, the life-style women adopt (including the influence of social norms, exposure to hazards of the environment, and changes in the modal personality), institutionalized sex-role expectations as they influence health services delivery, and genetic/biologic changes.

Two outcomes from changing health technology are possible. First, improved early detection and treatment methods for diseases of women such as breast cancer may contribute to a longer life-span and even more favorable sex mortality differences than exist now. Second, advancement of health technologies may bring on greater mortality and morbidity rates for women. Examples could include the appearance of vaginal cancer in daughters of women who had been given DES, a drug used to prevent pregnancy complications from about 1947 to 1970, and thrombophlebitis and increased risk of death from vascular diseases among women treated with birth control pills. Thus, one must carefully weigh the costs with the merits of each new development.

Likewise, the life-styles that women will adopt can improve as well as harm their health. As social norms change to allow more equal opportunity for women in the labor force and more emphasis is placed on self-actualization, women may be increasingly exposed to toxic substances and other hazards of the workplace that now account for work-connected disability and mortality among men. If women adopt health behavior, illness behavior, and sick-role behavior patterns more like those of men, it is possible that the advantage they now have from use of health services or self-care will be lost. On the other hand, if women maintain their previous patterns of self-health care, as well as utilization of services, they may be less affected than men by the hazards of the workplace. Furthermore, if sex discrimination in employment is finally abolished and women have equal opportunity to realize their ambitions in their jobs, their mental as well as physical health may improve. On the other hand, if more women adopt the personality patterns currently prevalent among men, such as aggressive competitiveness, the advantages accrued by improved opportunities in the work place may be erased.

As sex-role expectations among health professionals are erased, the reported high rates of some mental illnesses in females may decrease. However, the symptoms of mental illness reported by women and men may become more similar as these sex-role expectations merge. As the "roles" of the sexes grow more close, assumptions may be revised about appropriate therapies. For example, psychotropic drugs (such as tranquilizers) might not be given so readily to women as their work becomes more visible.

The self-health movement may make certain contacts with formal health services unnecessary; women may perform their own pelvic exams and Pap smears rather than having a nurse or physician do so. This may have both positive and negative effects on women's health. Positive outcomes may come from women's improved knowledge of their bodies, and the accessibility of health services may no longer be a barrier to health maintenance. Perhaps the single negative outcome of the self-health movement would be its incorrect application to problems that do require consultation with professionals in pathology. As clinicians come to realize that women are knowledgeable about their health, however, the social stratification between clinician and client is less likely to influence the process of health care. The demystification of health, which allows the dissemination of health information to women, is likely to result in consumers who are able increasingly to question decisions about treatment, explore alternative methods of healing, and carefully examine the effects of such procedures as surgery, drug therapy, and sterilization.

The change least likely to influence women's health in the future is our changing biology. Given current knowledge of genetics, major changes in the human organism are not likely to occur rapidly. It is, however, possible that health hazards will impinge on future generations as a result of contemporary environmentally induced exposures.

Black, E. Current estimates from the health interview survey, United States, 1976. *Vital and Health Statistics,* Series 10, No. 119, USDHEW, National Center for Health Statistics, Washington, D.C., November 1977.

Cole, P. Morbidity in the United States. In C. L. Erhardt & J. E. Berlin (Eds.), *Mortality and morbidity in the United States.* Cambridge, Mass.: Harvard Univ. Press, 1974, pp. 65–104.

Givens, J. Current estimates from the health interview survey, United States, 1978. *Vital and Health Statistics,* Series 10, No. 130, November 1979.

Johnson, A. Recent trends in sex mortality differentials in the United States. *Journal of Human Stress,* March 1977, 3:1, 22–32.

Wilder, C. S. Limitations of activity due to chronic conditions U.S. 1974. *Vital And Health Statistics,* Series 10, no. 111, USDHEW, National Center for Health Statistics, Washington, D.C., June 1977.

RUTH McCORKLE, R.N., Ph.D.

information exchange between women and health care providers

The getting and giving of information underlies all communication between patients and health care providers. Women who seek and obtain help for a symptom or ailment they see as threatening to their bodies go through a process of integrating messages into information, which subsequently they partially share with others. This intrapersonal communication does not occur unless a woman acquires and consumes some information about herself or the environment. This chapter presents an overview of the communication process that occurs from the time a woman recognizes something is wrong with her body and seeks help, to the time a decision is made and acted on for a specific treatment. For our purposes, this process is called *information exchange.*

the symptom

There are many events that may be seen as threatening to a woman and her relationships with others. The individual's perception of the event as threatening requires interpretation by the woman about the significance of the stimulus. This interpretation process is called "appraisal" by Richard Lazarus. A stimulus such as a symptom may be viewed as threatening by one individual and nonthreatening by another. The threat is not simply "out there" as part of the stimulus. Rather, it depends on the appraisal for its threat value, which in turn depends on the person's beliefs about what the stimulus means in relation to what is important in life (Lazarus, 1964).

When an event, such as the onset of a symptom, is perceived as personally threatening, stress occurs that shows itself in a state of disequilibrium. A crisis results when an individual's homeostatic state is overpowered by disequilibrium. During this time, the woman is faced with a problem that is of basic importance because it is linked with fundamental instinctual needs and is not quickly solved by normal problem-solving mechanisms (Caplan, 1956).

A symptom such as a breast lump that is associated with a life-threatening illness may have an additional effect on the person's perception of what is happening. The meaning of the symptom is a personal experience, and the meaning will determine what each woman does about the symptom. Nearly everyone delays taking any action at least for a short time when they first recognize the symptoms of a breakdown in the health of their own body. If the person perceives the threat as something that needs attention, she will seek medical help. But if the threat remains unperceived or perceived as so frightening that it paralyzes the person from acting, she may go to the extreme of denying the existence of any warning signs or symptoms in order to survive emotionally. Some delay in reporting symptoms is expected and permits a person to adapt to the threat and to realize her defenses for coping with it (Bard, 1973).

Denial is a protective mechanism that is used repeatedly in everyday life. It is a selective process whereby the informational content of certain internal and external stimuli is not acknowledged. When denial occurs, overwhelmingly threatening thoughts or facts are not allowed to reach the person's conscious awareness, and to all intents and purposes, they do not exist for that person (Mastrovito, 1974). It is important to remember that the distinctive quality of denying and denial is its occurrence in relation to certain people, but not all. The purpose served by denial in disease is not simply to avoid the threat of a diagnosis, but to protect and prevent the loss of a significant relationship (Weisman, 1972).

Some women realize they may have a symptom that warrants medical attention, but they delay seeking help for other reasons than denial. Most often this occurs with women who have children and place a higher priority on the welfare of their family in comparison to their own health. Traditionally, women have assumed primary responsibility for the maintenance of health of children, such as seeing that they get their immunizations. Some women minimize their own symptoms, confident they will go away with time, especially for common symptoms that are associated with an everyday ailment such as fatigue, cough, or headache. Few women have a good understanding that prompt attention to a symptom early may have a more sustaining effect on the welfare of their family if the symptom is a warning of a life-threatening illness such as heart disease or cancer. The majority of women eventually seek help if the symptom interferes with what they want to do on a day-to-day basis (Mechanic, 1968).

the diagnosis

The initial encounter with a person who has mobilized herself for help must be the beginning of an ongoing assessment of what alarmed the person in the first place. The physician takes a history and performs a physical examination as the person relates the symptoms or problem. This process continues until the physician diagnoses the person's problems with the assistance of sophisticated medical technology as well as expert knowledge.

Some problems are easier to diagnose than others, and the presence of symptoms does not necessarily mean the presence of a disease. The diagnostic period may take as long as a few days or months. Once the physician has confirmed or refuted what is suspected, the person must be informed of what is or is not wrong. If a disease is diagnosed, the woman must participate in decisions for a treatment plan and must understand the implications of the choice selected.

The purpose of establishing a diagnosis is to identify a reason for the person's symptoms and concerns, not to undermine the person. The actual conveying of messages to a person about the diagnosis and its implications is most effective as an ongoing process. One crucial factor involved in making treatment choices is that the consequences of some interventions, such as radical surgery, are irreversible. The effects of others, such as the use of medications or physical therapy, are gradual and usually reversible. For example, a woman with back pain may be told she needs a laminectomy (the surgical removal of one or more vertebral laminae that exposes the spinal cord to treat a herniated intervertebral disk). A more conservative approach might be for the woman to wear a back brace, sleep on a firm bed, or take muscle relaxants before resorting to surgery.

It is important that the woman has a clear understanding about the seriousness of what the physician is telling her about her body and what is being recommended. Information conveyed by the physician to that person can reduce her uncertainty. Everything that the physician says to the woman is potentially informative. Messages are informative if they are within the particular person's range of understanding, and if the message can be validated by that person. The message must also be comprehensible and have some use for the one who receives it (Thayer, 1968, pp. 189–190).

choice for treatment

For a person to participate in the decisions about treatment, the physician must share what is known about the disease and the options for therapy. This process assumes that patients receive messages from physicians and are asked for their input. But, in reality, some patients are denied these opportunities because physicians have been taught a particular perspective. One common example is recommending surgical treatment of back pain when other options are available, but not presenting these options unless the patient insists.

Information that the physician and other health care providers have about diseases and treatment options is an important source of power. The physician who controls such information has the ability to analyze it, process it, and assume responsibility for it (Claus & Bailey, 1977). Not only does the physician obtain and control information, but he or she also knows how to make it practically incomprehensible. Power is maintained by making the information as mysterious and inaccessible as possible, compiling it in such complex forms that only the physician can explain what (if anything) it means (Korda, 1975, p. 149). (See chapter 29—personal power assessment)

The task of helping a person make a choice for treatment is clear: to get complete information from the physician to the person with a disease in messages that are understandable and in a way that allows the person to make an informed choice. This process seems straightforward, but, in fact, it is often incomplete. Once the physician presents the person with the diagnostic findings and the available choices, the person must be responsible for sharing other data with the physician on how the options fit within her life. Together they need to weigh the pros and cons of the choices and their consequences, and come up with a treatment plan that is the best choice for that patient. Getting additional information from the patient about her life-style and how a treatment choice may affect day-to-day living has not been expected behavior from the physician. If doctors cannot handle this feedback from the person, or do not see it as their priority, other health care providers must participate in the process. This is especially important for patients who are intimidated by the presence of physicians.

the decision

In making a decision, shared information is essential between the physician and the woman. A decision is a choice among alternatives, designed to accomplish some goal. In disease, the primary goal is to get rid of or control the person's problem, but, unfortunately, that goal is not always reachable. Decision-making is a process of exploration and analysis that precedes a choice. The process includes: (1) defining the problem, (2) identifying alternative choice of actions, (3) evaluating alternative choice of actions for their consequences, (4) selecting a course of action, (5) implementing the decision, and (6) obtaining feedback about the results (Cooper, 1961).

Making a decision is a reciprocal process. Each participant has crucial information that the other needs to hear and integrate before an action is taken. Unfortunately, health care is complex and specialized, and rarely is information exchange confined to one patient and one physician.

factors influencing information exchange

There are many factors that influence effective information exchange among patient-provider systems. We will discuss four factors: (1) need for urgent action, (2) uncertainty, (3) specialization, and (4) common expectations for treatment goals.

need for urgent action

With some diseases, the physician conveys a sense of urgency, which may make the person feel that a decision should be made quickly. This occurs most frequently during a crisis period, such as the time of diagnosis or recurrence of symptoms thought to be successfully treated. As a result, some patients consent to decisions recommended by a physician before they have had an opportunity to realize what is happening. Discussions about some diseases such as cancer and the consequences associated with them contain fear-arousing messages for most people. The meanings of the messages conveyed may do little to decrease the person's fears; therefore, anxiety prevails. Anxiety is a formidable barrier among the person with the disease and the people with whom she relates. Bard found that anxiety interferes with the person's ability to hear, to understand, and to remember; therefore, it causes distortions and shifts on emphasis of what is said. For communication to be effective, efforts must be made to lessen disruptive anxiety. More frequently than not, anxiety decreases or diminishes when attention is focused on how messages are conveyed rather than what is said (Bard, 1973).

The choice of immediate medical intervention in a crisis such as that associated with cancer or other diseases needs to be weighed carefully in light of the ability of the patient and her family to participate in and understand the implications of a decision. The process is complex. For example, a physician informs a woman that he must operate immediately (within the week) to remove a cancerous growth on the larynx (the voice box), and the patient consents before she is fully aware, from the information given her by the physician, that the surgery will leave her without her voice. After the surgery, the patient is devastated by the postoperative problem of coming to terms with a permanent tracheostomy (an opening in the neck) and the fact that she no longer has her voice. The continued responsibilities of the surgeon to help this woman adjust to the consequences of the medical intervention are limited. There is no question that the surgeon will follow the patient to see if the incision heals and to monitor whether the cancer reappears. He will arrange for the woman to see a speech pathologist to determine if she can learn esophogeal speech, but routinely her rehabilitation will not include grief counseling to deal with the multiple losses she is experiencing or vocational guidance to assist her with returning to work. It is at this point that the patient learns the real meaning of the consequences of the decision to have the surgery.

One alternative is to give the person time before surgery to come to terms with the possible treatment choices, including the choice of no treatment. However, the delay to insure integration of information has the consequence of allowing the cancer to progress. No one person need be burdened with the sole responsibility of deciding to act rashly to have surgery or to delay over an extended time to integrate information. The decision must be seen as a reciprocal one where information is shared. For the person who insists that the physician's perspective is always best no matter what the consequences, resources must be provided that will help the patient to deal constructively with the outcomes of the surgery, the course of the disease, and the impact on life.

uncertainty

Another factor that influences the type of information exchanged between a patient and physician is the uncertainty associated with a particular disease and its course. There are two types of uncertainty that the patient may experience. The first is the uncertainty of *not knowing what is known* about a specific disease, its natural course, treatment choices, and effects. There are many aspects of diseases and treatments that are certain; providers must assume responsibility for making these aspects explicit when indicated by the patient's questions or behaviors. A series of contacts will allow the patient and primary care provider the freedom to share their concerns, validate their meanings, and develop a trusting relationship.

The second type of uncertainty is what remains unknown and uncertain about the many aspects of diseases, especially for chronic illnesses such as cancer, heart and kidney diseases. Davis coined the phrase "in limbo" for patients who knew the name of their disease and understood their treatment effects, but who were living with diseases that had no predictable, known end in sight. The patients were sensitive to and capable of interpreting symptoms and experiences in terms of favorable or unfavorable medical signs, indicating they had the necessary clues for thinking about and visualizing the course of their illness. They had to learn to live one day at a time, fully aware that each day may be the beginning of their final decline (Davis, 1966).

One approach that increases a person's ability to manage uncertainties surrounding a disease in which the actual length of survival is unknown is to provide consistent access to at least one provider. That provider can establish an ongoing mechanism for monitoring the patient's symptoms and activities. One of the primary purposes of this ongoing system is to lessen and prevent complicating crises that are predictable in specific diseases. Uncertainties surrounding some diseases cannot be elimi-

nated, but they can be managed. It is important that providers distinguish between the two types of uncertainties. Physicians along with other health care providers can play key roles in reducing the uncertainty of the situation by providing what information is known, by remaining available, and by establishing a trusting relationship with the patient in which whatever occurs will be faced together.

specialization

A third factor that influences information exchange between a patient and physician is technological advances in health care and the growth of medical specialization. A patient rarely sees only one physician for the diagnostic and therapeutic phases of a disease. Instead, an army of specialists may be needed. Specialists depend not just on factual data shared among their interdisciplinary team members, but also on access to special expensive equipment, such as cardiovascular monitoring devices, X-ray machines, and laboratory assistance for specimens that allow for a complete evaluation and combination of therapies for each person. Such equipment is expensive, nonportable and frequently centrally located in large cities with medical centers.

Krant describes the process of diagnosis as a routine evaluation starting with the person seeking help from a personal physician or internist. The patient is then likely to be referred to another specialist, usually a surgeon. If the patient is fortunate, and this is more likely so in smaller communities than in large cities, the two physicians will be associates, and the initial physician will be in close contact not only with the second, but also with the patient and family. If things do not go well immediately, or worsen at a later date, additional referring physicians may be necessary, frequently in another hospital or city, and depending on the seriousness of the illness and in what area of treatment the problem falls.

> With each successive movement to another specialist, the chance of continued close rapport with the initial physician diminishes. Each transition may well be discontinuous, requiring new relationships to be established . . . But with transitions, something gets lost, namely a closeness and dependency on a stable, continuous, medical figure. This discontinuous system works well to assure that good specialized professional talent is applied to the treatment of the disease, but the price for this conveyor belt can easily be an impersonalization and dehumanization of the individual suffering from the illness [Krant, 1966, p. 53].

common expectations
for treatment goals

In addition to the lack of personalized care that may occur because of the number of providers with whom the person comes in contact, messages may become distorted, conflicting, and confusing. A fourth factor that influences information exchange among all participants in the provision of care is the unspoken and sometimes unclear expectations of the treatment goals. Each participant, including the patient, family, and multidisciplinary health care team, has certain expectations of the other participants and of the outcome of the therapies. Communication breakdowns frequently occur in this complex patient-provider system because one or more participants have unrealistic or false expectations of each other and of the treatment outcomes.

Physicians expect themselves to be able to locate a specific cause for the patient's distress, but frequently this does not occur because symptoms are diffuse and cannot be readily classified. As a result, physicians may characterize the problems of such patients as trivial or label the patients as neurotic. In contrast, patients do not have a detailed perspective of disease processes, but they want to have their symptoms relieved so they no longer experience disruptions in their ability to perform their daily activities (Tressler & Mechanic, 1978).

One way to limit a communication breakdown is for each participant to make explicit what each expects and how that goal is to be achieved. This is especially important for the person who continues to complain of symptoms for which the physician has not been able to find a diagnosis. Patients need to be aware that if they are not satisfied with the care they are receiving that there are other providers who may be more attentive to their distresses. This does not mean necessarily that by changing physicians that the new doctor will find something that the first one did not, but it does mean that patients have a right to respectful treatment that assures that they will not be discounted for showing a description of what they are feeling.

Another approach to insure effective communication is to allow for degrees of flexibility in the patient-provider relationship. A decision for treatment that has proven to be ineffective and is reversible should be reversed, such as stopping an antihypertensive (high blood pressure) drug that is causing intolerable or unmanageable side effects.

Periodic assessment of the participants' perceptions of the treatment goals is invaluable data necessary to assure effective information exchange. If the participants' goals are incongruent, every effort should be made to clarify with each other their individual perceptions and meaning of what has happened and what each is planning. This ongoing process will minimize communication breakdown and enhance a shared decision-making process for which the provider feels professionally responsible and with which the patient can live on a day-to-day basis. At all times, the patient needs to remain a central figure in this process, where decisions are made within the context of what the patient wants, needs, or chooses to compromise. The degree of confidence with which a physician can present a treatment plan for an acute symptom with an established diagnosis that is curable is different than for a symptom that is difficult to diagnose and has persisted for months. This is important information for a person to know when participating in making a decision.

summary

Information exchange between a patient and provider is critical in helping people to understand what is happening and what options for therapy are available and recommended. Traditionally, women have sought help from physicians. More recently, women are seeking providers such as nurse practitioners and physician assistants, who are concerned not only with assisting people with their problems, but also with prevention and health maintenance. The process of information exchange assumes that a person who is experiencing a symptom and seeks help wants to be responsible for decisions affecting her life and has the mental capabilities to understand what is happening. Providers must assess not only the person's symptoms, but also the person's ability to take what is happening into account and the person's particular susceptibilities to hear and understand what to expect. The information exchange process is reciprocal. After the physician informs the person of a diagnosis and its treatment options, the person must be responsible to share how each of the options fits with her daily living. This is especially important if there are two equally effective treatments with different long-term consequences. No woman should be embarrassed to obtain a second opinion, whether she is satisfied with the information she has obtained or not. In fact, obtaining a second opinion should become customary rather than an exception.

It should be the responsibility of health care providers that all patients are consistently given opportunities for choice. Women who have been reluctant to participate as partners in making a decision among treatment alternatives are denying themselves an opportunity to be responsible for their own health. For many, the idea of shared decision-making may be new. Now is the time for women to assume their role in this process, for when they are faced with a problem and treatment alternatives, they should have a say about what happens to them and their bodies.

Bard, M. The psychological import of cancer and cancer surgery. *Proceedings of the American Cancer Society's national conference on human values and cancer.* New York: American Cancer Society, 1973, pp. 22–26.

Caplan, G. An approach to the study of family mental health, *U.S. Public Health Reports,* 1956, *71,* 10.

Claus, K. E., & Bailey, J. T. *Power and influence in health care.* St. Louis: C.V. Mosby, 1977.

Cooper, J. D., The art of decision making. New York: Doubleday, 1961.

Davis, M. Z., Patients in limbo. *American Journal of Nursing,* 1966, *66,* 746–748.

Korda, M. *Power: How to get it, how to use it.* New York: Ballantine, 1975.

Krant, M. J. *Dying and dignity: The meaning and control of a personal death.* Springfield, Ill.: Thomas, 1974.

Lazarus, R. A laboratory approach to psychological stress. In C. H. Grosser, H. Wechsler & M. Greenblatt (eds.), *The threat of impending disaster.* Cambridge, Mass.: M.I.T. Press, 1964.

Mastrovito, R. C. Cancer: Awareness and denial. *Clinical Bulletin,* 1974, *4,* 142–146.

Mechanic, D. *Medical sociology.* New York: Free Press, 1968.

Thayer, L. *Communication and communication systems.* Homewood, Ill.: Irwin, 1968.

Tressler, R. & Mechanic, D. Psychological distress and perceived health status. *Journal of Health and Social Behavior,* 1978, *19,* 254–262.

Weisman, A. *On dying and denying.* New York: Behavioral Publications, 1972.

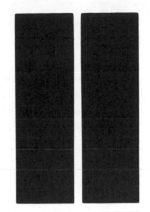

NANCY FUGATE WOODS, R.N., Ph.D.

WOMEN'S UNIQUE PHYSIOLOGY

Women have many special experiences related to their unique physiology. Only women menstruate, and only women can experience the human sexual response from a female perspective. Although these events are attributable to female biology, they are not only physiological in nature. Each woman is profoundly influenced by the sociocultural context in which events are experienced. Furthermore, these processes affect a woman's thoughts and feelings about herself as a woman. Being female and being sexual implies two somewhat opposing sides: women are "life-giving," rhythmically changing, and potentially highly orgasmic; women are also vulnerable.

Menarche, or the onset of menstruation, signals an important transition in a young woman's life. It is not merely a biological marker of sexual maturity, but also an event with social and cultural significance. For most women, menstruation is not especially disturbing or uncomfortable. For some, however, it may be most uncomfortable and even disabling. Fertility control becomes an important concern for most women, and some methods are associated with hazardous side effects.

Menopause, or the ending of menstruation, marks another important transition in a woman's life. Just as menarche and female sexuality are the object of myth and anxiety, so is menopause.

The physiological events discussed in this

37

section share many features. Often these events are the subject of myths and fears. Women may find that menarche, fertility control, their sexuality, or menopause cause them to seek health-related information or help from another woman or health worker. At times, the problems women experience are not related to their unique physiology, but to the social contexts in which they experience their bodies and their femaleness.

JOAN SHAVER, R.N., Ph.D.

female reproduction:
the menstrual cycle

The potential for a woman to conceive a child occurs in cycles, usually about once a month, during the childbearing years. There are profound physical adaptations of the reproductive organs occurring in each cycle. These changes are regulated by the brain, with hormones acting as messengers between the systems. In general, the female reproductive system is responsible for producing female germ cells, the *ova*, and for providing a hospitable environment for a new human being to grow when appropriate.

To understand the sequence of events associated with reproductive function, the menstrual cycle can be viewed in three phases. The beginning phase involves functional changes occurring in anticipation of the ovum uniting with a male germ cell, the spermatozoan, in a process called *fertilization*. The next phase involves changes in preparation for attachment of the fertilized ovum to the uterus, which is called *implantation*. These preparatory changes occur in every cycle. The nature of the final phase depends on whether the ovum is fertilized. If so, there are functional changes to support growth of the fertilized ovum, which constitutes the state known as pregnancy, or if not, the changes reflect withdrawal of the efforts to support pregnancy. In the latter instance, shedding of tissue lining the organ that was to house the pregnancy occurs. This creates the familiar menstrual bleeding, a sign known to most women. More commonly, the reproductive cycle is called the *menstrual cycle.* Menstrual blood flow heralds the failure of pregnancy to occur.

The purpose of this chapter is to review the important organs involved in reproduction, the adaptations that occur in each cycle, and the mechanisms for regulating the changes. This will help in understanding the objective signs and symptoms experienced by women as they go through the menstrual cycle, the complex sequence of events that provides the potential to become pregnant, and the general nature of some disorders that threaten women's health.

structure of the female reproductive tract

external structures

The female reproductive system is mainly a tract made up of several organs, the majority of which lie inside the body in the pelvic cavity. The tract opens to the outside of the body at the vaginal opening between the legs, in an area generally called the *perineum*. The opening from the urinary bladder to pass urine is close to the vaginal opening. Below these openings is the *anus*, through which the digestive tract passes waste materials (Fig. 4.1).

In the perineal area above the anus, the vaginal and bladder openings are encased by tissue forming the external genitalia. There is an outer fold of fatty tissue covered with skin and hair called the *labia majora*. This tissue continues upward toward the front to form a rounded pad of tissue over the pubic bones

figure 4.1
external structures of female reproductive tract

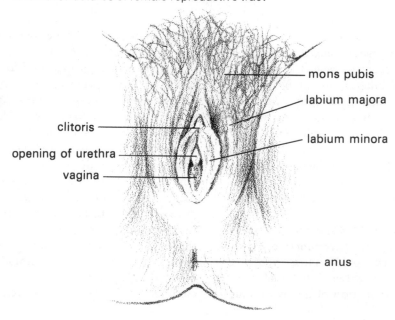

clitoris

opening of urethra

vagina

mons pubis

labium majora

labium minora

anus

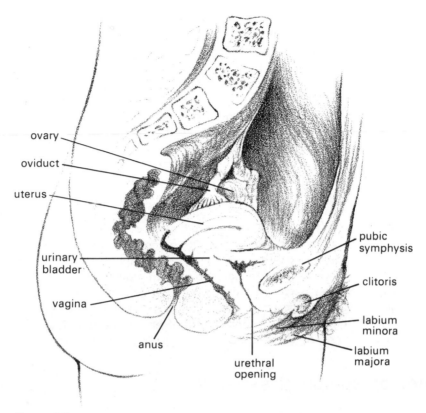

figure 4.2
structures of internal female reproductive tract

(the mons pubis). With maturity, the dense growth of hair known as pubic hair begins on the mons pubis and extends over the labia majora. Between the labia majora is another fold of delicate hairless tissue called the *labia minora*. At the convergence of the labia minora below the mons pubis is a small organ of erectile tissue called the *clitoris*. It is composed of hollow tissue that distends with blood during sexual arousal and plays an important role in female orgasm.

internal organs

The internal female reproductive tract (Fig. 4.2) starting from the external opening consists of the vagina, uterus, oviducts, and ovaries. The vagina (frequently called the birth canal) extends from the external opening as a hollow tube, which forms a pouch inside the female pelvis. The walls of the vagina are folded and are in contact in a relaxed state. The vagina has a large capacity to increase its volume by stretching during intercourse, vaginal examination, and especially during childbirth. During intercourse, sperm from the male are deposited in the vagina.

Protruding into the closed, pouch-end of the vagina is the neck of the *uterus*. The uterus is a hollow, thick, muscular, pear-shaped organ with a mucous lining (the *endometrium*). The bottom, narrow neck of the organ is called the *cervix*. It can be seen on vaginal examinations with a speculum, and cell samples are taken by the slight scraping of the cervix during a Pap test, designed to assure the presence of normal cell growth. The cervix tissue surrounds a small diameter opening between the vagina and the uterus, called the *os*. The uterus generally provides the appropriate environment for implantation of a fertilized ovum. It responds by producing the maternal part of the placenta, which is necessary to nourish a growing fetus. The uterus can grow markedly to accommodate an enlarging fetus and can contract very powerfully to push a baby out of the mother's body.

Toward the upper end of the uterus are two narrow tubes that protrude out from the body of the uterus. These tubes have muscular walls; cells lining the tubes secrete fluids. These tubes project backward to lie very close or partly wrap around two small almond-sized organs called *ovaries*. The tubes, called *oviducts* or *fallopian tubes*, have free ends that are funnel-shaped, have fine fingerlike projections called *fimbria*, and are responsible for collecting the female egg and for holding it in a certain segment of the tube for a few hours. Sperm, if deposited in the vagina, ascend through the uterus and on to the oviduct to interact with the ovum. Fertilization, thus, takes place in the oviduct. The oviducts, with fairly precise timing, eventually conduct the fertilized ovum to the uterus.

The ovaries are composed of thousands of immature female germ cells, the *ova*, or eggs, that mature, are released, and when united with a sperm can grow into a human being. The other important function of the ovary is to manufacture hormones, which in turn stimulate many types of cells to perform various functions. The ovaries are kept in place by a fold of fine connective tissue that holds them to a ligament attached to the uterus.

regulation of reproductive events

Reproduction cannot occur without properly functioning ovaries, but whether the ovaries function appropriately depends on complex interactions between the ovaries and the brain. The messages between these two organs are communicated by hormones, which are chemical substances secreted by certain cells of an organ into the blood and circulated to all tissues, but only certain cells within certain tissues respond to any one hormone.

The ovaries produce two important sex hormones, estrogen and progesterone. Brain areas, namely the hypothalamus and pituitary, respond to the amount of these hormones in the blood by "turning on" or "turning off" hormone secretions of their own. The brain hormones, when released into the blood, circulate to the ovaries and affect how they function. Although the cycle is continuous, one can begin by thinking of the state where the ovary has only immature eggs, and almost no sex hormones are being produced. Low blood levels of the sex hormones are sensed by the hypothalamus, which responds by sending a hormone messenger to the pituitary, causing it to secrete two brain hormones (follicle-stimulating hormone–FSH, and luteinizing hormone–LH). These brain hormones act on the ovary to induce at least one follicle (frequently more) to begin growing. As the follicle grows, more and more sex hormones are secreted from the ovary. Higher levels of sex hormones are sensed by the hypothalamus and perhaps the pituitary until eventually the brain hormones (FSH and LH) are turned off. This means that no new follicles

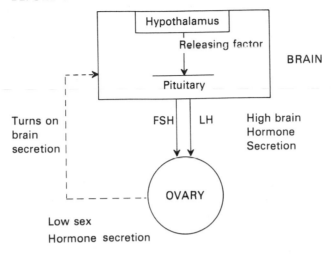

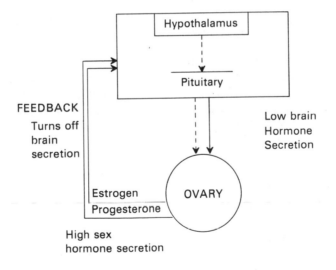

figure 4.3
regulation of reproductive events by the brain: a feedback system

are encouraged to develop for the time being. Later in the cycle, when the sex hormone levels wane, the brain hormones are again turned on. A system such as this (where low levels of ovarian hormones lead to higher levels of FSH and LH, which in turn cause ovarian hormones to be produced and, as they are, to turn off FSH and LH) is called a feedback system. It allows cell processes to remain within definite limits and, in this case, creates cycling of certain processes within organ functioning (Fig. 4.3).

details of the cycle

providing potential for fertilizing the ovum

OVARY FUNCTION. The ovaries at birth contain 300,000 to 400,000 follicles, each one a cluster of cells. Each follicle has one immature egg cell at the center, which is surrounded by layers of other cell types. As one follicle grows during a cycle, more and more estrogen is secreted by special cells. Although more than one follicle might begin to grow, all except one usually regress. The follicle grows larger because fluid accumulates between the cell layers, and the egg cell grows in size until eventually the follicle is a bulge on the ovary wall. After this time and in response to a surge of hormone (mainly LH) from the brain about two days prior, the ovum is expelled from the ovary by the fluid collected within the follicle. This activity is called *ovulation*. Occasionally, some women feel this as a cramp on one or the other side of the lower abdomen. There is sometimes a slight bloody vaginal discharge at this time.

In summary, this first phase produces a mature ovum ready for fertilization and is dominated by progressively increasing production of estrogen. Various cell types within the reproductive organs are responsive to estrogen, so higher levels of estrogen produced in this phase lead to other changes. These changes, as described below, facilitate the potential for having the sperm unite with the ovum.

OVIDUCT AND UTERUS FUNCTION. Fertilization, if it is to occur, takes place in the oviduct. The fimbriated end of the oviduct collects the ovum after release from the ovary and moves it only part of the way down the tube. Estrogen induces the muscle cells of the oviduct walls to contract more vigorously than when estrogen is low. This augmented contraction prevents the ovum from passing immediately to the uterus, but rather holds it in the tube. Under estrogen influence, fluid volume inside the tube increases in amount and becomes more dilute. This fluid likely contains important constituents that prepare the sperm to penetrate the protective coat surrounding the egg cell.

Also in response to estrogen, the uterus muscle contracts more vigorously, which assists any sperm that are present to ascend from the vagina through the cervix and uterus to the oviduct. The glands of the cervix secrete abundant thin, watery mucus, making it easier for the sperm to enter the uterus. In anticipation of pregnancy occurring, there is some growth of the uterus under the influence of estrogen. More protein for the muscular wall is manufactured and substances to be used for energy are stored in uterine muscle tissue. The lining of the uterus (the endometrium) increases in thickness about two to three times. More cells are present, their height is greater, and the glands increase in length. The blood supply enlarges in preparation for delivering more nutrients to the uterus should a pregnancy be implanted.

FERTILITY IMPLICATIONS. The major event of this first phase of the reproductive cycle is ovulation, or egg release. Failure to ovulate could be due to any number of difficulties with the sequence of normal events. Recall that there must be a normally functioning hypothalamus and pituitary to sense ovarian sex hormone levels, then synthesize and release FSH and LH. The hypothalamus is subject to influence from the higher brain centers, so emotional state and thought processes can alter its function. Particularly, if the surge of LH just prior to ovulation is not adequate, an ovum may not be released. This can happen frequently at the beginning of reproductive life (puberty) and at the end (menopause). These cycles are called *anovulatory* (no ovulation). In addition, the ovary cells must be capable of responding to LH and FSH.

Even though ovulation has occurred and there are adequate sperm in the tract, interaction between the two depends on complex events. Inability of the oviduct and/or uterus to respond to estrogen (in terms of movement and/or secreting adequate fluid) could lead to failure of: capture of the ovum by the oviduct, conduction to the proper part of the tube, retention of the ovum in the oviduct, adaptation of the sperm, or speed of sperm movement along the tract. It is possible to have the egg released and enter the pelvic cavity rather than the oviduct. It is also possible to have the ovum fertilized and begin growing in the tube with failure to have it conducted to the uterus. This state is known as ectopic pregnancy and results in loss of the pregnancy. Fertilization is a complex process that relies heavily on a time-ordered sequence. The released unfertilized ovum lives only about 24 hours. Sperm

live only about 48 hours, although some live up to 72 hours.

This preovulatory to ovulation phase of the reproductive cycle is dominated by increasing estrogen production. In actuality, there is a series of naturally produced estrogens, differing slightly from one another chemically and in potency. The most potent is b-estradiol, with estrone and estriol being slightly less effective. The ovary is the main source of estrogens in the nonpregnant female, although the placenta produces large amounts during pregnancy. Very small amounts are secreted by the adrenal gland. All natural estrogens are steroids having a chemical structure similar to cholesterol, from which they are synthesized. The liver converts estradiol to less active forms, and they are removed from the body in the urine.

As can be deduced from the previous discussion, the cyclic increase in estrogen stimulates muscle contraction of the uterus and oviducts, tissue growth in the uterus, and influences secretion within the tract. During sexual maturing, as the basal estrogen level is established, growth of mammary tissue and deposition of fat in the breast, as well as in the buttocks and thighs, leading to the female physique can be seen to occur. It causes the skin to be smooth and soft and affects bone activity so that the growth pattern in females is different from males. In general, there is a fairly consistent growth spurt at puberty, but growth ceases earlier in girls than in boys. After menopause, when estrogen production wanes, bone disorders like osteoporosis develop more frequently in females.

providing the potential
for implanting the fertilized ovum

OVARY FUNCTION. Following expulsion of the mature ovum from the ovary, the remaining follicle collapses, but it is transformed into a structure that now secretes the sex hormone *progesterone* in addition to estrogen. This follicle structure is called the *corpus luteum*, and its formation is dependent on the pituitary hormone, LH.

THE OVIDUCT AND UTERUS FUNCTION. This phase prepares the reproductive tract for implanting and nurturing of the possibly fertilized ovum. While estrogen acting alone augments muscle contraction of the oviduct, progesterone is thought to relax muscular activity to allow the potentially fertilized ovum to proceed to the uterus. The duration of time from egg release to its appearance in the uterus is 3 to 4 days. Progesterone also inhibits uterine muscle contraction, producing a quieted response so the fertilized ovum can attach to the wall. The lining of the uterus under its influence shows greatly increased secretion activity. The glands become prominent and secrete a sugar-rich solution. It has been suggested that these substances are necessary in helping the fertilized ovum adhere to the uterine wall and to nourish the cell complex that will become a human being. While estrogen alone leads to secretion of a thin watery substance from the glands of the cervix, progesterone leads to a decreased amount of mucus that is thicker and more viscous. This actually begins the protective sealing of the uterus to protect pregnancy.

IMPLANTATION DISORDERS. It is now clear that the activity of the ovaries can be viewed in two phases: (1) the *follicular* phase during which the follicle grows and estrogen secretion is dominant, culminating in ovulation, and (2) the *luteal* phase during which the corpus luteum secretes both estrogens and progesterone. Again, there are a number of processes leading to implantation. Inability of the corpus luteum to secrete adequate amounts of sex hormones or the inability of the uterus to respond to the hormones could lead to failure

to develop a hospitable environment for implantation. Progesterone especially is needed to sensitize the cells lining the uterus to receive the fertilized ovum. The effects of progesterone occur only if the estrogens have performed preliminary changes. The fertilized ovum must also be "activated" in the uterus in order to attach, although the sequence of events is not clear; it does, however, involve the sex hormones. Failure of implantation or inadequate implantation for these and other reasons can lead to spontaneous rejection (abortion) of a pregnancy before it is really established, and sometimes later in pregnancy as well. Most often, the exact reason for natural loss of a pregnancy is not apparent.

In the second phase of the reproductive cycle, the dominant hormones are estrogen and progesterone, which frequently act cooperatively. The corpus luteum of the ovary is the major site of progesterone production, although small amounts come from the adrenal gland. It is chemically similar to the estrogens and to other steroid hormones produced and secreted by the outer adrenal gland cells. The liver inactivates progesterone and it is removed from the body in the urine.

As mentioned, the effect of progesterone on the uterus is to increase secretions from the endometrial lining, augment the blood supply, and decrease motility. Progesterone acts cooperatively with estrogen to develop the breasts. Another major effect is on fluid balance. It causes the kidneys to retain water and body tissues to retain fluid. This retention is noted particularly in the last part of the menstrual cycle as perceived weight gain, and some women are aware of slightly enlarged breasts with some tingling sensation or tenderness.

In addition, progesterone increases body temperature. Normally, there will be a rise of one-half to one degree in body temperature in the 18 to 24 hours following ovulation.

WHEN PREGNANCY IS NOT ESTABLISHED. The corpus luteum of the ovary has a limited lifespan. It cannot maintain its production of estrogens and progesterone for longer than 8 to 10 days without the support that occurs only if a pregnancy has been established. When the ovum is fertilized in the oviduct, the cells immediately begin dividing so that a complex of cells (*blastocyst*) enters the uterus. Within a short time, the blastocyst attaches to the wall, and certain cells begin to embed in the endometrial lining to form the placenta. The placenta is the organ across which substances needed for growth are transferred from the mother's blood supply to the baby's blood supply. Early placental cells begin to secrete a hormone that sustains hormone secretion by the corpus luteum. Later, the placenta itself insures secretion of the sex hormones. In this manner, estrogens and progesterone remain high throughout pregnancy, and the reproductive cycle is held fixed in the secretory maintenance phase for varying lengths of time, but roughly in the vicinity of 280 days until a full-term baby is delivered.

When there is no pregnancy, the corpus luteum degenerates, causing estrogens and progesterone to diminish. The lower blood levels of these hormones signal the pituitary and hypothalamus to renew FSH and LH secretion so that another follicle will begin to mature, and the cycle begins again.

Withdrawal of estrogen and progesterone also removes growth support to the uterus, leading to sloughing off of the tissue lining it. The bloody discharge a woman recognizes as her "period" contains cells of the degenerating endometrium, many white blood cells, and actual blood. Substances in the discharge prevent the blood from clotting to any extent, unless flow is unusually heavy. Bleeding can last

from 2 to 8 days, with the usual being 4 to 5 days. Only about 50 to 100 milliliters (2 to 3 ounces) of blood normally are lost during a period.

summary of the menstrual cycle

Since menstrual bleeding is the most obvious indicator of reproductive system functioning, the practical approach in terms of assessing one's own cycle is to consider it as beginning with the first day of menstrual bleeding. Hence, we most often refer to the menstrual cycle. As review, consider a hypothetical 30-day cycle (Fig. 4.4). Days 1 to 5 constitute menstruation. Sex hormone secretion from the ovaries is low, the brain is beginning to secrete FSH and LH, and new follicle growth begins. Bleeding halts, and from days 6 to 15, FSH and LH progressively increase, the ovary follicle enlarges with the maturing egg cell and internal collection of fluid while progressively larger amounts of estrogen are released. This is sometimes referred to as the *follicular* phase of ovary function. The uterus responds to the estrogen by growth of the muscle wall and the endometrial lining. In terms of the uterus, this is called the *proliferative* phase. The oviduct increases motility and prepares the environment for fertilization.

About midcycle, for example, day 16, there is a surge of LH secretion leading to extrusion of the matured ovum from the surface of the ovary. The ovum is captured in the oviduct and held there temporarily. Following this, from days 17 to 26, the ruptured follicle becomes the corpus luteum, which secretes estrogen and progesterone. This is referred to as the *luteal* phase of ovary function. In response to both estrogen and progesterone, the oviduct has lessened contraction activity to allow passage of the ovum to the uterus. The uterus responds by quieted activity and increased se-

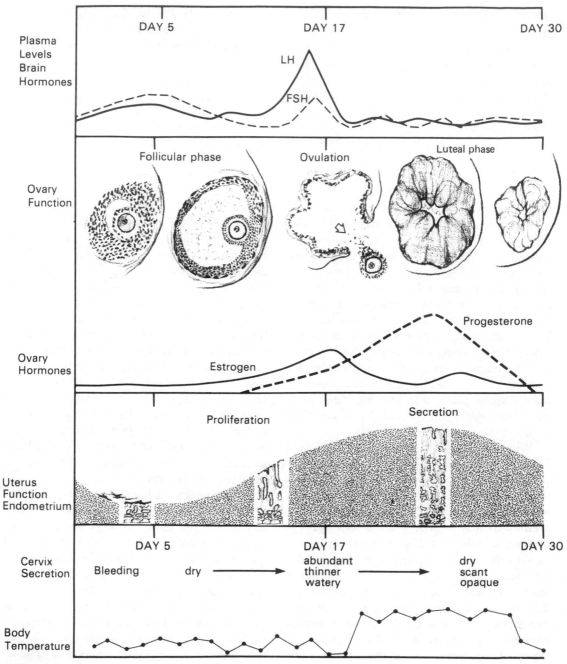

figure 4.4
physiological changes during a 30-day menstrual cycle

cretions to allow for nourishment of the possibly fertilized ovum and to facilitate its implantation. In terms of the uterus, this is called the *secretory* phase.

From days 27 to 30, the corpus luteum begins to break down if there is no fertilized ovum present, and its production of sex hormones turns off. In response to waning hormonal levels, the blood vessels to the lining of the uterus constrict, the cells are deprived of their nutrition, and the tissue begins to slough away. The blood vessels then dilate and bleeding begins, marking day 1 of a repeat cycle.

A popular notion is that a "normal" menstrual cycle is very regular and cycles every 28 days. Although this may be true for a small number of women, the range of normal cycle length is 20 to 40 days. Cycles are not perfectly regular in any one woman, but usually stay within 3 or 4 days of an average length. When the length of a woman's menstrual cycle varies by more than about 8 days, it is considered irregular. Bleeding between periods or after intercourse is indicative of the need to seek a health assessment. Cycles are frequently irregular in teen-agers, women moving into the menopause, and in some women who have just stopped taking birth control pills.

Some women have abundant periods where they experience blood-soaked underwear or bedsheets in spite of frequently changing sanitary napkins or tampons. Someone who has always had "heavy" flow may have no health problems, but regular checkups are a good idea in such cases. A woman whose periods suddenly become abundant should seek an immediate health examination from a professional.

control of fertility

Clearly, the frequent potential for becoming pregnant creates the necessity in our time and culture for controlling when and how often to have a child. An understanding of the female reproductive cycle is rudimentary to an informed choice regarding a birth control method or understanding how to maximize chances for pregnancy.

In the menstrual cycle, hormonal fluctuations regulate ovulation. Substantial levels of estrogen and progesterone inhibit release of the brain hormones that mature an ovum and cause its release from the ovary. Birth control pills consist of synthetically made estrogen and progesterone, which block the normal waxing and waning of the hormone levels, thus eliminating ovulation. They are taken on a 3-week-on, 1-week-off schedule so that when the pill is stopped, decreased estrogen and progesterone support of the uterus causes menstrual bleeding. There is much controversy regarding the safety of "the Pill," which is beyond the scope of this chapter. However, the Pill does generally provide a very high, although not perfect, level of contraception, but it also constitutes unnatural interference with the body's natural hormones, an interference not without risk. Most other methods of contraception involve chemical or mechanical interference with the admission of sperm to the tract or adherence of the fertilized ovum to the uterine wall.

There are circumstances when a woman prefers to abstain from intercourse at the time when she is fertile, and the same knowledge can be used to maximize the chances of pregnancy. Using the natural sequence of events as the main method for controlling pregnancy is a good example of applying the previously described knowledge about how the menstrual cycle works. When one wishes to predict the fertile period with some accuracy, there are generally three ways: (1) the calendar method, using the length of previous cycles, (2) the temperature method, using the fact that progesterone secreted following ovulation raises resting body temperature, and (3) the cervical mucus method, using hormone-modulated changes in consistency of mucus from the cervix. The combination of all three is often said to lead to a more dependable assessment (Cherniak, 1979; Shapiro, 1977).

The success of these methods is predicated on the following factors:

- Even though the time from menstruation to ovulation is variable from woman to woman, ovulation will occur 14 (plus or minus 2) days prior to the onset of menstrual bleeding.
- The unfertilized egg lives no longer than 24 hours following ovulation.
- Most sperm live only up to 48 hours, although some can live as long as 72 hours.
- Progesterone released by the corpus luteum raises resting body temperature within 24 hours after egg release, and it remains elevated until menstruation (about 14 days).
- Cervical mucus is scant, thick, and opaque when infertile, but as ovulation approaches, it becomes more abundant in amount of thin, watery, stretchable mucus.

From observing the length of each menstrual cycle for about 6 months, calculations can be made of the likely fertile days. It has been suggested that 18 be subtracted from the shortest cycle and 11 from the longest to determine the first fertile day and the first unfertile day following ovulation. A 30-day shortest and 35-day longest cycle would calculate to days 12 and 24. To prevent pregnancy, this method would suggest refraining from intercourse between days 12 and 24—the disadvantage, of course, being a rather lengthy period of abstinence.

A further means of detecting more definitely when ovulation has occurred is to record daily body temperatures. When the body temperature rises and remains elevated for 3 days, the fertile period is considered over. This method does not predict when ovulation occurs, but rather when it has occurred. The fertile time before ovulation can arbitrarily be considered as day 3 of the cycle or calculated by the calendar method. The temperature should be taken before arising, eating, smoking, or any other activity. Sometimes the temperature rise is gradual enough in some women to make the temperature graph difficult to interpret.

As a further refinement, a woman can use her fingers to assess her mucus from the cervix. After menstrual bleeding there will be a few dry days, some moist to wet days, followed by dry days. The first sign of wetness indicates the first fertile day. Ovulation is indicated by the last wet day, with the last fertile day being the third consecutive dry day.

There are other methods using an instrument to self-view the cervix and for testing the mucus stretchability. These brief descriptions accentuate the functional changes occurring throughout the female reproductive cycle and how they can be used to help a woman assess that cycle.

conclusion

The importance of understanding the functioning of the reproductive system is crucial to women's health. It is to a woman's advantage to be "in tune" with how her body is operating. Awareness of the normal events of the reproductive cycle improves self-assessment of, recognition of, and health-seeking behavior for disordered function so that health can be restored quickly if threatened. It can help a woman to understand what is expected in terms of alterations throughout the life-span and to accept the natural aging of the system.

Knowledge of the female reproductive system on the part of men can help eradicate mythical ideas that discredit a woman's intellectual abilities and claim emotional vulnerability due to menstrual functioning. As men are the sexual partners for most women, the knowledge they have regarding female sexuality and reproduction affects the mutual satisfaction of any relationship. Finally, such knowledge on the part of health workers will provide higher quality health care assessment and professional assistance in a partnership to support women in caring for and about themselves.

Boston Women's Health Book Collective. *Our bodies, ourselves: A book by and for women.* New York: Simon & Schuster, 1973.

Cherniak, D. *A book about birth control.* Montreal: Montreal Health Press, 1979.

Dalton, K. *The menstrual cycle.* New York: Pantheon, 1969.

Dalton, K. *The premenstrual syndrome and progesterone therapy.* Chicago: Year Book Medical Publishers, 1977.

Shapiro, H. I. *The birth control book.* New York: St. Martin's, 1977.

Strand, F. L. *Physiology: A regulatory systems approach.* New York; Macmillan, 1978.

Vollman, R. F. *The menstrual cycle.* Philadelphia: Saunders, 1977.

5

JEANNE BROOKS-GUNN, Ph.D.
DIANE N. RUBLE, Ph.D.

menarche:
fact and fiction

Puberty, marking the end of childhood and the beginning of adolescence, is a period of rapid and sometimes bewildering changes. As the adolescent female watches these changes occur, she may be alternately fascinated and terrified, pleased and disappointed, self-confident and self-conscious. Menarche, the onset of menstruation, is the most obvious sign of puberty for females; males have no such discrete and public marker, although in our culture some scientists see the boy's first ejaculation as comparable to the girl's first period.

Menarche is both a public and private event, one that the adolescent feels to be deeply personal but that is sometimes painfully evident to and broadly acknowledged by parents and friends. In her diary, Anne Frank

conveys the secretive nature of menarche and the ambivalent feelings about menstruation:

> Each time I have a period . . . I have the feeling that in spite of all the pain, unpleasantness, nastiness, I have a sweet secret and that is why, although it is nothing but a nuisance to me in a way, I always long for the time that I shall feel the secret within me again (1972, p. 117).*

The public nature of menarche is evident in the rites of passage in other societies and in peer and parental reactions in our society. Public reactions may be joyful, cruel, or

*Excerpt from *Anne Frank: The Diary of a Young Girl* by Anne Frank. Copyright © 1952 by Otto H. Frank. Reprinted by permission of Doubleday & Company, Inc. and Vallentine Mitchell & Co., Ltd.

52

terrifying. The movie *Carrie* begins with a locker room scene: Carrie, an awkward, unpopular, and sheltered teenager, begins to menstruate for the first time while showering after gym class. Not having been told about menstruation from her mother, girl friends, doctor, or teachers, she is terrified by the experience.

cultural customs and menarche

Just as cultural beliefs influence perceptions of menstruation, so do they affect beliefs about menarche. Crosscultural research indicates that menarche may elicit celebration, disdain, or no comment, depending on the culture (Delaney, Lupton, & Toth, 1976; Hays, 1964). The Apache Indians look upon a girl's first menstruation favorably, considering it an awesome, supernatural blessing. Eskimos isolate the girl from contact with people for 40 days, and in some South American cultures, a menarcheal girl is beaten or otherwise tortured (Delaney et al., 1976). Margaret Mead's description of the ceremony of the Arapesh illustrates the elaborateness and importance of the occasion in some cultural groups:

A girl's first menstruation and the accompanying ceremonial take place in . . . her husband's home. But her brothers must play a part in it and they are sent for; failing brothers, cousins will come. Her brothers build her a menstrual hut, which is stronger and better-constructed than are the menstrual huts of older women . . . The girl is cautioned to sit with her legs crossed. Her woven arm and leg bands, her earrings, her old lime gourd and lime spatula are taken from her. Her woven belt is taken off. If these are fairly new they are given away; if they are old they are cut off and destroyed. There is no feeling that they themselves are contaminated, but only the desire to cut the girl's connection with her past.

The girl is attended by older women who are her own relatives or relatives of her husband. They rub her all over with stinging nettles. They tell her to roll one of the large nettle-leaves into a tube and thrust it into her vulva: this will ensure her breasts growing large and strong. The girl eats no food, nor does she drink water. On the third day, she comes out of the hut and stands against a tree while her mother's brother makes the decorative cuts upon her shoulders and buttocks. This is done so gently, with neither earth nor lime rubbed in—the usual New Guinea method for making scarification marks permanent—that is is only possible to find the scars during the next three or four years. During that time, however, if strangers wish to know whether a girl is nubile, they look for the marks. Each day the women rub the girl with nettles. It is well if she fasts for five or six days, but the women watch her anxiously, and if she becomes too weak they put an end to it. Fasting will make her strong, but too much of it might make her die, and the emergence ceremony is hastened. (1950, pp. 80-81)*

What about our own society's rites of passage? Although we cannot compete with the Arapesh, some American families do celebrate the event. As one girl described her first period:

When I discovered it . . . (my mother) told me to come with her, and we went into the living room to tell my father. She just looked at me and then at him and said, "Well, your little girl is a young lady now!" My dad gave me a hug and congratulated me and I felt grown up and proud that I was a lady at last. (Shipman, 1971, p. 331)**

*Excerpts from *Sex and Temperament in Three Primitive Socieites* by Margaret Mead, pp. 92–93. Copyright©1935 by Margaret Mead. Reprinted by permission of William Morrow & Company.
**Excerpt from "The Psychodynamics of Sex Education," by Gordon Shipman in *Adolescent Behavior and Society: A Book of Readings*, Rolf E. Muuss, ed., Copyright©1971. Reprinted by permission of Random House, Inc.

Unfortunately, the event is not always acknowledged with pride. Another girl recalls her experience:

> I had no information whatsoever, no hint that anything was going to happen to me . . . I thought I was on the point of death from internal hemorrhage . . . What did my highly educated mother do? She read me a furious lecture about what a bad, evil, immoral thing I was to start menstruating at the age of eleven! So young and so vile! Even after thirty years, I can feel the shock of hearing her condemn me for

"doing" something I had no idea occurred. (Weideger, 1976, p. 169)*

In spite of our society's lack of a rite, adolescent girls learn a great deal about their society's attitudes and expectations during menarche. Cultural customs set the stage for menarche and puberty, specifically in terms of sociocultural beliefs and attitudes, acquisition of information, familial socialization, and physical changes.

menarche: a sociocultural and biopsychological phenomenon

sociocultural beliefs about menarche

Because of the large number of studies using self-report instruments to measure perceptions of the incidence or severity of menstrual-related symptoms, we have fairly extensive knowledge concerning cultural beliefs about menstruation. To explore the development of these beliefs, we asked females ranging from elementary school to college students to rate the severity of thirty symptoms during their intermenstrual, premenstrual, and menstrual cycle phases for themselves (self-reports) and others (general knowledge) as well.

In general, our cultural beliefs are mirrored in adolescent and adult self-reports about cycle changes and beliefs about the symptoms of females in general. Adolescent and adult females report approximately the same symptoms and cycle-phase changes, both believe that females in general experience the same (or even more severe) symptoms as they do themselves, and females who have not begun to menstruate expect to experience the same symptoms reported by their same-age peers who already are menstruating. In brief, there are remarkable similarities in the self-reports of global symptom changes across samples with different menstrual experience, suggest-

ing a likely impact of cultural beliefs on young adolescent girls.

Furthermore, these beliefs seem to be acquired early. Fifth- to sixth-graders knew about most culturally accepted cycle changes, although they had not learned all the specifics (for example, they did not know that water retention is more of a premenstrual than a menstrual symptom). Interestingly, the premenarcheal fifth- to sixth-graders expected to experience more severe changes than the premenarcheal seventh- to eighth-graders, probably because of differences in the nature of the information received and the way it is acquired (that is, the younger girls have less opportunity to discuss menstruation—fewer menstrual peers, less health knowledge, less maternal information).

The premenarcheal seventh- to eighth-graders expect to experience what their menstruating peers report. And severity of symptoms increases from junior to senior high school, with the older adolescents looking identical to college samples. This increase may be due to more cultural information being

*Excerpt from *Menstruation and Menopause: The Physiology and Psychology, the Myth and Reality* by Paula Weideger. Reprinted by permission of Alfred A. Knopf, Inc.

acquired or to more experience with menstruation itself (and having more opportunity to experience more symptoms).

To give a concrete example from these data, let us look more closely at the findings for pain and water retention, the two most commonly reported symptoms in adult women. Like the majority of adults studied, all groups of girls reported experiencing or anticipating cycle-phase differences for the two Menstrual Distress Questionnaire (MDQ) scales. Sample comparisons indicate that the premenarcheal fifth- to sixth-graders expect to experience more water retention (but not pain) than their premenarcheal seventh- and eighth-grade counterparts. The premenarcheal junior high school students expect to experience more pain than the postmenarcheal junior high school students report. Finally, the senior high school and college students (all postmenarcheal) report more severe pain and water retention than the junior high school girls who are menstruating.

acquisition of menstrual-related beliefs

Adolescent girls, even those who have not begun to menstruate, have acquired many of the cultural beliefs about cycle-related symptoms. Where do adolescents learn about menstruation and what type of information is actually transmitted? In this section, we examine the sources of menstrual-related information, the type of information actually given by various sources, and the amount of preparation given to girls prior to the onset of menarche.

SOURCES OF INFORMATION. The family has traditionally been the major information source for young girls, with the mother providing most of the information (Abel & Joffe, 1950). In one study, Haft (1973), fifty percent reported that their mother was their first source of menstrual information. Sisters, especially older ones, are potentially good sources of information. Other than the mother and older sisters, family members seem to contribute little information. The father's contribution to girls' knowledge about menstruation seems to be minimal, and most studies do not even mention fathers as sources of this kind of information. Female friends are a major source of information. And health education classes comprise another primary source of information. Over three-quarters of the subjects learned something about menstruation in a health class (Ruble & Brooks-Gunn, 1977; Whisnant & Zegans, 1975). This is not surprising, since approximately three-quarters of all adolescents currently receive some form of health education in elementary or junior high school (Whisnant, Brett, & Zegans, 1975).

The last major source involves the media. Within media sources, the booklets prepared by the sanitary products industry provide the bulk of the information. Most health classes use these booklets, sometimes in conjunction with films, in the explanation of menstruation, and most girls list books or booklets as a source of information (Ruble & Brooks-Gunn, 1977; Whisnant & Zegans, 1975).

Finally, the onset of menarche seems to result in an increase in information-seeking. In our studies of seventh- to eighth-grade pre- and postmenarcheal girls, postmenarcheal girls reported learning more from some sources than did the premenarcheal girls (Brooks-Gunn & Ruble, 1980; Clarke & Ruble, 1978). This increase may be due to the increased interest of adolescent girls or to an increased concern of family and friends.

PREPARATION FOR MENARCHE. In general, preparation for menarche has involved familial and sociocultural practices. In most European cultures (for example, Germany, Poland, Ireland) at the beginning of this century, girls were given no advance warning; in contrast, adolescents in Italy were likely to have heard their female relatives discuss menstruation, which was a topic of great importance and, therefore, discussed freely. After the onset of menstruation, mothers in all of these cultures explained menstruation to their daughters. However, the completeness of the explanations varied greatly. As an extreme, Polish peasants did not tell their daughters how to wear sanitary cloths nor how to keep them in place; the girls were expected to know how to do this.

When these cultural groups immigrated to America, adolescents were more likely to be given information prior to the event, since it was thought to be "old-fashioned" not to do so. Also, families wanted their girls to learn their own culture's customs and beliefs, not those of another group. Often sisters or other female relatives provided this information. The value of advance preparation in America is reflected in changing trends; in a sample of adults interviewed in the late 1950s, one-third of the girls had no advance warning (Shainess, 1961), while in the late 1970s, only a few (less than 5 percent) had no advance warning (Brooks-Gunn & Ruble, 1980).

TYPES OF INFORMATION. The contents of booklets distributed by the personal products industry and used in health classes and were examined because these booklets probably mirror the attitudes and beliefs of our society (Whisnant, et al. 1975). Menstruation was characterized both as a normal, natural part of life as well as an embarrassing event that needs to be concealed, and as a hygienic crisis that needs to be combated by frequent bathing and napkin changing. As one states, menstruation is "a natural, normal part of life. Treat it naturally, normally, and you won't be embarrassed or upset each time it comes." Another booklet states: "It's absolutely impossible for anyone to know you are menstruating unless of course you act stupid about the whole thing" (Whisnant et al., 1975, p. 817).

The booklets also give fairly explicit and rigid instructions for combating any physical changes that may occur, and by doing so they seem to deny that such changes might happen in at least some women. For example: "Mild cramps are often caused by factors other than menstruation. These factors include constipation, poor posture, insufficient exercise, and a poor mental attitude" (Whisnant et al., 1975, p. 817). Girls are urged to compensate for any bodily changes (another inconsistency) by having a positive mental attitude and plunging into activities. In short, the booklets reflecting cultural beliefs send the readers mixed messages about the meaning of menstruation.

menarche as a biological event

SEQUENCE OF PHYSICAL CHANGES. Puberty is universally seen as a period of rapid physical growth and sexual maturation, even though the definition of puberty is in dispute. The sequence of events during this time of physical change has been extensively studied, with a general picture of development emerging.

Before the advent of sexual maturation, a growth spurt typically occurs, with rapid increases in height and weight between 7½ to 11½ years of age. After a very rapid spurt, physical growth continues at a slow pace for several years (Tanner, 1970). After the growth spurt, usually the first sign of sexual maturation is breast budding, with the breasts becoming elevated and the nipples enlarged. The second sign is usually the appearance of pubic hair. The breasts and pubic hair develop gradually. The third sign involves the growth of the uterus and vagina and the enlargement of the labia and clitoris. Only after these changes have occurred does menstruation begin. Finally, axillary hair appears, hips broaden, and fat deposits increase (Conger, 1973; Tanner, 1970).

As is obvious from this description, it is difficult to pinpoint the precise onset of puberty, since the physical changes occur gradually and overlap within and across individuals. For example, pubic hair sometimes appears prior to breast budding. However, menarche is almost always one of the last physical changes. To complicate matters, the different signs of sexual maturation do not seem to appear systematically, perhaps because they may be controlled by different hormones. For example, research seems to indicate that age of menarche is independent of the growth spurt (Damon, Damon, Reid, & Valadian, 1969; Tanner, 1970).

HORMONAL CHANGES. In addition to sexual maturational changes, hormonal changes occur at the time of puberty (see chapter 4 for a description of hormonal changes associated with menstruation). An increase in hormone production happens around the age of 11, although it is not clear exactly when the pattern of female hormonal cyclic fluctuations is established. In the past, hormonal fluctuations were thought to occur at the onset of menarche, but recent studies show cyclic variation in hormone production prior to menarche, at least in some girls (Hansen, Hoffman, & Ross, 1975).

AGE OF MENARCHE. One of the most well-known facts about menarche is the change in age that has occurred through the nineteenth century. In Europe and the United States, the age of menarche has declined about four months per decade since 1850 (Sherman, 1971). Attempts at explaining the downward trends have not been entirely successful. The most well-documented factor in the downward trend is nutrition; heredity and general state of health may also play a part (for example, Tanner, 1970).

In summary, menarche involves an intriguing interplay of individual experiences, physiological changes, cultural beliefs, and trans-mission of knowledge. General cultural attitudes concerning negative aspects of menstruation and the symptoms associated with it are acquired at a young age, but they may be acquired or provided differently between elementary and junior high school. A young girl infers from the cultural beliefs what she can expect to experience when she begins menstruating. She may also receive specific preparatory information from significant others, such as mothers or health classes, which affect the nature of her expectations.

These factors—general cultural stereotypes, expectations for self, and specific information received from others—jointly contribute to the postmenarcheal girl's self-reported experience of menstruation. Finally, the postmenarcheal girl's direct physical experience of symptoms is also likely to be a contributing factor to her responses, although social expectations have also been shown to affect self-perceptions of physiological states (Schacter & Singer, 1962).

If the menarche is as important an event as many psychologists and physicians believe, a girl's early experience of menstruation may affect other aspects of her life as well. Therefore, it is necessary to acknowledge the fictions that have arisen about menarche and replace them with fact.

Abel, T., & Joffe, N. F. Cultural background of female puberty. *American Journal of Psychotherapy*, 1950, 4, 90–113.

Brooks-Gunn, J., & Ruble, D. N. *The social and psychological meaning of menarche*. Paper presented at the meeting of the Society for Research in Child Development, San Francisco, March 1979b.

Brooks-Gunn, J., & Ruble, D. N. *Dysmenorrhea during adolescence*. Paper presented at the meeting of the American Psychological Association, New York, September 1979a.

Brooks-Gunn, J., & Ruble, D. N. Menarche: The interaction of physiological, cultural and social factors. In A. J. Dun, C. M. Graham, & C. Beecher (Eds.). *The menstrual cycle: Synthesis of interdisciplinary research*. New York: Springer, 1980.

Clarke, A., & Ruble, D. N. Young adolescents' beliefs about menstruation. *Child development,* 1978, *49,* 231–234.

Conger, J. S. *Adolescence and youth: Psychological development in a changing world.* New York: Harper, 1973.

Damon, A., Damon, S. T., Reid, R. B., & Valadian, I. Age at menarche of mothers and daughters with a note on accuracy of recall. *Human Biology,* 1969, *41,* 161–175.

Delaney, J., Lupton, M. J., & Toth, E. *The curse: A cultural history of menstruation.* New York: Dutton, 1976.

Englander-Golden, P., Whitmore, M. R., & Densthbier, R. A. Menstrual cycle as a focus of study and self-reports of moods and behaviors. *Motivation and Emotion,* 1978, *7,* 75–86.

Frank, A. *The diary of a young girl.* New York: Pocket Books, 1972.

Haft, M. H. An exploratory study of early adolescent girls; body image, self acceptance, acceptance of traditional female role, and response to menstruation. Unpublished doctoral thesis, Columbia University, 1973.

Hansen, H. R., Hoffman, H. J., & Ross, G. T. Monthly gonadotropic cycles in premenstrual girls. *Science,* 1975, *190,* 161–163.

Hays, H. R. *The dangerous sex: The myth of feminine evil.* New York: Putnam, 1964.

Mead, M. *Sex and temperament in three primitive societies.* New York: Mentor, 1950.

Ruble, D. N. Premenstrual symptoms: A reinterpretation. *Science,* 1977, *197,* 291–292.

Ruble, D. N., & Brooks-Gunn, J. *Adolescents' attitudes about menstruation.* Paper presented at the meeting of the Society for Research in Child Development, New Orleans, March 1977.

Ruble, D. N., & Brooks-Gunn, J. Menstrual symptoms: A social cognition analysis. *Journal of Behavioral Medicine,* 1979, 2, 171–194.

Ruble, D. N., Brooks, J., & Clarke, A. Research on menstrual-related psychological changes: Alternative perspectives. In J. E. Parsons (Ed.), *The psychobiology of sex roles and sex differences.* Washington, D. C.: Hemisphere, 1980.

Schacter, S., & Singer, J. E. Cognitive, social and physiological determinants of emotional state. *Psychological Review,* 1962, *69,* 379–399.

Shainess, N. A re-evaluation of some aspects of femininity through a study of menstruation: A preliminary report. *Comparative Psychiatry,* 1961, *2,* 20–26.

Sherman, J. *On the psychology of women: A survey of empirical studies.* Springfield, Ill.: Thomas, 1971.

Shipman, G. The psychodynamics of sex education. In R. E. Muuss, (Ed.) *Adolescent behavior and society.* New York: Random House, 1971.

Tanner, J. M. Physical growth. In P. H. Mussen (Ed.), *Carmichael's manual of child psychology.* New York: Wiley, 1970.

Weideger, P. *Menstruation and menopause.* New York: Knopf, 1976.

Whisnant, L., Brett, E., & Zegans, L. Implicit messages concerning menstruation in commercial educational materials prepared for young adolescent girls. *American Journal of Psychiatry,* 1975, *132,* 815–820.

Whisnant, L., & Zegans, L. A study of attitudes toward menarche in white middle-class American adolescent girls. *American Journal of Psychiatry,* 1975, *138,* 809–814.

BARBARA SOMMER, Ph.D.

menstrual distress

are menstruation and its accompanying events stressful? facts vs. fallacies

Historically, menstruation has a negative reputation, and it continues to be viewed by many people in many cultures as a malevolent force in a woman's life. There are several theories of why menstruation is viewed negatively. One belief is that menstruation is inherently problematic, that the biology of the menstrual cycle is disruptive to the person. Psychoanalytic theories have focused on the

symbolic significance and fear associated with a monthly discharge of blood. At a sociological level, the role and status of woman may influence how people view events that are uniquely female. All of these beliefs may contribute to the development of expectations and stereotypes that in turn influence people's attitudes and behavior toward menstruation. The purpose of this chapter is to examine the *scientific* evidence concerning the existence and incidence of menstrual distress, taking into account, where appropriate, physiological, social, and psychological factors.

The author wishes to express gratitude to Patricia Rozee Koker and Robert Sommer for their critical reading and suggestions.

incidence of stress

It is difficult to determine the number of women who find menstruation debilitating. Reviewing the literature from the United States and Western Europe, Sommer (1978) found that a majority of women report unpleasant or uncomfortable symptoms associated with the premenstrual and/or menstrual phase of the cycle. However, one-fourth of the women report severe menstrual symptoms. The most common are pelvic and back pain, water retention, and negative moods, particularly irritability, nervousness, depression, and fatigue. Less than one-third of women surveyed markedly changed their routine during the days surrounding menstruation.

performance measures

Researchers looking at performance measures—tests of perceptual and cognitive ability (including intellectual tasks), athletic performance, and job performance—found that although many women *expect* a decline in ability associated with menstruation, this does not occur (Bernstein, 1977; Creutzfeld, Arnold, Becker, Langenstein, Tersch, Wilhelm, & Wuttcke, 1976; Gamberale, 1975; Golub, 1976; Sommer, 1973). Munchel (1977) and Altenhaus (1978) attempted to exaggerate the belief with lectures on menstrual disability for some of the women they studied. They still found no effect on the women's performance in a variety of perceptual-motor and arithmetic tasks and puzzle-solving. Rodin (1976) found that in a high-anxiety test situation, high-symptom menstruating women performed better than moderate-symptom menstruating women and nonmenstruating women.

Despite a long history of reasonably well-designed studies going back to Lough's 1937 study of "functional periodicity" that fail to document a menstrually produced decrement in ability, the belief persists. Dalton (1960, 1968) reported two studies supporting the idea of debilitation. The first was a study of the weekly marks of a group of English school girls. In the second study, she examined the grades on standard examinations. Both of the studies are seriously flawed in the statistical analysis of the data. Even as presented, the degree of difference in performance seems attributable to chance. In the first study, 27 percent of the students showed a drop in marks from the preceding week during their premenstrual phase. What the users of this data failed to point out is that 17 percent showed an increase in their marks and 56 percent showed no change. Such differences are more likely due to chance than menstruation. The second study provides similarly unclear results. Dalton's findings have been presented uncritically, despite her own assertion that the alleged handicap was not evenly distributed among the young women taking the tests. In the same paper she pointed out that the stress of the exams changed the cycle length in 42 percent of the young women and that more than expected by chance were menstruating during the examination week. If test anxiety brought about menstruation, it does not make sense to claim that being in the normal premenstrual or menstrual phase was the cause of the poor performance. If, in fact, performance was lower, it seems more likely that a third factor—anxiety—produced both the menstruation and the poor test performance. The fact that these studies have been acknowledged (Barash, 1979; Hutt, 1972) and the larger number of better controlled and more correctly analyzed studies have been ignored illustrates the power of menstrual myths.

Those who believe in the existence of menstrual debilitation cite studies of accident rates, psychiatric admissions, and suicide attempts to show that the premenstrual and menstrual phases are times of high risk of mental derangement. However, it is quite possible that the stress of strong emotion may lead to changes in the endometrium, resulting in menstrual bleeding. In other words, rather than the menstrual cycle phase causing antisocial or self-destructive behavior, such behavior may contribute to the onset of menses (Parlee, 1975). The necessary test is to have a record of prior menstruations. Furthermore, these studies have been few in number and involve small groups from selected populations, and are, thus, of limited use for a general theory.

mood

There are many beliefs concerning changes in mood believed to precede or accompany menstruation. Common ones are that women become moody, irritable, hostile (or bitchy), cannot engage in a rational argument, are prone to tears, easily fatigued, and subject to bouts of anxiety and depression. Many studies have been made on mood and the menstrual cycle. Their general form is to compare self-reports of mood or behavior over three segments of the cycle—premenstrual, menstrual, and midcycle. Earlier studies supported their results.

More recent studies provide evidence *against* a simple relationship between mood and the menstrual cycle. Swandby (1978), studying daily self-reports of anxiety, hostility, and depression for 35 days in 10 women with normal cycles and 10 women using oral contraceptives, found no difference in mood scores across cycle phase. Lee and Lewinsohn (1978) studied daily mood reports of 18 women, eight of whom had a history of clinically diagnosed depression. They also assessed behavior at four weekly group interview sessions. The nondepressed women did not show significant phase-related mood changes. However, the depressed group did show a premenstrual increase in depression, fatigue, and confusion, but *not* anxiety, anger, and vigor. An additional characteristic of these last two studies was the inclusion of males. They were assigned arbitrary menstrual-cycle designations. Lee and Lewinsohn included eight males and found that two of the 38 variables studied showed significant phase effects. In other words, false findings will occur by chance. Even the men experienced such things as depression, which in women is attributed to the menstrual cycle. A major flaw in many past studies was that had these subjects been women, the two phase effects probably would have been presented as evidence of the effect of the menstrual cycle on mood or behavior. (Figure 6.1 on page 62 shows commonly used phase designations.

Other studies have taken into account additional factors such as daily events, life changes, and stereotyped beliefs or expectations about menstruation. These factors seem to have more influence on mood than do the hormonal changes of the menstrual cycle.

A few investigators have looked at positive factors associated with the cycle. The behavior of 24 middle-class women was compared with that of their husbands; the 17 women who were not using oral contraceptives reported an increase in activities during the phase between the end of menstruation and ovulation (follicular phase), compared with their husbands and the rest of women, who were using the pill. The men, however, showed as much variation in activity levels, although not a consistent pattern. The distribution of energy devoted to any given activity (work, social, family, home) remained proportionately the same across the ebb and flow of activity for both women and men (Dan, 1976). Looking at positive mood as indicated on daily checklists by 29 non-pill users, this author found a midcycle increase in degree of positive mood. There was no indication of a

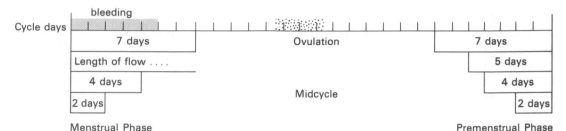

Figure 6.1   Phase designation used in behavioral research studies

premenstrual or menstrual increase in negative mood.

Other researchers have found no changes in either moods or enjoyment of activities, based on daily logs, as a function of the menstrual cycle phase. However, scores on the Menstrual Distress Questionnaire (MDQ), which was completed twice by the participants, showed the usual cycle-related differences, for example, indications of discomfort and distress prior to and with menstruation. The MDQ is a frequently used assessment checklist where one indicates the occurrence of specified symptoms premenstrually, menstrually, and midcycle. My studies found a similar contradiction when comparing twice-weekly mood reports of 20 women over a five-week span with a one-time MDQ symptom list.

A possible explanation for the discrepancy between daily reports and retrospective checklists is that many women at some time experience mild to moderate negative symptoms associated with menstruation. Because of a clear set of cultural expectations and beliefs about the effects of menstruation, these symptoms become fixed attributes of the menstrual cycle. When asked about her menstrual experience, a woman may indicate discomfort even though it does not recur each month. When the possibility for general or stereotyped answers is reduced, as when keeping a daily log over time, the negative moods previously associated with menstruation disappear. There is also evidence that negative moods are more likely to be attributed to the menstrual cycle when they occur during the premenstrual or menstrual phase. When they occur midcycle, they are attributed to some other cause. This attribution is made by both men and women. Thus, even if an individual woman does not perceive the source of her mood as menstrually related, those around her might.

In an attempt to clarify how biochemical fluctuations and psychosocial factors (such as anticipation of menstruation and fear of pregnancy) relate to menstrual mood changes, four groups of women were studied: 19 normally menstruating women (menses, cyclic hormones, possible fear of pregnancy), 24 women with tubal ligations (menses, cyclic hormones, no fear of pregnancy), 17 contraceptive users (highly predictable menses, less cyclic hormones, no fear of pregnancy), and 15 women who had undergone simple hysterectomies (no menses, cyclic hormones, no fear of pregnancy). These groups assessed their feelings of depression, energy level, irritability, anxiety, headache, and back pain on a daily basis for three months. There were no differences in complaints among the four groups. Thus, neither the hormonal changes, nor the event of menstruation, nor absence of fear of pregnancy appeared to contribute in a distinctive way to the pattern of menstrual symptoms. The data also failed to confirm the assumption that mood changes are cyclic, that is, that they show a gradual increase and decrease in pattern following the hormonal fluctuations of the menstrual cycle. The mood changes that did occur were more aptly described as phasic or episodic. They were present at some times and absent at others. They did not show a rhythmic pattern. Looking at the sample as a whole, there was a trend for greater anxiety and back pain, but *not* depression, increased energy, or headache around the time of menstruation (Vingilis, 1979).

From this overview of the material on mood change, some conclusions can be drawn. Mood changes in women cannot be predicted on the basis of the hormonal fluctuations of the menstrual cycle alone. The fact that a considerable number of earlier studies found evidence of mood change, while others have not, suggests that factors other than, or in addition to, the biological play a role in mood change. These factors may be related to learning, expectation, and perhaps personality. Biological factors might contribute, but be less powerful than social or psychological factors. Potential hormonal effects may be either enhanced or reduced by a variety of other characteristics, of the person and of the environment. Recent studies take into account other contributors to mood and separate them from menstrual factors. They also have been designed to reduce the likelihood of stereotyped responses. Finally, improved attitudes about menstruation may contribute to a decrease in reports of negative effects.

Despite the negative history associated with menstruation, improved research and education are producing a more positive view. When 191 college undergraduates were surveyed, they indicated an acceptance of menstruation as routine, and they felt fairly positive about it, agreeing, for example, with the statements "menstruation provides a way for me to keep in touch with my body" or "menstruation is a recurring affirmation of womanhood." Less than one-third indicated that it was debilitating, for example, "women are more tired than usual when they are menstruating." (Brooks, Ruble, and Clark, 1977)

Are menstruation and its accompanying events stressful? The answer is not an unqualified yes or no. For some, it is not at all stressful; for others, mildly or moderately so; for a small percentage of the population, it is highly stressful.

symptoms, causes, and treatment

categories of menstrual distress

Menstrual symptoms have traditionally been relegated to two general categories: premenstrual syndrome or tension, and dysmenorrhea (pain). Symptoms associated with the premenstrual syndrome are water retention (swelling, edema), weight gain, headache, other aches and pains, negative affects, including depression, irritability, crying spells, hostility, insomnia, difficulties in concentration, increased appetite, constipation, acne, and others ranging from vertigo to alcohol excess.

DYSMENORRHEA—MENSTRUAL PAIN. Dysmenorrhea comes from the Greek: *dys* means difficult, painful, bad, disordered; *menorrhea* means discharge of the menses. Dysmenorrhea generally covers menstrual cramps, backaches, headaches, and any of the discomfort and negative moods accompanying menstrual flow. Premenstrual tension and dysmenorrhea are very broad categories. Symptoms overlap and may contribute to one another. For example, in some cases anticipation of menstrual flow and associated pain may bring on premenstrual anxiety or irritability. Further, the same hormonal factors may contribute to both premenstrual and menstrual symptoms.

Unfortunately, the term "premenstrual syndrome" has come to represent a distinct entity. In fact, there is no such thing as a "premenstrual syndrome." It does not constitute a reliable, predictable entity. Clinical entities, such as pneumonia and tuberculosis, follow a relatively clear and predictable course of genesis, development, and outcome. They have a characteristic group of signs and symptoms that are quite consistent from person to person. This is not to say that premenstrual and menstrual symptoms do not exist. They do, but there is no consistent, clear pattern of symptoms that occur together in all individuals. A person showing premenstrual water retention may not show any of the other symptoms. The same criticism applies to treating dysmenorrhea as a single entity. When a large number of women were surveyed, seven different clusters of symptoms were relatively independent of one another. These were pain, concentration, behavioral change, autonomic reactions (nausea, dizzyness, sweats), water retention, negative affects, and arousal (Moos, 1968). Given the current level of understanding, we should refer to specific symptoms instead of using broad syndrome-type labels.

Estimates of the incidence of menstrual pain vary from 30 to 75 percent. However, in several studies where the degree of pain was specified, the occurrence of severe pain ranged from 8 to 13 percent. There was one notable exception. Fifty-five percent of an adolescent sample from Helsinki reported severe pelvic pain accompanying menstruation. Ratings of backache, headache, and premenstrual pain fell below 13 percent in this group. In most cases, the pain is uterine cramping and/or lower backache. Other discomforts are headache and breast tenderness, both reported at much lower frequencies than cramps and backaches.

MENSTRUAL CRAMPS. One of the most recent breakthroughs in the area of menstrual distress is the discovery of the role of prostaglandins in menstrual cramps. Prostaglandins are minute substances produced in many body tissues, and they cause contraction of smooth muscle. Those produced in the uterus cause the smooth muscle of the uterine walls to contract, and they are the initiators of labor contractions as well as menstruation. Cramps result from a diminished flow of blood to the uterine muscle when it has been contracting, a situation brought about by excess prostaglandins. Drugs that inhibit prostaglandin activity reduce menstrual cramps. It has been known for some time that menstrual pain is related to ovulation. The use of oral contraceptives, which inhibit ovulation, is associated with a decrease in cramping. Oral contraceptives do not directly inhibit prostaglandins, but they contribute to a reduction in prostaglandin production by the uterus. The prostaglandin excess may also account for nausea, vomiting, diarrhea, headaches, and other symptoms due to the effects of prostaglandins on the smooth muscles of the stomach, intestines, and blood vessels (Marx, 1979).

A variety of prostaglandin-inhibiting drugs are generally available. Although using a drug for treatment always poses potential side effects, prostaglandin inhibitors need be used only when cramping is most likely, that is, the first two days of flow. Thus, one can avoid possible damage to an embryo in the case of early pregnancy.

Prostaglandin research has uncovered an important contributor to dysmenorrhea, but it does not rule out other potential contributors. Some women with normal concentrations of prostaglandins suffer from painful menstrual symptoms. However, prostaglandins and hormonal factors seem most often responsible for such symptoms as pain, nausea, fever, and water retention. Whether psychological factors contribute to the hormonal imbalance is still unknown. Furthermore, physical symptoms such as nausea and pain may bring about such psychological outcomes as negative mood and difficulties with concentration.

There is no evidence to support the belief that one cause of dysmenorrhea is a uterus that is too small or too poorly developed to accommodate the menstrual substance. But general debilitation and chronic illness may contribute to dysmenorrhea.

Other drug treatments for menstrual cramps are aspirin, ethyl alcohol, amphetamine, and progesterone. Aspirin is a weak prostaglandin inhibitor. Ethyl alcohol, often taken as a glass of wine, has been effective for some; Lydia Pinkhams, an old remedy for "female problems," was 40-proof before Prohibition! Amphetamine leads indirectly to the reduction of prostaglandins. However, both the alcohol and amphetamine solutions pose potential problems of addiction. Progesterone is now considered unsuitable because of side effects (Dickey, 1976).

The area of nondrug intervention for the treatment of dysmenorrhea is promising. One approach is to use the techniques of behavioral therapy, a combination of relaxation training and systematic desensitization. Women are taught, either by a therapist or through the use of a tape, techniques for deep muscle relaxation. A variety of techniques may be used. One is to systematically tense and relax the muscles of the body, beginning with the toes, moving up the legs, through the body and arms, and finally to the shoulders, neck, and head. Imagining oneself in a very relaxed position, such as being in a warm pool of water in a very beautiful place, is another

technique. Breathing with the entire diaphragm to a slow count can bring relaxation. The prescribed techniques are practiced on a daily basis.

Progressive desensitization is a technique described by Wolpe (1969) for overcoming phobias (irrational fears). The first step is to construct a hierarchy of the least to the most feared aspect of the phobia. With the help of the therapist, a person confronts the least fearful situation repeatedly until it no longer elicits fright. Then, the person progresses to the next item on the hierarchy, eventually overcoming fear at the highest level. The underlying principle is for the person to unlearn the fear reaction by confronting the fearful stimulus in small doses with the support of the therapist. In other words, the person learns to be "unafraid" of the phobia stimulus.

These principles have been adapted to treating menstrual problems. The woman, who has been taught relaxation techniques, is advised to imagine that she "looks at the calendar and realizes that her period is due to begin in 10 days." After doing so, she tries to maintain a relaxed state. When she is able to do that repeatedly, she moves on to the next step. The final image is that she "begins to feel severe pain and cramping." The aim of this type of therapy is to learn how to maintain muscle relaxation in the face of anticipated pain. The underlying rationale is that fear and subsequent muscle tension contribute to menstrual distress.

Lamaze childbirth education methods, which also emphasize relaxation and breathing techniques, have been used with success to alleviate menstrual pain. Cramps involve the uterine muscle, and as muscle relaxation in general is accompanied by dilation of the blood vessels and a subsequent rise in temperature, it is believed that women might relieve cramps by learning relaxation techniques. Using a tele-thermometer to give feedback on vaginal temperature, Heczey (1977) trained women how to relax. They learned to change their vaginal temperature. Heczey's hope was that alteration in the blood flow in the vaginal region would also occur in the uterus. Another group of women was individually taught relaxation techniques without the feedback. Both groups showed improvement when compared with a similar, but nontreated group. The most effective treatment was relaxation in combination with biofeedback.

BACKACHE. Backaches associated with menstruation were reported by 15 to 54 percent of the women studied. The specific cause of lower back pain has not been explored in detail. It may result from a temporary relaxation of the joints in the pelvis due to the action of a hormone called relaxin, which is produced by the corpus luteum. Lower back pain has long been viewed as a stress-related disorder. Other discomforts such as diarrhea, nausea, or stomach pain may contribute to increased muscular tension, felt more directly in the lower back.

OTHER DISCOMFORT. Tender breasts probably result from changes in prolactin concentration. Prolactin is a hormone produced by the pituitary and plays a role in milk production. Swelling due to increased water retention results from alterations in electrolytic balance brought about by a variety of hormonal changes. Acne also reflects changes in hormonal patterns. As discussed earlier, nausea, vomiting, diarrhea, and headaches may be linked to prostaglandin production.

PREMENSTRUAL PROBLEMS—DISORDERS OF MOOD. Many women report only mild to moderate mood change, or none at all, around the time of menstruation, but when changes are reported, they tend to be negative—anxiety and nervousness, depression, hostility, or irritability—particularly occurring premenstrually. However, attempts to explain the occurrence of these symptoms have met with remarkably little success. A variety of theories has been developed and tested. The explanations and treatments have been effective for some women. However, there are no instances where a single explanation holds up for a large group of symptomatic women. Perhaps there are many causes for the complaints, a recognition that may have been delayed by premature acceptance of the idea of a single "premenstrual syndrome." What may be required is a more precise delineation of symptoms, each with a different set of causes and a different treatment.

For some women, hormonal factors may be the major source of menstrual distress. For others, psychological factors may be the chief contributor. Furthermore, hormonal and psycho-social factors are likely to interact. Recognition and acknowledgement of the disturbance may in itself have a beneficial effect in reducing symptoms. This is not to suggest that complaints are imaginary or unreal. Recognition and a framework for describing a physical reaction or set of feelings often serve to reduce the anxiety and concern that might contribute to distress. This powerful effect, sometimes called the placebo effect, may occur along with hormonal changes. Unfortunately, psychological contributors are often recognized only by the exclusion of physical factors. A physician (or patient) failing to find hormonal abnormality may only then conclude that psychological factors are the cause. Conversely, finding a hormonal abnormality may result in dismissing possible psychological contributors. But psychological and hormonal factors are not mutually exclusive. Finding one contributor does not eliminate the possible action of other contributors. Assuming only a single cause may contribute to the lack of consistent research results and may lead to ineffective treatment.

interrelationship of emotions and hormones

The possible interaction between psychological and physiological factors has been emphasized repeatedly. There is evidence for direct neural and hormonal pathways connecting the various parts of the brain with the controlling mechanisms of the menstrual cycle.

EMOTIONS AND HORMONES. The hormonal fluctuations of the menstrual cycle stem from a very delicate and exact set of positive and negative feedback systems among the hypothalamus, pituitary gland, and the ovaries, referred to as the hypothalamic-pituitary-ovarian axis. The following example illustrates the finely tuned nature of this system.

Estrogen, produced by the ovary under the stimulation of FSH (follicle-stimulating hormone) from the pituitary, stimulates a pituitary surge of LH (luteinizing hormone), which in turn brings about ovulation: FSH→ ovary → estrogen → hypothalamus → LH surge → ovulation. If there is *too little* estrogen, the LH surge is blocked (Check, 1978). The hormones exert both enhancing and inhibiting effects on one another, depending on the amount produced as well as the rate of secretion, that is, the speed as well as level of their increase or decrease. The system is not a closed one, and here is where emotions play a part. Connections, both neural (actual nerves) and hormonal (via the circulation) exist between the hypothalamus and both the cerebral cortex and the limbic system (Figure 6.2).

The cerebral cortex is the part of the brain involved in thinking, learning, and perception. The nearby limbic system governs emotional responsiveness, with influences from the cerebral cortex. Thus, the pathways exist for the influence of higher brain centers, via the hypothalamus, on the menstrual cycle.

Here is a more specific example. The cerebral cortex and the limbic system produce at the nerve endings substances called *biogenic amines.* Three major ones are dopamine, norepinephrine, and serotonin. The secretion of these substances appears related to emotional states. All three influence releasing factors produced by the hypothalamus. These releasing factors affect other body hormone levels. Dopamine, by its effect on the hypothalamic releasing factor, suppresses LH from the pituitary. Recall that the LH surge is essential for ovulation. Thus, an increase of dopamine blocks ovulation and, if continued, leads to amenorrhea (absence of menstruation). Continuing work is likely to produce evidence of other relationships between the biogenic amines and menstrual function. The biogenic amines and their effects are the means by which environmental and situational factors experienced by the individual are translated from the psychological to the physiological. Although mind and body are experienced as quite different from one another, connections between the two clearly exist.

The ovarian hormones, estrogen and progesterone, as well as a host of other hormones produced in other endocrine glands, circulate through the bloodstream and are picked up by receptor cells in various parts of the body and brain (see Figure 6.3). There are specific receptors for estrogen and progesterone in the pituitary gland, the hypothalamus, and the limbic system. At present, there is no evidence of similar cells in the cerebral cortex. However, the hypothalamus and limbic systems influence the cerebral cortex, probably by the differential secretion of biogenic amines, again via direct nerve transmission and through the blood system.

The evidence is more clear for psychological processes affecting the reproductive hormones via the cerebral cortex than for the reverse (reproductive hormones affecting the cerebral cortex). Thus far, there are no indications that the cerebral cortex is particularly sensitive to ovarian hormones. However, there is a tendency (strong in the past, remaining in the present) to place a heavy emphasis on the role of hormones in female psychology—the "anatomy is destiny" notion. The evidence leans more toward the "mind over matter" cliché. However, in contrast with the

figure 6.2
schematic representation of connections from the brain to the ovaries

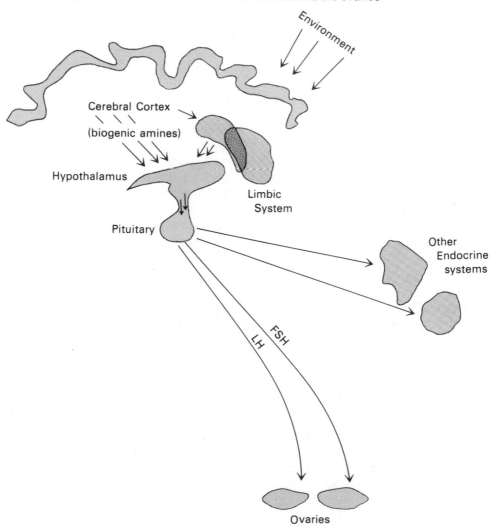

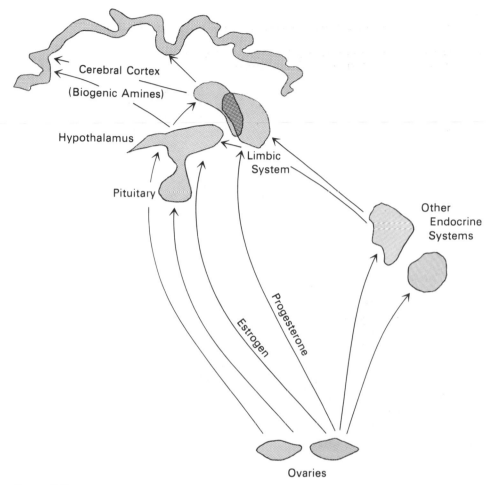

figure 6.3
schematic representation of connections from the ovaries to the brain

cerebral cortex, the limbic system does contain specific receptors for hormones such as estrogen, progesterone, and testosterone. Here may lie a partial explanation of the clear findings on performance and the more contradictory results on mood. Learned and skilled performance of complex motor, perceptual, and cognitive tasks primarily involve the cerebral cortex. Hormonal effects, if at all, would be indirect. The cerebral cortex also plays a very important role in mood, feelings, and emotions. How we perceive things based on our appraisal of the immediate situation, as well as our experience in the past, will determine in large part our emotional response. However, that emotional response *also* involves the limbic system, which does contain specific receptors for ovarian hormones. Thus, it is at the limbic levels that there is an opportunity for hormones to influence emotion.

table 6.1
nature of support for suspected causes and treatments for menstrual disorders

+ = scientific support; - = scientific evidence against; ? = equivocal scientific results;
A = anecdotal support, e.g., physicians' claim of success in practice; S = speculative

DISORDER	SUSPECTED CAUSE	RATING	TREATMENTS SUGGESTED FOR DISORDER	RATING
Menstrual cramps	Hormonal imbalance related to ovulation	+	Prostaglandin inhibitors	+
	Prostaglandins	+	Muscle relaxants	+
	Psychogenic	?	Antispasmodics	+
			Analgesics (pain relievers)	+
			Behavioral therapy (relaxation, desensitization)	+
			Psychotherapy	?
			Tranquilizers	A
			Dietary alteration (increased liquids, natural laxatives, increased iron intake)	A
Backache	Calcium deficiency	A	Application of heat	+
	Relaxin (produced by corpus luteum)	S	Vigorous exercise	+
	Stress produced by other symptoms	S	Calcium supplements	A
			Girdle or adhesive strapping	A
			Increasing flexibility and strength through exercise	A
Breast engorgement	Estrogen/Progesterone ratio	+	Pyridoxine (Vitamin B6)	A
	Prolactin	+		
Premenstrual disorders	Estrogen/Progesterone ratio	+	Natural progesterone	+
	Prolactin	+	Oral contraceptives (combination type)	+
	Environmental stress	+	Diuretics	?
	Situational stress	+	MAO inhibitors	?
	Expectation	+	Prolactin inhibitors	?
	Personality	?	Pyridoxine (Vitamin B6)	?
	Water retention	?	Tranquilizers	A
	Monoamine oxidase (MAO)	?	Dietary alterations (reduced salt intake, reduced carbohydrates, increased protein, increased natural laxatives)	A
	Hypoglycemia	A		
	Calcium deficiency	A		
	Aldosterone excess	-	Reduction of environmental and situational sources of stress	A
	Progesterone excess	-	Synthetic progestogens	-
			Estrogen	-
			Behavioral therapy (relaxation, desensitization)	-

HORMONAL FACTORS IN MENSTRUAL DISORDERS OF MOOD. A long-held theory has noted an imbalance between estrogen and progesterone during the premenstrual phase. A review of the literature found an excess of estrogen, relative to progesterone, in the latter phase of the cycle associated with symptoms of premenstrual irritability, anxiety, and hostility. If this is so, something more than a simple ratio must be involved, such as a rapid change over time, because just prior to ovulation, estrogen levels are high and progesterone levels are very low. Hypoglycemia (low blood sugar) resulting from hormonal factors has been suggested as a possible cause of premenstrual irritability and nervousness.

The hypothesis of an imbalance between estrogen and progesterone has not held up in predicting premenstrual depression. Increases in prolactin, a pituitary hormone, have been implicated in complaints of depression (Smith, 1975).

Water retention resulting from changes in the potassium/sodium balance in body cells is a popular theory of premenstrual mood change. Several other studies have documented the presence of water retention without other complaints and have found severe complaints occurring in the absence of water retention (Smith, 1975).

Although a wide variety of treatments have been effective in some cases, none has proven totally effective when tested in well-controlled studies (see Table 6.1).

personality

Reactions to a biological event such as menstruation might be conditioned by personality, which refers to the characteristic way a person thinks and behaves in adjusting to environment. By personality, we also mean the person's traits, values, motives, attitudes, emotional reactivity, and self-image. A reasonable hypothesis is that personality factors contribute to menstrual distress. Menstruation is a distinctive female characteristic and, therefore, is an apt symbol and focus for feelings and attitudes surrounding feminine identity and sexuality. Unfortunately, it is difficult to make clear predictions about menstrual problems from personality factors. For example, menstrual discomfort is often a part of the female stereotype. Thus, women who score high on the *CPI* feminity scale might report a higher incidence of menstrual distress. On the other hand, it could be argued that highly feminine women might be very accepting of female biology, and thus experience fewer menstrual problem than less feminine women. Gough (1975) found that women who scored high on the femininity scores of the California Personality Inventory (CPI) reported more severe symptoms than those who scored low on the index. However, Berry and McGuire (1972) found a negative relationship between femininity scores and menstrual symptoms.

Given the current state of findings, personality does not appear to be a major contributor. Our means of assessment may be inadequate and lacking in the necessary sensitivity to pick up relationships that might exist between personality and menstrual distress. Should there be such a relationship, the direction of cause and effect would have to be studied. Experiencing severe menstrual problems, particularly in the pubertal years, may in itself influence personality development.

expectation

Both men and women have a clear set of expectations about symptoms and the menstrual cycle. In many cases, these expectations were learned prior to puberty. In an attempt to separate expectation and actual experience, Ruble (1977) devised an ingenious experiment. Volunteer participants were taken into a laboratory and connected, by electrodes on the scalp, to an EEG (electroencephalogram) machine, which measures brain waves. They were told by an official-looking person in a white laboratory coat that the brain-wave patterns would predict the onset of menstruation. Ruble found an increase in reports of water retention and pain by the women who were led to believe that they were in the premenstrual phase of their cycle.

One interpretation of these results is that women's symptom reports are stereotyped and culturally determined expectations. Another interpretation is that continued or prolonged association between symptom and cycle phase leads to a conditioned perception. If cultural beliefs alone were responsible for attributing negative symptoms to menstruation, self-reports of mood should be affected, as well as the more physical symptoms of water retention and pain. Ruble did not find differences in the reports of negative mood or other behavioral changes between women led to believe they were premenstrual and those led to believe they were midcycle. Nevertheless, Ruble's findings do support the theory that expectation plays a part in menstrual problems. It is very difficult to separate expectations and experience, and it is reasonable to expect that one affects the others. Expectation may affect both the *perception* of body state (sensing or feeling a symptom) and the *reaction* to it. What one feels and what one does about it reflect two different levels of response, and each is likely to be influenced by past experience and expectation, as well as by situational and environmental factors.

general health and environment influences

Vitamin or mineral deficiency, improper posture, lack of exercise, and other general health factors may contribute to menstrual distress. These more obvious considerations highlight the observation that menstrual distress in many cases should be treated as a problem of public health education.

An increase in the number of life changes, desirable and undesirable, may be related to reports of increased menstrual discomfort. It may be that women undergoing the stress of life changes may develop both a physical susceptibility to menstrual problems and a psychological inability to cope with discomfort. The association was found only among nonusers of oral contraceptives. Oral contraceptive use has been long associated with diminishing menstrual symptoms and may provide a protection against stress effects on hormone secretion, at least with regard to the development of menstrual symptoms. It is difficult to see that oral contraceptive use would contribute to better coping. Thus, the group differences lend support to the involvement of hormonal factors in the development of menstrual symptoms. On the other hand, women who use oral contraceptives and those who do not may differ in other ways that affect their responses to life stress. Inadequate nutrition would be expected to play a role, and it is a major contributor to amenorrhea (absence of menstruation) and delayed menarche (first menstruation).

summary

Many hormonal and psychological factors have been implicated in menstrual distress. An excess of prostaglandins may account for pain, nausea, vomiting, and headache ac-companying the early stages of menstruation. The sources of negative mood, particularly in the premenstrual phase, require more complex explanations involving both psychological and physiological mechanisms. Hormonal, social, and psychological factors may interact to produce distress. Their relative contributions probably vary from person to person and from period to period. Individuals are likely to experience different disorders or combinations of symptoms that require different therapies. Treatment that is effective for water retention and lethargy may be of no use in reducing anxiety and nervousness. Improving general health and taking a critical look at situational and environmental factors that aggravate symptoms may make any remaining discomfort more manageable.

Altenhaus, A. L. The effect of expectancy for change on performance during the menstrual cycle. Doctoral dissertation, Rutgers Univ., 1978.

Barash, D. (quoted by Lacitis, E.). Women's place is in their genes? *Seattle Times*, September 20, 1979, p. A15.

Berry, C., & McGuire, F. L. Menstrual distress and acceptance of sexual role. *American Journal of Obstetrics and Gynecology*, 1972, *114*, 83–87.

Berstein, B. E. Effect of menstruation on academic performance among college women. *Archives of Sexual Behavior*, 1977, *6*, 289–296.

Brooks, J., Ruble, D. & Clark, A. college women's attitudes and expectations concerning menstrual-related changes. *Psychosomatic Medicine*, 1977, *39*, 288–289.

Check, J. H. Emotional aspects of menstrual dysfunction. *Psychosomatics*, 1978, *19*, 178–179.

Creutzfeldt, O. D., Arnold, P. N., Becker, D., Langenstein, S., Tersch, W., Wilhelm, H., & Wuttcke, W. EEG changes during spontaneous and controlled menstrual cycles and their correlation with psychological performance. *Electroencephalography & Clinical Neurophysiology*, 1976, *40*, 113–131.

Dalton, K. Effect of menstruation on schoolgirls' weekly work. *British Medical Journal*, 1960, *1*, 326–328.

Dalton, K. Menstruation and examinations. *Lancet*, 1968, *2*, 1386–1388.

Dan, A. Patterns of behavioral and mood variation in men and women. Variability and the menstrual cycle. Unpublished doctoral dissertation, University of Chicago, 1976.

Dickey, R. P. Menstrual problems of the adolescent. *Postgraduate Medicine*, 1976, *60*, 183–187.

Gamberale, F., Strindberg, L., & Wahlberg, I. Female work capacity during the menstrual cycle: Physiological and psychological reactions. *Scandinavian Journal*

of Work & Environmental Health, 1975, *1*, 120–127.

Golub, S. The effect of premenstrual anxiety and depression on cognitive function. *Journal of Personal & Social Psychology*, 1976, *34*, 99–104.

Gough, H. G. Personality factors related to reported severity of menstrual distress. *Journal of Abnormal Psychology*, 1975, *84*, 59–65.

Heczey, M.D. Effects of biofeedback and autogenic training on dysmenorrhea. In A. J. Dan, E. A. Graham, and C. P. Beecher (eds.), *The Menstrual Cycle: A Synthesis of Interdisciplinary Research*, Volume 1, New York, Springer, 1980.

Hutt, C. *Males & females*. Middlesex, Eng.; Penguin, 1972.

Lee, W. M., & Lewinsohn, P. M. Depression and the menstrual cycle: A preliminary report. Unpublished manuscript, Psychology Dept., University of Oregon, 1978.

Marx, J. L. Dysmenorrhea: Basic research leads to a rational therapy. *Science*, 1979, *205*, 175–176.

Moos, R. The development of a menstrual distress questionnaire. *Psychosomatic Medicine*, 1968, *30*, 853–867.

Parlee, M. B. Menstruation and crime, accidents, and acute psychiatric illness: A reinterpretation of Dalton's data. Paper presented at the annual meeting of the *American Psychological Association*, Chicago, 1975.

Rodin, J. Menstruation, reattribution and competence. *Journal of Personal & Social Psychology*, 1976, *33*, 345–353.

Ruble, D. Premenstrual symptoms: A reinterpretation. *Science*, 1977, *197*, 291–292.

Russell, G. F. Psychological and nutritional factors in disturbances of menstrual function and ovulation. *Postgrad. Med. J.*, 1972, *48*, 10–13.

Smith, S. L. Mood and the menstrual cycle. In E. Sachar (ed.), *Topics in Psychoendocrinology*. New York: Grune & Stratton, 1975.

Sommer, B. The effect of menstruation on cognitive and perceptual-motor behavior: A review. *Psychosomatic Medicine*, 1973, *35*, 515–534.

Sommer, B. Stress and menstrual distress. *Journal of Human Stress*, 1978, *4*, 5–10, 41–47

Swandby, J. R. A longitudinal study of daily mood self-reports and their relationship to the menstrual cycle. Paper presented at the Second Annual Interdisciplinary Conference on the Menstrual Cycle, May 25–26, 1978, St. Louis.

Vingilis, E. Feeling states and the menstrual cycle. Unpublished manuscript, York University, Canada, 1979.

Wolpe, J. *The practice of behavior therapy*. New York: Pergamon, 1969.

MARIE ANNETTE BROWN, R.N., Ph.C.

fertility control

For virtually all women sexually involved with men in the 1980s, contraception is an issue. Actively or passively, they choose whether to use some form of birth control.

There has been significant progress in the development of effective contraception since the early 1960s. Birth control pills and IUD's, which gained widespread use in the 1960s, were refined and made safer in the 1970s. Prior to these developments and to the legalization of abortion in the 1970s, motherhood was practically inevitable; fertile women who were sexually involved with men became pregnant.

Today, however, women must make a very different kind of adjustment as they struggle to take more responsibility and to make choices about their reproductive functions—and about their sexuality. Some women find planning for sexual intercourse and deliberately controlling contraception either unmanageable or undesirable; instead, they prefer "letting nature take its course." But others find that their increasing ability to control their reproductive functions has had a dramatic, positive impact on their life-styles, relationships and self-concepts. However, there is discouragement associated with birth control, too. As far as the science has advanced, it falls short of satisfying the demands made of it. An ideal contraceptive would be 100 percent effective, 100 percent safe, conveniently easy to understand and to use, physically unconnected with the act of intercourse, inexpensive, easy to distribute widely—*and* completely reversible! There is no such contraceptive method. So, a woman's "freedom of choice" is limited by the many limitations of the methods available.

More discouraging news is that contraceptives are not necessarily readily available to all women. Some rural areas do not have family planning facilities. Many women still hesitate to seek health care because of the possibility of hurried, impersonal, moralizing, or disapproving attitudes. Where sound, supportive guidance and competent medical care are relatively inaccessible, women cannot feel wholly free to choose whether, or how, to practice birth control.

attitudes affecting contraceptive success or failure

One's attitudes and feelings toward contraception are an integral part of one's life. A woman or a man may feel uncomfortable and uncertain about contraception due to his or her own personal moral confusions as well as to conflicting messages from society. Although women do experience considerable physical discomfort with various methods of contraception, it is the social attitudes pertaining to birth control in general that seem to determine contraception effectiveness.

feelings about sex and pregnancy

Our society has ambivalent feelings about sexuality. Discomfort and embarrassment cause many people great difficulty in dealing with birth control openly and straightforwardly. A woman may feel ambivalent about her sexual involvement, and thus have difficulty acknowledging it to herself, to her partner, or to anyone else. To view contraception realistically, and thus to use it effectively, a woman needs to confront her feelings about having intercourse.

To become pregnant or not is a conflict of motivations that underlies many women's difficulty with the idea of contraception, let alone the individual method. Contraception cannot be wholeheartedly practiced when a woman is struggling to discover and to coordinate her dreams, her values, and her sexual behavior.

relationship with partner, parents, peers, and professionals

Of course, the effectiveness of any contraceptive method depends on its regular use, and regularity is not always a feature compatible with a man-woman relationship. And the most "regular" stable couples may be unable to cooperate in order to use contraceptives effectively because they disagree about who is responsible for birth control, or about the best time for pregnancy and child-rearing. The partner who is eager for a child may subtly sabotage the use of contraception.

Women faced with a personal decision about contraception may turn to a variety of "authorities." For example, adolescent women are especially affected by their parents' great concern about their sexuality. Peers can be mutually influential in increasing or decreasing each other's confidence in contraception in general, as well as in the safety, ease, and effectiveness of a particular method.

People considering birth control also are confronted with conflicting information about newsworthy contraceptive issues, such as risks and side effects, in magazines, on the radio or TV, and from their health care provider. The authority that an individual decides to accept, and to trust, will influence future contraceptive decisions.

identity and will

Especially since the early 1970s, women have been learning to value themselves and their bodies, to take care of themselves. This attitude contributes dramatically to contraceptive success. But many women still have low self-esteem. Lack of assertiveness also prevents some women from obtaining contraception. To get a prescription for birth control pills or a diaphragm, a woman must go through a decision-making process, then act on her choice by going to a doctor, hospital, or clinic, and following through with what is prescribed for her. Furthermore, contraception may require that a woman adopt a new kind of assertiveness about the frequency of intercourse, that she straightforwardly state that she does not want to have sex right now. This kind of strength and self-possession can be difficult for some women, especially those who are young or who do not feel secure about themselves.

men and contraception

The willingness to use birth control, especially among younger women, is strongly influenced by the attitude of the male partner. Some men are reluctant to discuss contraception with their partners, some feel uncomfortable talking specifically about their sexual activity, and some women fear their partners may be "turned off" or think them unfeminine if they are knowledgeable and prepared in sexual matters. But many women are finding that discussion of contraception with a man who truly accepts his responsibility for preventing pregnancy enriches a relationship rather than causes difficulties. This open discussion often increases respect and intimacy, so a woman can use birth control and feel comfortable doing so.

Most women now expect their partners to participate in contraception in some way. A man can accompany his partner to the Planned Parenthood clinic or private physician's office and share the financial costs of examinations and contraceptive supplies. Prior to each intercourse, he can ask her if her diaphragm or foam is in place or participate in its insertion. Occasionally he himself can assume the responsibility for contraception by using condoms. If no contraceptive is available, he can explore lovemaking activities that do not involve intercourse. Most of all, men can be aware that the responsibility to prevent pregnancy, like the pleasure of sexual intercourse, is a shared one.

contraceptive methods and birth control practices

Each contraceptive method has distinct advantages and disadvantages that require thoughtful reflection. A woman needs to become informed about each of the available choices so that she can select the one most appropriate for her body, feelings, and life-style. She must assess the risks and benefits of each method and interpret them according to her own values (see Table 7.1 pp. 77-84)

effectiveness

Most people selecting a contraceptive method want to know how well it will work.

table 7.1   a comparison of contraceptive methods

Oral Contraceptives

MECHANISM OF ACTION

Estrogenic agents influence normal patterns of ovulation, ovum transport, implantation, or placental attachment.

Progestational agents influence ovulation, sperm penetration of the ovum, ovum transport, implantation, and alter cervical mucus.

Minipills alter the uterine lining and cause thickening of the cervical mucus.

INSTRUCTIONS FOR USE

Note: Combination-type birth control pills come in two variations:

1. The 28-day series has 3 rows (or 21 pills) of actual contraceptive pills and 1 row (or 7 pills) that are inert, containing no medication. These 7 "spacer pills" are designed to maintain the woman's habit of daily pill-taking.

2. The 21-day series has only 21 pills (or 3 rows), all containing contraceptive medication. No spacer pills are included.

GENERAL DIRECTIONS

1. With the very first package of pills *only*, take the first pill in the package on the fifth day of your menstrual flow (counting the first day of bleeding as day #1), or after the baby is one month old, if postpartum. Take 1 pill daily until the package is finished.

2. To begin all subsequent packages of pills:

   a. If you have the 28-day kind, start a new package *immediately* after finishing the present package.

   b. If you have the 21-day kind, take no pills for 7 days and on the eighth day, begin a new package of pills.

3. Follow these instructions, regardless of when your menstrual period occurs or how long it lasts:

   a. If you should continue your menstrual flow when you have finished the spacer pills, begin a new package anyway as scheduled.

   b. Your period probably will occur: on 28-day pills, sometime during the week you are on the last 7 pills (the spacer or inert ones); on 21-day pills, sometime during the 7 days while you take no pills.

   c. Most women have a shorter, lighter flow on pills. Only a half-day of dark spotting is not unusual.

   d. Occasionally you may miss a period entirely. If you have taken the pills regularly as directed, the chance of a pregnancy is very, very small. If you miss 2 periods in a row, see your health care provider for a checkup.

4. Take your pills at approximately the same time (morning, afternoon, evening) each day in order to maintain a fairly constant level of the hormones in your blood. Take the pills immediately after a meal if you have problems with nausea or upset stomach.

MISSED PILLS

1. If you miss *1 pill*, take the pill you forgot as soon as you remember, and take your regular one at the usual time. Or if you do not notice the forgotten pill until your usual time, take both pills at once.

2. If you miss *2 pills*, take 2 pills each day for the next 2 days. (You can take either 2 at a time or 1 in the morning and 1 at night.) Use a backup method of protection (foam and condoms) until your next period. If you miss 1 or more pills and skip a period, call your health care provider to ask about a pregnancy test.

3. If you miss *3 or more pills*, begin using another method of protection and call your health care provider for advice. Some people advise discontinuing pills for 4 to 6 weeks until you have a regular period. Other people suggest stopping pills for 1 week and then resuming a new package while using a backup method during the first 2 weeks of that package.

FOLLOW-UP INSTRUCTIONS

If you have a new pill prescription, see your health care provider after 3 months. He or she will want to check your weight and blood pressure and discuss your adjustment to pills. Have a complete gynecologic exam once a year to insure the safe continuation of your birth control pill program.

ADVANTAGES

1. Convenient use.

2. Does not interrupt physical act of intercourse.

3. Highly effective.

4. Decreased incidence of benign breast growths, heavy menstrual cramping and flow, premenstrual tension, acne, ovarian cysts, and iron deficiency (anemia).

5. Majority of women have no significant side effects or serious health problems from the pill.

DISADVANTAGES

Serious risks include higher incidence of:
1. Thromboembolic effects (blood clots), interaction of oral contraceptives, and smoking increase risk of heart attack.
2. Information of benign tumors.
3. Gallbladder disease.
4. Elevated blood pressure.
5. Danger to fetus if taken while pregnant.
6. Fluid retention with aggravation of migraines, asthma, epilepsy, kidney or heart disease for some women; growth of pre-existing fibroid tumors, liver problems, accentuation of depression.

SIDE EFFECTS

1. Nausea.

2. Breast changes, tenderness.

3. Spotting, bleeding between periods.

4. Decreased menstrual flow.

5. Missed periods.

6. Increased vaginitis, itching, or discharge.

7. Acne.

8. Chloasma (mask of pregnancy).

9. Corneal edema.

10. Depression, fatigue, mood changes.

11. Decreased sex drive.

12. Postpill amenorrhea.

13. Decrease in quality and quantity of breast milk in breastfeeding mothers.

14. Vitamin deficiency— B_{12}, B_6, folic acid, ascorbic acid.

CONTRAINDICATIONS
ABSOLUTE

1. Thromboembolic disorder (blood-clotting disorder) or history thereof.

2. Cerebrovascular accident (stroke) or history thereof.

3. Impaired liver function.

4. Coronary artery disease or history thereof.

5. Liver tumor or history thereof.

6. Malignancy of breast or reproductive system or history thereof.

7. Pregnancy (known or suspected).

STRONG

8. Woman has given birth within past 10–14 days.

9. Severe vascular or migraine headaches.

10. Hypertension (high blood pressure) with resting diastolic BP of 110 or greater.

11. Diabetes, prediabetes or strong family history of diabetes.

12. Gallbladder disease or previous gallbladder problems during pregnancy.

13. Mononucleosis, acute phase.

14. Sickle cell disease or sickle cell trait.

15. Undiagnosed, abnormal vaginal bleeding. (Many physicians strongly feel this should be listed as an absolute contraindication to pill use. It remains here since we cannot in a simple, straightforward manner define "abnormal." The authors would definitely concur that if the clinician feels that the woman's bleeding pattern is "abnormal," she should not be provided with birth control pills.)

16. Elective surgery planned (for example, hysterectomy or elective orthopedic procedures). Discontinue pills 4 weeks before surgery.

17. Long-leg casts or major injury to a lower leg.

18. Over ages 35–40 (risk is even greater if the woman is obese, hypertensive, a heavy smoker, diabetic, or has high cholesterol levels).

19. Breast tumors or fibrous breast lumps.

OTHER

Women should probably *not* start taking birth control pills if they have:

20. Irregular menstrual cycles or profile.

21. Heart or kidney disease (or history thereof).

22. History of heavy smoking.

23. Conditions likely to make patient unreliable at following pill instructions, such as mental retardation, major psychiatric problems, history of alcoholism, history of repeatedly taking pills incorrectly, or extreme youth.

24. Breastfeeding (oral contraceptives may be initiated as weaning begins and may be an aid in decreasing the flow of milk).

May start pills but observe very carefully for change (worsening or improvement) of the problem:

25. Depression.

26. Hypertension (high blood pressure) with resting diastolic BP of 90–100.

27. Chloasma (brown facial spots) or hair loss related to pregnancy (or history thereof).

28. Asthma.

29. Epilepsy.

30. Uterine fibroids.

31. Acne.

32. Varicose veins.

33. History of hepatitis, but now normal liver-function tests.

Intrauterine Device (IUD)

MECHANISM OF ACTION

Acts as a foreign body, altering the uterine lining to create a sterile inflammatory response; this makes the uterus less receptive for implantation.

INSTRUCTIONS FOR USE

1. Check strings regularly with each menstrual period.

2. Report *any* unusual symptoms or warning signs to your clinician immediately.

3. Have IUD checked three months after insertion.

4. Have yearly pelvic examinations.

5. For extra protection against pregnancy, use a backup method (foam, condoms, diaphragm) midcycle, i.e., days 10–18 of the average 28-day cycle.

ADVANTAGES

1. Simple to use; no preparation or interference with intercourse.

2. No systemic effects.

3. Requires little ongoing attention except to check string to ensure that it is in place.

4. Excellent effectiveness.

DISADVANTAGES

1. Discomfort and cramping accompanying the insertion of an IUD.

2. Women wearing an IUD may have longer, heavier menstrual flow, increased menstrual cramping, and additional spotting.

3. Risk of pelvic infection.

SIDE EFFECTS

1. Risk of pelvic inflammatory disease increased; they may lead to serious infections, infertility.

2. Pregnancy may occur, with a high risk of miscarriage and infection if IUD is left in place; higher incidence of tubal pregnancies.

3. Perforation of the uterus by the IUD.

4. Expulsion of the IUD.

5. Cramping and bleeding may increase.

6. Rare allergic reactions to the copper in the IUD have been reported.

CONTRAINDICATIONS

ABSOLUTE

1. Active pelvic infection (acute or subacute), including known or suspected gonorrhea.

2. Pregnancy.

STRONG

1. Recent or recurrent pelvic infection.

2. Acute cervicitis or vaginitis.

3. History of ectopic pregnancy.

4. Valvular heart disease.

5. Single episode of pelvic infection if patient desires subsequent pregnancy.

6. Abnormal Pap smear, cervical or uterine malignancy or premalignancy.

7. Impaired response to infection (diabetes, steroid treatment, etc.)

8. Impaired blood-clotting response.

9. Impaired access to emergency medical care.

OTHER RELATIVE

10. Uterine irregularities (such as small uterus, bicornate uterus, cervical stenosis).

11. Menstrual or bleeding problems (such as heavy menstrual periods, anemia, abnormal uterine bleeding, severe menstrual cramps).

12. Irregular growths (such as endometriosis, fibroids, endometriosis polyps).

13. Allergy to copper.

14. Psychological or intellectual problems (such as inability to check for IUD strings).

15. Multiple sexual partners (because of the statistically increased risk of gonorrhea).

16. Past history of gonorrhea.

17. Past history of severe vaso-vagal reactivity (fainting may be a warning).

18. Concern for future fertility.

19. Recent pregnancy.

Diaphragm

MECHANISM OF ACTION

Provides a physical barrier to sperm and holds the contraceptive jelly or cream in place.

Contraceptive cream inactivates sperm and prevents them from passing into the uterus.

INSTRUCTIONS FOR USE

1. Empty bladder of urine and wash your hands.

2. Apply contraceptive jelly-cream to the diaphragm: use approximately 1 tablespoon (or ¾ inch if it comes in a tube) in the center of the diaphragm cup.
   a. Use more cream all the way around the outside rim.
   b. Smear additional cream or jelly on the outside of the cup for extra protection.
   c. Do *not* use vaseline or cold cream, as they damage the rubber and have no contraceptive effect.

3. Assume one of the number of possible positions: lie down or squat on the bed or floor; sit on the toilet; stand with one leg propped up, as if to insert a tampon.

4. Squeeze the rim of the diaphragm together; push and slide it into the vagina downward and back as far as it will go. It will then open up inside the vagina in the proper place, covering the cervix, with front rim behind the pubic bone.

5. Once the diaphragm is in place, it is immediately effective. If intercourse does not occur *within 2 hours,* an additional application of cream or jelly should be inserted. Note: Some authorities believe that 2 hours is unnecessarily restrictive and that it is safe to allow up to 6 hours to elapse before intercourse. At present, research data supporting either position is not available.

6. If intercourse is repeated, leave the diaphragm in place and insert an extra application of cream or jelly.

7. After the last act of intercourse, the diaphragm must be left in place 6–8 hours. (It should be removed and washed at least once every 24 hours to avoid an unpleasant odor.)

8. Douching is unnecessary. If douching is desired, wait until after the diaphragm is removed.

9. Remove the diaphragm by inserting one finger into the vagina, hooking it up behind the rim, and pulling down and out. If it is difficult to hook your finger behind the rim, use a squatting position and push down with the abdominal muscles.

10. You may want to urinate more regularly while wearing a diaphragm. The rim often presses against the bladder and can be uncomfortable if the bladder is full.

11. Care of the diaphragm:
    a. Wash in warm water, rinse, and pat dry.
    b. Dust with cornstarch to preserve rubber (no baby or bath powders).
    c. Test periodically by gently stretching rubber, especially around the rim, and examining for holes.
    d. Do not use vaseline, as it may cause the rubber to deteriorate. If more lubrication is desired, use additional spermicidal jelly; K-Y jelly can be used without harming the diaphragm, but it is *not* a spermicide.
    e. Store away from heat.
    f. Don't worry—rubber normally will discolor over time.
    g. With proper care, the diaphragm may last several years. However, see h.
    h. Have your diaphragm checked routinely *each* year during your annual pelvic exam, and immediately if you have a pregnancy, pelvic surgery, weight loss, or gain of more than 15–20 pounds, or if the diaphragm causes you discomfort or pain.

ADVANTAGES

1. Ease of use.

2. No health risks other than pregnancy.

3. Decreases messiness if intercourse during menstruation.

4. High effectiveness rate.

5. Woman (and her partner) can become better educated about her body.

6. Diaphragm is necessary only for occasions when the woman is having intercourse.

DISADVANTAGES

1. Must be used with each act of intercourse.

2. Requires preplanning.

3. Use of jelly or cream, which some consider messy.

SIDE EFFECTS

1. VAGINAL IRRITATION. Jelly or cream may cause ir-

ritation; allergy to the rubber is also possible, but rare.

2. PRESSURE FROM DIAPHRAGM. Wearing a diaphragm may increase bladder symptoms, irritation, or infections; improper fit may also cause pelvic cramping or pressure.

3. DISCHARGE. Leaving the diaphragm in place too long can cause increased discharge with strong odor.

CONTRAINDICATIONS

1. PHYSICAL PROHIBITIONS—pelvic abnormalities. A few women may not be able to use a diaphragm because they cannot be satisfactorily fitted. Certain pelvic abnormalities, such as severely displaced uterus or relaxed vaginal walls, can prohibit a stable and satisfactory diaphragm placement.

2. DISCOMFORT OR AVERSION. Most motivated women can learn to insert the diaphragm properly. Occasionally, however, a woman who has an intact hymen because she has never had intercourse may experience too much discomfort with insertion. Also, a woman who has an aversion to manipulation of her genitals may not be able to tolerate the insertion procedure.

Contraceptive Creams and jellies

MECHANISM OF ACTION

Traps, collects and destroys sperm cells. Forms a mechanical barrier over cervix; immobilizes sperm.

INSTRUCTIONS FOR USE

Each brand of cream or jelly may have slightly different instructions for use. Fill the applicator tube, insert it into the vagina like a tampon, and push in the plunger. Most clinicians recommend two applications for each act of intercourse. All brands must be inserted prior to intercourse; some recommend a short waiting period of 2–3 minutes between insertion and the beginning of intercourse to allow the cream or jelly to disperse more completely in the vagina. Several kinds suggest that intercourse should occur within 15 minutes after insertion of the jelly.

IMPORTANT: For dependability of spermicide alone, select the type of cream or jelly that is designed to be used *alone*, rather than the kind specified for use with a diaphragm.

ADVANTAGES

1. Usually produce less vaginal irritations than foam.

2. Packaging provides another advantage, as a woman can more effectively monitor her supply.

3. Some women find that cream or jelly can be an excellent vaginal lubricant for intercourse.

DISADVANTAGES

1. Lower effectiveness rate than foam. Pregnancy rates vary considerably, depending on the source quoted, but the most recent *Population Reports* has noted the following comparative rates of pregnancy per 100 women per year; foam 3.98; cream 6.19; jelly 23.1.

2. Jellies do not disperse evenly or rapidly and tend

to remain in the location where inserted. It is, therefore, important to insert the jelly exactly in front of the cervix.

SIDE EFFECTS

None.

CONTRAINDICATIONS

There are no health problems that would make it inadvisable for a woman to use cream unless she has demonstrated an allergy in the past. However, people who would view an unplanned pregnancy as a major health risk or life-style difficulty would be advised to use foam with condoms, or to use a more effective barrier method, the diaphragm.

Foam

MECHANISM OF ACTION

Traps, collects, and destroys sperm cells. Forms a mechanical barrier over cervix; immobilizes sperm.

INSTRUCTIONS FOR USE

1. Keep stored in cool area.

2. Shake can vigorously before use (to insure mixing of spermicide with foam).

3. Fill applicator. (Each brand of foam has a slightly different technique for fillings.)

4. Lie down. Insertion is similar to putting in a tampon. Spread apart lips around vagina and insert applicator as far as possible (approximately 3–4 inches).

5. Press in plunger to deposit foam around cervix.

6. Remove applicator from vagina.

7. Repeat process if another application of foam is desired. Different brands of foam have different size applicators, some requiring two applications. Delfen and Koromex applicators hold only 5 cc of foam, and at least 10 cc are necessary to provide protection. Emko, Because, and Clakon applicators hold 17 cc.

8. You may want to insert foam after oral sex due to its unpleasant taste and smell.

9. If more than 15–30 minutes elapse before intercourse, a new applicator full must be inserted; and an additional application of foam is necessary for each act of intercourse.

10. Do not douche for 6–8 hours after intercourse.

11. Wash applicator with soap and water before storing for future use.

12. Keep an extra supply of foam on hand. It is difficult to know exactly when a bottle is going to be empty.

13. If you are going to resume daily activities immediately after intercourse and want to avoid discharge that may soil clothes, use a tampon or sanitary pad.

14. If you or your partner experience irritation, try a different brand of foam, or switch to another form of vaginal spermicide.

15. Again, make sure you have *contraceptive foam*, and not a vaginal hygiene product.

ADVANTAGES

1. Effective immediately after insertion—no "waiting period" necessary.

2. Available in preloaded applicators.

3. May produce less discharge after intercourse than other spermicide products.

DISADVANTAGES

1. Improper preparation and insertion (i.e., not high enough into the vagina) may decrease effectiveness.

2. Requires exacting preparation (i.e., first filling applicator, then inserting into vagina).

3. Shelf life of approximately one year.

4. Consecutive acts of intercourse, requiring multiple applications of foam in one lovemaking session, can become messy.

SIDE EFFECTS

1. Allergy or irritation.

CONTRAINDICATIONS

There are no health problems that would make it inadvisable for a woman to use foam, unless she has demonstrated an allergy in the past. However, people who would view an unplanned pregnancy as a major health risk or lifestyle difficulty would be advised to use foam with condoms, or to use a more effective barrier method, the diaphragm.

Withdrawal (coitus interruptus)

MECHANISM OF ACTION

Sperm not ejaculated in or near vagina. Male removes penis from partner's vagina when he feels he is approaching orgasm.

INSTRUCTIONS FOR USE

1. Rely on withdrawal for contraception only when your self-control and reflexes are not affected by alcohol, drugs, etc.

2. Wipe off the tip of penis immediately before inserting it into the vagina.

3. The man should withdraw his penis clearly before ejaculation occurs.

4. Make sure the ejaculate fluid has no contact with the woman's genitals.

5. Use positions that make it easy to withdraw the penis rapidly.

ADVANTAGES

1. Medically safe and always available as a method of birth control.

2. An excellent back-up method in emergency situations, and a reasonable choice for couples who can deal with a moderate pregnancy risk.

3. Some couples may find their sexual relationship enhanced by the de-emphasis on ejaculation inside the vagina. Mutual stimulation to orgasm following withdrawal often increases both partners' satisfaction with this method.

DISADVANTAGES

1. A man who has premature ejaculation, difficulty controlling his ejaculations, or little forewarning when he is about to ejaculate would be a poor risk to use this method effectively.

2. Unreliable for couples who do not feel they would have the self-control necessary, or who would be frustrated by the method.

SIDE EFFECTS

None.

CONTRAINDICATIONS

See Disadvantages.

Condoms

MECHANISM OF ACTION

The condom covers the penis during intercourse so that the man ejaculates into the condom rather than into the woman's vagina. Since no sperm travel up into the uterus, an egg cannot be fertilized.

Condoms prevent sexually-transmitted diseases by preventing direct contact of the penis with the mucous membranes of the vagina, contact that is usually necessary for organisms to be passed from one person to another.

The theoretical effectiveness of condoms ranges from 96–98% when used properly every time. The possibility of manufacturing defects leading to breakage or pinhole leaks accounts for the 2–4% theoretical failure rate. The actual use effectiveness of condoms is about 90%.

Lack of reliable use is the most common reason for the high 10% failure rate for this method.

INSTRUCTIONS FOR USE

1. Buy good quality condoms.

2. Stored away from heat, condoms should last about two years. Do not use old or used ones, or ones of questionable age.

3. For maximum reliabil-ity, use a condom with every act of intercourse.

4. The condom must be rolled onto the penis *before* any penis-vagina contact.

5. Use condoms with a reservoir tip, or leave about ½" of empty space at the tip of the condom to collect the semen and help prevent breakage.

6. If you desire additional lubrication, do not use vaseline, which weakens the rubber. A sterile lubricant such as K-Y jelly or a contraceptive cream or jelly will provide excellent lubrication.

7. Hold the condom at the base of the penis when withdrawing it from the vagina.

8. Remove the penis from the vagina soon after ejaculation to prevent the condom from slipping off as the size of the penis decreases.

9. Do not re-use a condom.

ADVANTAGES

1. No medical risks.

2. Widely available, and at least expense among the barrier methods.

3. Small and convenient, easy to carry and store.

4. The man takes active responsibility for his sexuality and its possible consequences.

5. After intercourse, the condom can provide reassuring evidence that it has worked; and by containing the ejaculate, it decreases the woman's excess vaginal discharge.

6. May help prolong intercourse in the situation where the man ejaculates sooner than he or his partner prefers. Or, the tight-band sensation from the elastic holding the condom in place may provide increased pleasure or help maintain an erection.

7. Prelubricated condoms may help reduce a problem of vaginal or penile irritation.

8. Condoms help prevent sexually transmitted disease and reinfection of the reproductive tract when one or both partners are receiving treatment for such a problem.

DISADVANTAGES

1. Men or women, or both, may object to the inconvenience of preplanning or disruption of lovemaking.

2. Some object to an unpleasant smell or uncomfortable feel of the condom.

3. If there is not enough lubrication, friction from the condom can cause vaginal irritation.

4. There is a risk of the condom's slipping off the penis during intercourse, or as the man withdraws after intercourse.

5. It may reduce the man's pleasurable sensations during intercourse.

SIDE EFFECTS

None.

CONTRAINDICATIONS

1. Either partner may be allergic to latex rubber, although such an allergy is rare, and switching to skin condoms will solve this problem.

2. Some men are unable to maintain an erection while using a condom.

Natural family planning methods

MECHANISM OF ACTION

Sexual intercourse is avoided during the fertile time surrounding ovulation. The woman uses a bodily sign such as temperature or cervical mucus to identify her fertile time.

INSTRUCTIONS FOR USE

See page 90.

ADVANTAGES

1. Natural family planning is completely safe, with no risks or side effects (except the chance of pregnancy).

2. It can be practiced with very little cost, if any.

3. The project of natural family planning can provide a couple with the feeling of working together for a common goal.

4. It can provide a woman useful feedback about her reproductive processes and health, and a sense of control over her body.

5. Natural family planning is acceptable to religious groups that prohibit other birth control methods.

DISADVANTAGES

1. Natural family planning requires considerable knowledge and preparation, sincere commitment, and self-control from both partners.

2. Requires several months of record-keeping before beginning actual use, and careful, continuous record-keeping during use.

3. Some women do not seem to have clearcut mucus or temperature patterns, despite careful record-keeping.

4. Women with irregular cycles may have problems with the temperature and calendar methods.

5. Health problems (such as vaginal infections) or significant life stresses may interfere with cyclic patterns or scrupulous record-keeping.

6. Some researchers believe that pregnancies that result from intercourse in the later half of the cycle will produce more fetal abnormalities because of fertilization of an old egg (Jongbloet, 1971).

SIDE EFFECTS

None.

CONTRAINDICATIONS

None.

It is important when comparing methods to be consistent in quoting either theoretical or use-effectiveness rates. Table 7.2 gives the failure rates for each method, considering both theoretical and use effectiveness. The failure rate is the percentage of women who would become pregnant within one year after beginning to use a particular method. Theoretical effectiveness refers to the method used perfectly, with no errors, *exactly* according to instructions. Use effectiveness, on the other hand, is more representative of the "real world." It includes users who are careless as well as those who are conscientious. All the methods except coitus interruptus, rhythm, and lactation have an excellent theoretical effectiveness rate. That is important, for many people erroneously believe that the effectiveness of methods such as foam or condoms is so low that one might as well not use any method.

oral contraceptives

Some 80 to 100 million women throughout the world, and 10 to 15 million American women, use oral contraceptives regularly. Yet, today, there is a considerably more cautious position about oral contraceptives than in the 1970s. Several decades of research have demonstrated that their effects extend to virtually every organ system in a woman's body and create complex endocrine alterations. Furthermore, they may have disruptive side effects and provide potential risks to the safety and health of some women. Birth control pills continue to be the overwhelmingly popular choice among young, healthy, sexually active

table 7.2

method effectiveness: theoretical and actual use rates (number of pregnancies during the first year of use per 100 nonsterile women initiating method)*

METHOD	USED CORRECTLY AND CONSISTENTLY	AVERAGE U.S. EXPERIENCE AMONG 100 WOMEN WHO WANTED NO MORE CHILDREN
	THEORETICAL EFFECTIVENESS	ACTUAL USE EFFECTIVENESS
Abortion	0	0+
Abstinence	0	?
Hysterectomy	0.0001	0.0001
Tubal ligation	0.04	0.04
Vasectomy	0.15	0.15+
Oral contraceptive (combined)	0.34	4[a]–10[b]
I.M. Long-acting progestin	0.25	5–10
Condom plus spermicidal agent	Less than 1[c]	5
Low-dose oral progestin	1–1.5	5–10[b]
IUD	1–3	5[a]
Condom	3	10[a]
Diaphragm (with spermicide)	3	17[a]
Spermicidal foam	3	22[a]
Coitus interruptus	9	20–25
Rhythm (calendar)	13	21[a]
Lactation for 12 months	25	40[d]
Chance (sexually active)	90[e]	90[e]
Douche	?	40[a]

[a]Ryder, Norman B., "Contraceptive Failure in the United States," *Family Planning Perspectives* 5:133–142, 1973.

[b]Oral contraceptive failure rates may be far higher than this, if one considers women who become pregnant after discontinuing oral contraceptives, but prior to initiating another method. Oral contraceptive discontinuation rates as high as 50–60% in the first year of use are not uncommon in family planning programs.

[c]Data are normally presented as Pearl indices. For conversion to the form used here, the Pearl index was divided by 1,300 to give the average monthly failure rate n. The proportion of women who would fail within one year is then $1-(1-n)$.

[d]Most women supplement breast feedings, significantly decreasing the contraceptive effectiveness of lactation. In Rwanda, 50% of nonlactating women were found to conceive by just over 4 months postpartum. It might be noted that in this community sexual intercourse is culturally permitted from about 5 days postpartum on (Bonte, M., and van Balen, H., *J. BioSoc Sci* 1:97, 1969).

[e]This figure is higher in younger couples having intercourse frequently, lower in women over 35 having intercourse infrequently. For example, MacLeod found that within 6 months 94.6% of wives of men under 25 having intercourse 4 or more times per week conceived. Only 16.0% of wives of men 35 and over having intercourse less than twice a week conceived (MacLeod, *Fertility and Sterility* 4:10-33, 1953).

*Reprinted from *Contraceptive Technology*, 1980-81.

women (approximately 30% of women in their childbearing years use the pill).

Oral contraceptives contain two female hormones as basic ingredients: progestin (a synthetic progesterone) and estrogen. There are two major types of oral contraceptives: combination and mini-pills (a third type called sequential pills was removed from the market by the FDA). Combination-type oral contraceptives contain a particular level of both estrogen and progestin. Mini-pills contain only a progestin.

The effectiveness of oral contraceptives may be decreased if taken simultaneously with the following drugs: Dilantin, phenobarbital, rifampicin, ampicillin, antihistamines, phenylbutazone, meprobromate, and other sedatives and tranquilizers. A woman should discuss these medications with her health care provider.

Birth control pills differ in the kind, strength, and amount of the synthetic estrogens and progestins used in each brand or type of pill. There are twenty-two different types of oral contraceptives presently available, with several new brands to be released soon. All brands have similar basic physiological effects and similar rates of effectiveness in preventing pregnancy. Many women, however, react to each different brand of pill in a somewhat different way as different compounds are used by pharmaceutical companies to create the estrogen and progestin in their pills. Furthermore, each company makes several different strengths of pills. Often a woman who experiences side effects on one type will feel much more comfortable after a change to a different strength or brand of pill.

An important warning suggested by a number of recent studies is that stronger pills (with more than 50 micrograms of estrogen) are associated with higher circulatory risks. Therefore, these pills should be avoided unless there is a strong rationale for using them. They include Ortho-Novum 1/80, Ortho-Novum 2, Norinyl 1/80, Ovulen, Enovid E. (See Table 7.3 for symptoms related to problems with oral contraceptives.)

The majority of women taking birth control pills today are using one of the "standard pills" with approximately 50 mcg. of estrogen. These include Ortho-Novum 1/50, Norinyl 1/50, Demulen, Norlestrin 1, Norlestrin 2.5, Ovral, and Zorane 1/50.

In the past few years, a group of pills with less than 50 mcg. estrogen has appeared. They include Modicon, Brevicon, LoOvral, Loestrin 1.5/30, Loestrin 1/20, Zorane 1.5/30, Zorane 1/20, Norinyl 1/35 and Orthonovum 1/35. The disadvantage of these pills is that some users seem to have more irregular spotting and missed periods. The advantage is that some women had less trouble with side effects, such as nausea, water retention, or breast symptoms, because of the lower level of hormones. At this point, there is no evidence that these new lower dose pills have less serious risks, such as circulatory disorders.

"Mini-pills" is the term used by most people to refer to progestin-only pills. Mini-pills contain no estrogen and do not usually prevent ovulation. Researchers suspect that their primary effects are changes in the cervical mucus that inhibit sperm migration and changes in the lining of the uterus that make it an unsuitable environment for implantation. Many clinicians believe that mini-pills may be safer because they contain no estrogen and one-third the amount of progestin. However, they are otherwise similar to regular and combined pills, so all risks, problems, warnings, and contraindications apply. At present, there is no completed long-term research that confirms any decreased health risks of mini-pills compared to others.

Mini-pills are taken differently from regu-

table 7.3
symptoms that suggest serious problems with oral contraceptives

SIGNAL	POSSIBLE PROBLEM
1. Abdominal pain (severe)	Gallbladder disease, hepatic adenoma, blood clot.
2. Chest pain (severe) or shortness of breath	Blood clot in lungs or myocardial infarction.
3. Headaches (severe)	Stroke or hypertension.
4. Eye problems: blurred vision, flashing lights, or blindness	Stroke or hypertension.
5. Severe leg pain (calf or thigh)	Blood clot in legs.

symptoms that suggest serious problems with iud's

SIGNAL	POSSIBLE PROBLEM
1. Pelvic pain, severe cramping; pain with inter course; fever or chills; flulike symptoms, such as fatigue, general body ache, headaches; unusual vaginal bleeding or unusual vaginal discharge, particularly with foul odor.	Pelvic inflammatory disease; perforation of the uterus.

lar combination pills. They are begun on day 1 of a menstrual period and continued without stopping until protection from pregnancy is no longer desired.

intrauterine device (IUD)

The IUD continues to be chosen as the most appropriate method of contraception for 60 million women throughout the world and 3 to 4 million American women (Hatcher et al., 1980).

The IUD is a small white device made of inert plastic placed inside the uterus by a clinician. Newer models have added copper or progesterone hormones to enhance their effectiveness. All IUD's have a nylon string that extends out of the uterus, through the cervix, and into the vagina. IUD's also contain a minute amount of barium, which makes it possible for the IUD to be found on X-ray. There are five types of IUD's available in the United States—Lippes Loop, Saf-T Coil, Copper 7, Copper T, and Progestasert.

The best time to insert or remove an IUD is during the menstrual period—when the cervix (opening to the uterus) is dilated, when the bleeding and cramping can occur simultaneously with the menstrual period, and when the woman can be certain that she is not pregnant. The removal of an IUD usually involves some strong cramping, which subsides rapidly. Insertion, however, can be particularly painful for some women and may cause dizziness, faintness, nausea; consequently, it is wise for a woman to have a friend or partner accompany her to have the IUD inserted, in case she needs someone to drive her home. The copper and progesterone IUD's must be periodically replaced, while the plastic ones can be left in the uterus indefinitely. Manufacturers presently recommend that the copper IUD's be replaced every 3 years, and the progesterone IUD's every 1 to 1½ years. These recommendations may change if studies indicate that the time period can be safely increased.

IUD's have become so controversial in the

past several years that many clinicians either refuse to insert them or take a strong negative attitude toward them because of pelvic infection and subsequent infertility risks (see Table 7.3). Other professionals feel that the IUD continues to be the optimal method for the woman over 30 in a monogamous relationship who desires no further children. IUD users themselves are divided.

diaphragm

The diaphragm is a round, dome-shaped, soft rubber cup with a flexible rim around the edge. For 100 years, millions of American and European women have successfully avoided or spaced pregnancies with this simple device combined with contraceptive jelly. With the concern about side effects and risks associated with other methods, the diaphragm is regaining popularity. Particularly, women who are secure in their sexual relationships find the diaphragm method of birth control appropriate to their life-styles. The main factors determining a woman's effective use of the diaphragm are her level of motivation to follow all the instructions correctly and her comfort with planning for intercourse and touching her genitals.

The diaphragm and spermicidal cream or jelly are always used together. The diaphragm is flexible and can be compressed and passed easily into the vagina. It is released in the upper widening canal of the vagina, where it covers the entrance to the cervix like a dome-shaped lid. It forms a physical barrier to sperm and holds the jelly or cream in place. The spermicidal cream inactivates the sperm and prevents them from passing into the uterus. The diaphragm fits snugly in the vagina at the time of insertion. Then, during intercourse, when the vagina expands, the diaphragm is able to move around somewhat.

The correct size for each woman is easily determined by the health care provider during a pelvic exam. The distance from the back wall of the vagina to the pubic bone varies from woman to woman, so this distance is determined and the correct size of diaphragm is prescribed. With a proper fit and proper insertion, it is not felt by either the woman or the man during intercourse. The health care provider who fits a woman's diaphragm will give her an opportunity to practice insertion and removal several times, until she feels confident that she will be able to use it correctly. Most women insert the diaphragm with their hands, although a special insertion device is available.

cervical cap

The cervical cap is a thimble-shaped rubber dome similar to a diaphragm. The cap is a popular method in England and Europe, but has not been in general use in the United States since about the 1940's. Apparently, the cap's popularity in America declined with increased use of the diaphragm, so American manufacturers stopped making them. Recently, it has been reintroduced in the United States by a number of women's clinics responding to interested consumers. These cervical cap devices, however, must still be ordered from manufacturers in England and can be obtained only in research studies. Research is now underway to determine effectiveness, procedures for use, and potential problems. Like the diaphragm, the cervical cap must be fitted by a clinician. It is used with spermicidal cream, inserted prior to intercourse, and left in place for eight hours afterward. Some clinicians believe the effectiveness of the cap is equivalent to that of the diaphragm; others feel it is slightly lower.

Unlike the diaphragm, the cervical cap uses

strong suction to fit snugly over the cervix and hold the cream right at the cervical opening. In contrast, the diaphragm spreads out over the entire length of the vagina. Some people believe that the cap can be inserted a longer period of time before intercourse occurs, making it more convenient and less tied to the actual act of sex. Others warn that if a period of time elapses between insertion and actual intercourse, additional jelly must be inserted. In general, the cervical cap requires more expertise on the part of the user for insertion and removal. Therefore, it is important that the woman have ample opportunity to practice insertion and removal.

vaginal spermicides

Vaginal spermicides are a convenient and readily available contraceptive used by 4 million American women. One of the forms of spermicides can be used alone, with a diaphragm or condom, or as an emergency back-up method of contraception in situations such as forgotten pills or a lost IUD string.

Vaginal spermicides now come in the form of foams, creams, jellies, and suppositories. These various forms can be confusing. Warning: *Make sure you have contraceptive products* and not vaginal hygiene or feminine deodorant products!

Foam is the most frequently recommended and used of the vaginal spermicides, as it is considered most effective. It is sold in a small aerosol bottle with a plunger-type plastic applicator. The foaming action distributes the spermicide, which has the appearance and consistency of shaving cream, evenly over the cervix, contributing to its effectiveness.

The *Encare Oval* is an effervescing suppository that begins to work in the presence of warmth and moisture. It is an approximately 1-inch oval containing the same spermicide

(Nonoxynal-9) as foam. Encare Oval's pre-packaging in a small fingertip size and shape eliminates the need for applicators, large tubes, and filling procedures.

The efficacy of the Encare Oval in preventing pregnancy is controversial. A survey of Encare users in West Germany reports a rate of only 1 pregnancy per 100 women per year. The U.S. Food and Drug Administration, however, has posed some questions about the reliability of the methods used in the German study. Consequently, the National Medical Committee of Planned Parenthood has suggested that, until further study, the Encare Oval be categorized effective equivalently to contraceptive foam.

Instructions for use require that the Encare Oval be inserted at least 10 minutes before intercourse, and if intercourse does not occur within one hour, a new suppository must be inserted. It is extremely important that the Encare Oval be inserted as high up in the vagina as possible so that it will dissolve directly in front of the cervix. A woman should not douche for 6 to 8 hours after the last act of intercourse.

The Encare Oval creates heat as it effervesces in the moist vaginal environment. The sensation of warmth and heat may be either pleasant or unpleasant to either the woman or her partner, depending upon their personal preferences.

withdrawal

Withdrawal, called coitus interruptus, "pulling out," "being careful," or "taking care," has been practiced for birth control since ancient times when it was first discovered that semen and pregnancy were related. Withdrawal probably is the most frequently used contraceptive method in the world. It requires the man to remove his penis from his partner's vagina when he feels that he is approaching orgasm, before he "comes." Ejaculation of the semen then occurs completely away from the woman's genitals so that the sperm cannot enter the vagina and eventually fertilize an egg. Even if a couple practices this method faithfully, pregnancies occur. Sperm can be stored in the man's prostate, urethra, or cowper's glands. These sperm enter the small amount of clear lubrication, called "precoital" or "pre-ejaculatory" fluid, that is discharged from the penis during sexual arousal, prior to actual ejaculation. The likelihood of the presence of sperm in the precoital fluid increases if intercourse occurs more than once in close succession.

abstinence, and sex without intercourse

Abstinence means no sexual intercourse, the only 100 percent effective method of birth control. Abstinence need not exclude sexual interaction. Sexual pleasuring without intercourse may be used as a periodic alternative to traditional intercourse using another contraceptive, or as the couple's consistent primary method of birth control.

To use abstinence as a reliable contraceptive method, the couple must, of course, be consistent.

condoms

A condom is a sheath of thin rubber or animal tissue that covers the man's penis during intercourse. Historically, condoms were designed to protect men from venereal disease, rather than women from pregnancy. Ironically, today it is men who most often express the greatest objections to their use. Many men, however, are concerned enough about the health risks their partners may undergo—with either contraceptive methods or pregnancy—

that they are more than willing to share the responsibility for birth control. Couples often use condoms as a second method to insure a higher effectiveness, or to alternate with other barrier methods.

Recent attention to condoms has resulted in an increase in variety. Condoms can be lubricated or nonlubricated, latex rubber, or animal tissue. The natural skin condoms are more expensive; they are said to provide much more sensitivity for the male during intercourse. They are also particularly good for the man with a very large penis, as they tend to run larger. The latex condoms now come in different shapes to provide increased pleasure with pressure areas on the penis, and some are ribbed for extra stimulation of the woman.

natural family planning— fertility awareness

Natural family planning was previously called "the rhythm method" and used mainly by couples whose religion prohibited other contraceptive measures. More recently the consumer movement, and increasing interest in the body's healthy functioning, have stimulated interest in fertility awareness.

During their cycles, women can record a variety of subtle and overt signs directly related to their fertility: temperature patterns, cervical mucus patterns, pain or spotting with ovulation, breast tenderness, mucus ferning patterns, position and consistency of the uterus, mood, and sex drive (Hatcher et al., 1980).

The three main forms of natural family planning are the calendar method, the basal body temperature method, and the mucus method. The calendar method can help signal the first fertile day, while the temperature and mucus changes can identify the time of ovulation and the end of the fertile period.

The principle of natural family planning is basic: a couple must avoid sexual intercourse during the fertile time surrounding ovulation, the release of the woman's egg, when it is available to be fertilized by a sperm. The woman uses one or more of the bodily signs to indicate whether she is in the fertile phase of her cycle. Because the egg lives approximately 24 hours and the sperm live up to 72 hours (perhaps longer), the fertile period lasts about a week.

calendar method

The calendar method of natural contraception relies on a prediction based on a woman's menstrual-cycle history. She must know the number of days in her shortest and longest cycle. To calculate the length of a cycle, she counts from the first day of her menstrual period up to (but not including) the first day of her next period. This is recorded for six months. The next step is to pinpoint the probable day of ovulation, according to both the longest and shortest recorded menstrual cycles.

Ovulation usually occurs about 14 days (plus or minus 2 days) *before* the beginning of the next menstrual period. Regardless of the length of the menstrual cycle, the length of time between ovulation and the beginning of menstruation is the same for all women. It is the time period before ovulation that varies considerably. A woman must calculate her longest and shortest cycles because almost no one has exactly the same length cycle each month. The shortest cycle will tell the woman the earliest day on which she might ovulate; the longest cycle predicts the latest day she may ovulate. Then, to allow for egg and sperm survival, 3 to 4 days must be added on each side of the "outside" estimated days of ovulation. This calculation gives the unsafe

"fertile period" when the couple must abstain from intercourse. Table 7.4 shows a precalculated summary of the first and last fertile days for different cycle lengths.

temperature method

The temperature method can add more precision in pinpointing the time of ovulation. The woman charts her basal body temperature (BBT), the temperature of her body when completely at rest. The temperature is taken for five full minutes, either rectally or orally. It must be taken consistently, immediately upon awakening, before getting out of bed, drinking, eating, or talking. Women have a slightly lower BBT of 96–98 degrees right before ovulation, rising to 97–99 degrees after ovulation. The characteristic pattern is a drop about 24 hours before ovulation and a rise that remains elevated until the next menstruation. The rise at ovulation may be sudden, may be a gradual climb, or may climb in steps over several days. Some women do not experience the temperature drop before ovulation—just a steady rise. An individual woman's pattern may differ each month.

Most clinicians feel that the safe period begins only *after* the temperature has dropped and then been elevated for three full days. The first part of the cycle—all the days between the beginning of the menstrual period and the third day of the next temperature rise—is considered unsafe time for intercourse. If intercourse should occur several days before ovulation, there is a possibility that a sperm could survive to fertilize a newly released egg.

A woman's temperature patterns are quite sensitive to a variety of events. Physical and emotional stresses, changes in daily schedule and sleep patterns, even electric blankets may cause variations. If BBT patterns are unclear, it is advisable for a woman to consult a family

table 7.4

how to calculate the interval of fertility

IF YOUR SHORTEST CYCLE HAS BEEN (NUMBER OF DAYS)	YOUR FIRST FERTILE (UNSAFE) DAY IS	IF YOUR LONGEST CYCLE HAS BEEN (NUMBER OF DAYS)	YOUR LAST FERTILE (UNSAFE) DAY IS
21	3rd Day	21	10th Day
22	4th Day	22	11th Day
23	5th Day	23	12th Day
24	6th Day	24	13th Day
25	7th Day	25	14th Day
26	8th Day	26	15th Day
27	9th Day	27	16th Day
28	10th Day	28	17th Day
29	11th Day	29	18th Day
30	12th Day	30	19th Day
31	13th Day	31	20th Day
32	14th Day	32	21st Day
33	15th Day	33	22nd Day
34	16th Day	34	23rd Day
35	17th Day	35	24th Day

Day 1 = First Day of Menstrual Bleeding

planning clinician before relying on this method.

mucus method

The mucus method relies on observation of changes in the character and appearance of the cervical mucus during the menstrual cycle to determine the time of ovulation and maximum fertility. This has also been called the Billings Method, after an Australian husband-wife team of doctors who identified the link between hormone levels, which affect ovulation, and mucus secretion. To use this method, the woman is trained to know the changes in cervical mucus that occur with ovulation and to avoid intercourse (or use backup methods) during that time.

Basically, the mucus pattern goes through the following predictable phases:

1. Menstruation. Menstrual flow disguises the mucus patterns so it is not possible to detect changes. The last several days of the period are considered *unsafe*, particularly in women with short cycles.

2. Early dry days. *Safe.* Immediately after the period, a woman may have dry days when no mucus in present.

3. Early preovulatory days. *Unsafe.* As egg starts to ripen, the secretions are cloudy and sticky, generally whitish or yellow.

4. Ovulation. *Very unsafe.* Immediately before, during, and after ovulation, mucus is clear, watery, profuse. This clear slippery discharge resembles egg white in consistency.

5. Late dry days. *Safest.* Between the fourth day following ovulation and the next menstrual period, women have either thick, cloudy, sticky mucus, or none at all.

A woman using this method must check herself several times a day. She can check her mucus by wiping with toilet tissue before urination, by observing the discharge on her underpants, or by putting a finger in her vagina to obtain mucus.

Douching, semen, natural lubrication from intercourse, foam, jelly, lubricants, medication, and vaginal infection all can change the amount and quality of the mucus observed, and thus obscure the natural mucus pattern. Consequently, many clinicians recommend abstinence until the fourth day after ovulation, as nearly as that can be determined.

sympto-thermal method

The combination of all the natural methods is often called the sympto-thermal method. Theoretically, this should be much more effective in preventing pregnancy than any one method alone.

"morning after" treatment

If a couple has intercourse without contraception regularly (at least twice a week), within one year 80 percent of the women will become pregnant; if a couple has intercourse on one occasion only, estimates range from 2 to 30 percent. A safe, simple method of contraception that could be administered after intercourse is an appealing idea, but no such treatment exists. A woman can immediately insert spermicidal foam, cream, or jelly into her vagina, or if a spermicide is not available, she could try a vinegar-water (2 tablespoons to 1 quart) douche. However, these measures may well be too late, as sperm move extremely fast from the vagina into the uterus.

At this time, options for morning-after birth control are very limited. Furthermore, because of the accompanying risks, morning-after measures must be considered in emergencies only, not as primary methods.

High doses of estrogen given within 72 hours of unprotected intercourse theoretically interfere with conception and/or implantation of the egg. The woman takes the hormones for five days to increase chances of its being effective. DES is presently the only estrogen officially considered and approved by the FDA for morning-after treatment (see chapter 19).

The primary concern about all estrogens is the effect these hormones might have on a developing fetus. If the morning-after treatment is unsuccessful, and the woman continues to be pregnant, the fetus is exposed to a very high dosage of estrogen. The past experience of women who took DES during pregnancy (1947-1970) to prevent miscarriage has revealed a higher incidence of reproductive organ and breast cancers among their daughters as they reached adulthood. Consequently, many strongly consider aborting a pregnancy that has been exposed to unsuccessful morning-after treatment.

Preliminary research shows that the insertion of an IUD immediately after unprotected intercourse will prevent pregnancy. However, further study and FDA approval is necessary before this becomes a widely available option for women.

sterilization

Sterilization procedures—vasectomy and tubal ligation—seal or completely obstruct the tube or passageways that make the egg or sperm available for fertilization.

In the male, two tubes, the vas deferens, carry the sperm from the testicles, where they are made, to the urethra, which transports them outside the body. If a vas deferens has been blocked, as in a vasectomy, the sperm do not travel anywhere and are reabsorbed by the body. The ejaculatory fluid is produced in other areas along the man's genital tract; consequently, the body keeps making ejaculatory fluid in proportion to the frequency of orgasm. The only difference is that there are no sperm in this fluid. Because the sperm comprise such a minute portion of the fluid, the man notices no difference in the amount of his ejaculation.

A tubal ligation is the parallel operation for women. When the fallopian tube has been closed, as in a tubal ligation, the egg cannot travel to the uterus to meet with sperm, and it therefore is reabsorbed by the body. Because a woman's hormones and ovaries function normally after a tubal ligation, she continues to release an egg each month and have menstrual periods like those before her surgery.

Even though sterilization is the most effective method of contraception, there have been cases of failure. Very rarely the tubes (vas deferens or fallopian tubes) can grow back together spontaneously. No one knows how this is possible. Reported pregnancy rates after sterilization vary, depending on the procedure and probably on the skill of the surgeon. For vasectomy and laparoscopic tubal ligations, pregnancies have occurred at the rate of 1–2.5 per 100,000 procedures. Translated into the kind of effectiveness rates discussed for other methods, if 1,000 couples underwent vasectomy or laparoscopic procedures, one or two of the women would become pregnant in a five-year period.

Belsky, R. Vaginal contraceptives: A time for reappraisal? *Population Reports*, Ser. A, No. 3. Washington, D.C.; George Washington Univ., 1975.

Beral, V. Morality among oral contraceptive users. *Lancet*, 1977, *2*, 727–731.

Boston Women's Health Book Collective. *Our bodies, ourselves.* New York: Simon & Schuster, 1976.

Edmondson, H.A. Liver cell adenomas associated with use of oral contraceptives. *New England Journal of Medicine*, 1976, *294 (9)*, 470–472.

Family Planning Perspective Digest. 7 year prospective study of 17,000 women using pill, IUD and diaphragm. *Family Planning Perspectives*, 1976, *8*, 241–248.

Green, C. R., Sartwell, P. E. Oral contraceptive use in patients with thromboembolisms following surgery, trauma or infection. *American Journal of Public Health*, 1972, *62*, 680.

Hatcher, R. A. et al. *Contraceptive technology 1980–81.* New York: Irvington, 1980.

Johnson, V. E. et al. The physiology of intravaginal contraceptive failure. In (Ed.) M. S. Calderone, *Manual of Family Planning Practice*, 2nd ed. Baltimore: Williams & Wilkens, 1970, pp. 232–245.

Jongbloet, P. H. Mental and physical handicaps in connection with overripe ovopathy. M. A. Ross, P. T. Piotrow, Birth control without contraceptives, *Population Reports*, Ser. 1, No. 1, June 1974. Washington, D. C., George Washington Medical Center.

Klaus, H. et al. Use effectiveness and satisfaction levels with Billings ovulation method: Two year pilot study. *Fertility and Sterility*, 1977, 28, 1038–1043.

Martin, L. L. *Health care of women.* Philadelphia: Lippincott, 1978.

Oral Contraceptives and Health, *Report of the Royal College of General Practitioners.* London: Pittman, 1974.

Oral contraceptives and health: An interim report for the oral contraceptive study of the Royal College of General Practitioners. New York: Pittman, 1975.

Org, H. et al. Oral contraceptives reduced risk of benign breast diseases. *New England Journal of Medicine*, 1976, *8*, 294, 419, 422.

Phillips, J. et al. Laparoscopic procedures: A national survey for 1975. *Journal of Reproductive Medicine*, 1977, *18*, 219–225.

Physicians' desk reference, ed. 32. Oradell, N.J.: Medical Economics, 1978.

Roe, R. et al. Female Sterilization: Vaginal approach. *American Journal of Obstetrics and Gynecology*, 1972, *112*, 1031–1036.

Ross, M. A., & Piotrow, P. T. Birth control without contraceptives. *Population Reports*, Ser. I, No. 1. Washington, D. C.: George Washington Univ., 1974.

Shapino, H. I. *The birth control book.* New York: Avon, 1978.

Stewart, F. et al. *My body my health: A concerned woman's guide to gynecology.* New York: Wiley, 1979.

NANCY FUGATE WOODS, R.N., Ph.D.

menopause

The average age at which American women experience menopause is 51 years; changes in our bodies, however, begin much earlier. Women in the United States generally stop menstruating between the ages of 45 and 55 years. Although it was once assumed that women who had an early menarche would have a late menopause, current evidence suggests no relationship between age at menarche and age at menopause (Treloar, 1974).

Women in the late thirties and early forties ovulate less frequently than in their twenties. The number of ovarian follicles is fixed at birth and decreases gradually over the life cycle, but the effects of the decreasing number may not become evident until the fifth decade of life. Loss of estrogen seems to be a direct result of fewer ovarian follicles to produce it.

The remaining follicles in the ovaries are less sensitive to messages received from the pituitary gland. These messages usually lead to the development and release of an ovum from the follicle. Because the remaining follicles do not produce the same amount of estrogen as did the follicles that were already ovulated, the endometrium of the uterus is no longer prepared for implantation every month, and, therefore, the menstrual periods change in frequency and subsequently diminish. There are, however, some follicles that will develop and produce an ovum; for this reason, some women become pregnant during the transition to menopause.

In an attempt to stimulate the ovary to produce more estrogen, the pituitary gland secretes more follicle-stimulating hormone (FSH) and luteinizing hormone (LH). Because the ovary no longer produces the same amount of estrogen in response to FSH and LH, the levels of these hormones, especially FSH, increase. Over time, however, a new steady state is achieved.

The decreasing production of estrogen by the ovaries is a gradual process, and the ovaries continue to produce small amounts of estrogen even after menopause. The adrenal glands also continue to produce estrogen, as well as androgen, which is converted to estrogen in the fatty tissues of the body.

Over time, less estrogen leads to some changes in estrogen-dependent functions: the waning and stopping of the menstrual periods, changes in the vagina, vulva, and breasts. These changes are apparent with aging in all women, but each woman's response to the changes is unique.

transition to menopause

The occurrence of menopause is somewhat analogous to the occurrence of ovulation: you cannot determine that you have experienced either one until after it has happened. Absence of a menstrual period for one year is a good indication that the menopause has occurred. However, some women do have a period after a year of none at all, which makes it difficult in some cases for women to determine whether they have actually experienced menopause.

Each woman's situation is unique, although there are usually some characteristic changes in the menstrual periods prior to menopause. In many women, the interval between menstrual periods becomes irregular and usually the length of the entire cycle becomes shorter. The shorter cycle length is due to a shorter follicular phase; increased production of FSH is believed responsible for beginning the maturation of ovarian follicles at more frequent intervals (Sherman, Wallace, & Treloar, 1979). Shorter menstrual cycles become interspersed with long periods of time during which no menstrual period occurs. For example, a woman whose menstrual periods occurred about every 29 days when she was in her thirties may find that in her late forties she menstruates every 22 days for a few cycles and then skips several months. Some women keep a menstrual calendar on which they record the date, duration and amount of menstrual flow, and days between cycles, and this allows them to see their transition to menopause.

Once the changes in menstrual cycle characteristics associated with menopause begin, it is not possible to predict when they will end. For some women, the cessation of menstruation occurs abruptly. For others, menstrual periods may be very irregular for several years before they cease.

menopause: what does it mean?

Although we can define menopause as a normal physiological process, it has many meanings for women throughout the world. For many, menopause means loss of fertility and aging. The restricted role definitions of wife and mother for many women, and the loss of a valued role in society (the reproducer), may be associated with negative feelings. Some women welcome the freedom from pregnancy afforded by the lack of ovulation. In a youth-oriented culture, it is not easy to age, and since menopause marks aging, some women consider it a disease to be survived.

Yet, not all women respond negatively to menopause. Some women responded with positive or neutral reactions when asked what came to mind when they first saw the word *menopause*. Older, particularly postmenopausal, women were matter of fact about menopause; younger women expressed more fear and negative feelings. There are several explanations for the differences in younger and older women's feelings about menopause, and they include myths and attitudes toward aging women.

Women's positive and negative attitudes about menopause may be attributed to the conflicting information they receive about what to expect during this period. Some women, when asked to state the worst thing about menopause, indicated not knowing what to expect. Currently, menopausal women are often portrayed as tragic or comic figures, for example, in medical journal advertisements for tranquilizers or estrogens. The language of menopause is riddled with negative images: senile vaginitis, atrophic breasts, and estrogen starvation, to name only a few. (Reitz [1979] includes an extensive list of these images, which she terms her "cringe list.") When such phrases are used in professional publications, it indicates that changes must be made to erase the negative images that pervade society. Women themselves can help by changing the language they use to describe their experiences. For example, Reitz recommends replacing the phrase "atrophic vaginitis" with the phrase "venerable vagina."

effects of menopause on women's health

A number of symptoms are ascribed to menopause in both professional and lay literature: hot flashes, melancholia, muscle aches and pains, cold sweats, weight gain, flooding, joint pains, palpitations, crying spells, insomnia, dizziness, headaches, fatigue, constipation, and diarrhea. But most of these symptoms are experienced by women throughout their lives and, indeed, even by men.

There are many myths about menopause, but some research is also inaccurate. Much of the data on menopausal symptoms has been compiled from women who seek help for those symptoms. Using their menopausal problems to characterize the experience of all women can distort documentation of the menopausal experience. In some studies, the symptoms of menopause are commonly reported to medical care providers who are trained to believe that numerous symptoms are attributable to menopausal hormone changes or that these symptoms are a result of the woman's "empty nest syndrome," not her biology.

Women are subject to the simultaneous effects of biological and social forces on their behavior and health. Thus, it would seem imperative for researchers to take into account not only the biological changes women experience in the transition to menopause, but also social and role changes. The symptoms women experience at menopause cannot be attributed solely to hormonal or social changes.

One alternative to clinicians' reports about women's menopausal symptoms is to interview women who are *not* seeking medical help for their symptoms and who are not institutionalized. Although it is often assumed that women will experience some form of distress during the transition to menopause, major studies of women residing in the community (not institutions) have shown that this is not the case. In every study for which such information was recorded, there was always a group of women who experienced no symptoms. The size of the "no distress" group ranged from 16 to 38 percent (Woods, in press). Usually little attention was given to these women—especially what may have *prevented* their symptoms.

These same studies showed that many women, on the other hand, *were* distressed by the symptoms that occurred during their transition to menopause. Hot flashes were reported by 43 to 93 percent of women during the year after their last menstrual period. Some women experienced difficulty with severe hot flashes for as long as 15 years, whereas some had only occasional hot flashes for a short period of time. Many of the women who had hot flashes also reported sweats, and some reported night sweats. For some women, night sweats disturbed their sleep as they awakened drenched with perspiration. Insomnia was often reported by women after menopause. Headaches, dizziness, joint pains, tingly sensations of the skin, and irritability were also noted frequently during these same periods.

Symptoms that did *not* seem to coincide with any particular time surrounding menopause were weight gain, palpitations (pounding of the heart), depression, suffocation, breast discomfort, and flooding. (Flooding describes menopausal bleeding in amounts that are much greater than the woman's usual menstrual flow; this symptom is common among women during the transition to menopause, but may also be a signal of disease and should be discussed with a physician or nurse practitioner.) Although some women *do* report these symptoms, they are not associated with any specific time period surrounding the menopause.

On their own, women did not frequently report symptoms of vaginal changes, such as pain or burning during intercourse, vaginal discharge, or feelings of tightness in the vagina, nor did they report symptoms characteristic of relaxation of the pelvic muscles, such as loss of urine during coughing or sneezing, or feelings of urgency to urinate. When women were asked about these symptoms, however, many found them troublesome.

Although women do report a variety of menopausal symptoms, two seem to be particularly troublesome and are believed to be a result of the decreasing levels of estrogen produced by the ovaries. These two symptoms are hot flashes and changes in the vagina.

the hot flash

A hot flash (sometimes referred to as a hot flush) is the sudden sensation of being very warm, sometimes described by women as roasting, burning, or heated up from the inside. Hot flashes can begin anywhere on the body and radiate to other parts of the body. Often they begin on the chest, neck, or face.

Women may have only a few hot flashes every day or may have as many as 20 to 30. Some women experience hot flashes both day and night, while others seem to be more troubled at either one or the other of these times. The hot flashes may last only for a few seconds or for as long as an hour. Some women have mild or moderate flashes, but others have severe hot flashes that cause them to interrupt their usual activity and leave them drenched in sweat (Voda, 1981).

Although the precise mechanism causing the hot flash is unknown, it is believed that changes in the brain's temperature regulation center in the hypothalamus probably are responsible for initiating the hot flash. The sympathetic nervous system (the part of the autonomic nervous system responsible for the flight part of the fight-or-flight mechanism) is responsible for the increase in skin temperature and sweating on the outside of the body. No one understands the mechanism that causes the hypothalamic temperature regulating set-point to change, but it has been suggested that the hypothalamic release of LHRH (luteinizing hormone releasing hormone) may be involved. A third and yet unknown factor may be responsible for the release of LHRH as well as alteration in the hypothalamic set-point. The set-point is analogous to the setting that one may adjust on a furnace. Body temperature is regulated in relation to this set-point, with certain actions designed to release excess heat, for example, sweating, and some to gain heat, as shivering or moving about (Meldrum, Tataryn, Frumor, Erlik, Lu, and Judd, 1980).

For many years, the customary treatment for women who had severe or moderate discomfort from hot flashes was estrogen replacement therapy (ERT). However, the growing evidence associating ERT with endometrial cancer (Weiss, Szekely, & Austin, 1979) has promoted alternative ways to cope with hot flashes. There are many self-health approaches women can try. These include:

1. Wearing clothing that breathes, such as natural fabrics instead of polyesters.
2. Cooling off by removing layers of clothing, using a fan, swimming, opening a window, sipping a cold drink.
3. Vitamin "E" (Reitz, 1979).
4. Genseng, an herb used in the Orient for thousands of years.

Estrogen replacement therapy seems to postpone, not avert hot flashes. Once ERT is discontinued, the hot flashes usually reappear (Seaman & Seaman, 1977).

menopausal vaginal changes

Menopause affects the vagina. Lubrication is commonly regarded as the hallmark of sexual arousal in women. As women age, the amount of time needed to respond to sexual stimulation increases. Masters and Johnson's (1966) work on human sexual response revealed that aging women who had sustained regular patterns of sexual activity did not experience the vaginal problems commonly attributed to the menopause.

In addition to problems with lubrication, some women find that the vagina feels constricted. The capacity for vaginal expansion, in response to sexual arousal, may diminish at menopause. The lack of expansiveness of the vagina and the delayed production of vaginal lubrication may make intercourse uncomfortable. If the sexual stimuli are sufficiently arousing, however, intercourse may be quite comfortable.

Instead of resorting to ERT for vaginal changes, there are several less risky measures that women can explore. Seaman and Seaman 1977 recommended:

- Tender and imaginative lovemaking to enable the woman to experience her full capacity to respond to sexual stimulation.
- Regular orgasms (although the mechanisms by which these lead to a healthy vaginal condition are unknown, the orgasmic response is accompanied by a dramatic increase in vaginal blood supply).
- Lubricants such as KY jelly or other water-soluble lubricants to supplement the woman's own vaginal lubrication.

Although estrogen-containing vaginal creams are sometimes recommended, the degree to which the estrogens are absorbed into other parts of the body makes them somewhat risky.

Another change that occurs with decreased estrogen production is a thinning of the fatty tissues around the vaginal opening and the opening to the bladder (urethra) and the relaxation of the pelvic muscles. These changes may cause some women to experience discomfort during intercourse as well as having difficulty with stress incontinence (losing urine with a cough or sneeze). One way of limiting discomfort during intercourse is through gentleness, plus a supplementary lubricant. To cope with accidental loss of urine, women can practice a set of exercises to improve their pelvic muscle tone and thereby limit accidental loss of urine (see Table 8.1). Incidentally, many women who do these exercises regularly find that an added effect is improvement of their sexual responsiveness.

coping with menopause

For some women, menopause is *not* a troublesome life experience, but for other women, it presents new and challenging situations. In some instances, these challenges threaten previously held self-images and life-styles. Many women will not need to re-examine their feelings about themselves and their lives; others may find it helpful to talk about these new challenges with other women or, in some instances, with a therapist.

Women have formed support groups to help one another cope with the experiences of menopause and other life changes that occur. Some women's groups are also concerned with decision-making about the use of various treatments. One concern is whether to use estrogen replacement therapy. Although ERT does seem to help some women cope with hot flashes and vaginal changes, its helpfulness has not been demonstrated for all women.

table 8.1
exercises to improve urine control

Do these exercises while sitting on the toilet. Start and stop the flow of your urine.

Once you know how it *feels* to contract your pubococcygeus muscle (this feels as it did when you stopped the flow of your urine), you can proceed with the following exercises each day. Gradually increase the frequency of the exercise at intervals throughout the day.

1. Contract the pubococcygeus muscle and hold for 3 to 5 seconds.
2. Contract the pubococcygeus muscle very rapidly several times in a row.
3. As you breathe in, contract the pubococcygeus muscle.
4. Bear down as if you were going to have a bowel movement. Then relax. Now, as you are relaxing, tighten the pubococcygeus muscle.

It is usually recommended that these exercises be done 10 to 20 times a day to maintain good muscle tone.

And because of the growing concern about the risk of endometrial cancer, women are frequently faced with trying to decide whether to risk ERT use.

The decisions you make about coping with menopausal symptoms are highly individual. Until safe and effective alternatives are available, there may be some women who will choose to take ERT in face of known risks. Clearly, these decisions are difficult. There are, however, some questions women can consider before deciding to use *any* therapy.

1. Does my problem disrupt my life?
2. Do I have information about treatment or management?
3. What are the advantages and disadvantages of the alternative?
4. What do I get for what I risk?

Masters, W., & Johnson, V. *Human sexual response.* Boston: Little, Brown, 1966.

Meldrum, D., Tataryn, A., Frumar, A., Erlik, J., Lu, K., and Judd, H. Gonadtropins, estrogens, and adrenal steroids during the menopausal hot flash. *Journal of Clinical Endocrinology and Metabolism*, 1981, *3*, 73–90.

Reitz, R. *The menopause: A positive approach*. Radnor, Pa.: Chilton, 1979.

Seaman, B., & Seaman, G. *Women and the crisis in sex hormones*. New York: Ramson, 1977.

Sherman, B., Wallace, R., & Treloar, A. Menopausal transition: Endocrinological and epidemiological considerations. *Journal of Biosocial Science*, 1979, *6*, 19–35, suppl.

Treloar, A. Menarche, menopause and intervening fecundability. *Human Biology*, 1974, *46(1)*, 89–107.

Voda, A. Climacteric hot flash. *Maturitas*, 1981, *3*, 73–90.

Weiss, N. S., Szekely, D., & Austin, D. "Endometrial cancer in relation to patterns of menopausal estrogen use." *JAMA*, July 20, 1979, *242(3)*, 261–264.

Woods, N. F., Menopausal distress: A model for epidemiologic investigation. Tucson, Ariz.: Proceedings of the Interdisciplinary Research Conference on Menopause, in press.

NANCY FUGATE WOODS, R.N., Ph.D.

HEALTH-DAMAGING BEHAVIORS

Women can promote and maintain their own health, and in addition many women can promote and maintain the health of their families. They also can choose to engage in behaviors that potentially are health-damaging. Although women's main nutritional problems are likely to be related to overeating or eating too much of the wrong thing, undernourishment also has significant hazards for two age groups—adolescent women who are subject to anorexia nervosa (self-starvation) and elderly women who may lack sufficient money to buy food.

Smoking has become a major threat to women's health. It is predicted that lung cancer will become the leading cause of cancer deaths for women in the 1980s.

Women have traditionally been discouraged from engaging in physical activity, particularly vigorous exercise. This inactivity probably contributes to a number of women's health problems—obesity, heart disease, and osteoporosis. One means of coping with the problems that people face is escaping from them. Women not only use psychoactive drugs to escape, but they also are consuming more alcohol. Women today are more likely to drink than ever before in history and at younger ages.

Health-damaging effects cannot always be attributed to behavior. We increasingly are aware of the effects of the social and biophysical environment on our health. Although stress is a universal condition of existence, the

103

biological responses to it have variable effects. The biophysical environment constantly affects women and can alter health status. Exposure to infections or to toxic substances in air, food, water, or soil can result in serious illness or death. Also, the home environment contains potential health hazards.

BONNIE METZGER, Ph.D.

over- and under-nutrition

Less than 1 percent of all Americans can be considered undernourished, while the prevalence of obesity is increasing. Both conditions can be dangerous to your health.

obesity

According to the National Center for Health Statistics, 35 percent of women ages 45 to 64 with incomes below poverty level and 29 percent of the same age group with incomes above the poverty level are classified as obese. Obesity is most simply defined as an excess quantity of fat in the body. However, what constitutes an excess quantity is a matter of controversy. In general, the average young adult woman's body weight is composed of 20 to 27 percent fat. Of this, 12 percent or less is essential to body structure; the remaining fat serves as a reservoir of stored energy. Total body fat gradually increases during middle age and is followed by a sudden reduction during the seventieth decade.

The average percentage of body fat differs in women and men. The average young adult male's body is composed of only 15 percent body fat, of which 2 percent is essential to body structure.

Women appear to be metabolically more

efficient and conserve energy more readily than men. Under conditions where food is plentiful, women store energy more readily than men and seem more resistant to nutrient deprivation. Although pregnancy is not the average state, it is a normal state for women and clearly demonstrates these evolutionary sexual differences in nutrient conservation and metabolism. The average healthy woman, eating according to dictates of appetite, gains 27.5 pounds of body weight during pregnancy; of that, 7.7 pounds is stored fat. This stored fat is gained before the final three months of pregnancy and provides a reserve energy store that would maintain the developing fetus despite sudden severe food deprivation (Hytten, 1979).

The primary question that arises, then, is how does this incredibly efficient organism, which can systematically respond to the internal mechanism of appetite, become at times a calorie-consuming, energy-conserving organism apparently out of control? Most researchers freely admit they do not know, although physical, psychological, and social theories abound.

Some researchers suggest the size and number of fat cells themselves are the major regulatory features of body weight and that these regulatory factors are influenced at critical times in human development by specific dietary factors (Faust, 1977). Other biological theories suggest that food intake may be influenced by the effect of certain hormones and/or nutrients on specific parts of the brain. Still others imply that obesity is not the result of excessive caloric intake and failure of appetite control, but due to an unusual reduction in or resistance to the expenditure of energy.

In general, there is currently as much evidence for psychological or social thories of obesity as there is support for biological proposals. Fat parents tend to have fat children. However, this relationship does not appear to be totally due to genetics, since it can also be observed in adopted children, as well as the family dog! Widely held beliefs about the causes of obesity are either not scientifically established or not true. For example, investigations comparing obese to nonobese individuals find no consistent psychological differences. Other studies suggest that the eating behavior of obese people does not significantly differ on a large scale from those who are not fat; they do not necessarily eat faster, eat more at one sitting, or select different types of food (Kolata, 1977).

The only real consensus appears to be that obesity is most likely a highly complex, individual disorder, probably reflecting unique etiological patterns. This complexity and lack of scientific fact are probably reflected by the few (5 to 20 percent) obese people who can lose weight and maintain the weight loss in response to treatment. There are no easy or sure treatment programs for obesity. Indeed, those programs with the highest probability of success acknowledge the complexity of the problem and approach its resolution by a combination of many different methods—dieting, exercise, support groups, family therapy, and behavior modification.

The difference between the terms *ideal* and *average* weight is essential to a discussion of women's health problems. Ideal body weight is based on the Metropolitan Life Insurance Company's prediction of the weight, at a certain height and age, that is most likely to be associated with the lowest incidence of chronic illness and the highest rate of longevity. It is, thus, the weight at which you might be considered the healthiest; on the other hand, average weight is the weight you are most likely to obtain and maintain if your exercise and eating patterns are more similar to, than different from, those of your neighbors. Average weights are based on the sum total weight of all persons weighed, divided by the number of persons weighed.

Average weight is the basis for the statement that obesity is on the uprise in the United States. On the other hand, the health effects of obesity are most generally estimated by determining the individual's percentage above ideal body weight. This percentage is the basis for judging the potential health risk of obesity. Percentage above ideal weight is determined by dividing the total of your current body weight, minus your proposed ideal weight, by ideal weight, and multiplying the result by 100 (Current Weight − Proposed Ideal Weight ÷ Ideal Weight) × 100 = Percentage Overweight).

obesity and health

Obesity is associated with many major health problems. The results of a long-term study conducted with a sample of 5,209 adults in Framingham, Massachusetts, suggest that in both men and women obesity is strongly correlated with heart disease and stroke. For example, women who are 35 percent above their ideal body weight have a two-time greater chance of developing stroke or chronic heart disease. Indeed, women 50 percent above their ideal body weight increase the probability of developing a debilitating cardiovascular disease by at least three times that of comparable-age women of ideal weight. A report from the Framingham study proposed that if everyone above ideal weight had been at ideal weight, the incidence of stroke and congestive heart failure would have been reduced by 35 percent (Gordon & Kannel, 1973).

The exact mechanism that affects the relationship between obesity and cardiovascular disease is unclear, but it is known that weight increase above "ideal" is strongly associated with high blood pressure and elevated blood cholesterol levels. The Framingham study also

suggested that individuals whose weight is 50 percent above ideal levels have on the average a systolic blood pressure that is 14 millimeters (mm) of mercury higher than those persons of ideal weight. (Blood pressure is recorded in millimeters of mercury; the systolic, or upper number, records the highest arterial blood pressure of the heart cycle, and diastolic, the lower number, records the lowest pressure.) Women with systolic blood pressure consistently above 160 mm are three times as likely to have a stroke as women with systolic blood pressures of 140 or lower.

Both hypertension and elevated blood cholesterol levels are implicated in the formation of atherosclerotic plaques (fat deposits) in artery walls, and a systematic loss of weight is usually accompanied by a decrease in those atherogenic agents. But, despite the strong relationship between obesity and hypertension and elevated blood cholesterol levels, other convincing evidence suggests that cardiovascular problems due to obesity can occur without these atherogenic factors. These disease-producing mechanisms, like so many other aspects of obesity, have yet to be identified and explained.

Overweight has also been implicated in the formation of gallstones. Again, the mechanism is not implicit. Although the excessive intake of high fat and carboydrate foods may seem like the most likely villains, recent research would suggest that the relationship is not with food type but with obesity itself and the resulting lack of regular moderate exercise, frequent periods of fasting, and reduced dietary fiber intake.

This same type of relationship is suggested between obesity and diabetes. It is not the excessive intake of a specific type of nutrient that shows up as related positively with diabetes, but, instead, the amount of fat tissue itself. In addition, there are significant implied relationships between weight, the degree of obesity, and estrogen levels in women. Fat tissue plays an important role in the production of estrogen. Thus, obesity may create a situation in the obese woman of long-term exposure to high blood levels of estrogen. These levels are thought to be high-risk factors for endometrial cancer (Vermeulen & Verdonck, 1978).

Obesity seems to have potent effects on the hormones of women. Women who weigh more than 280 pounds are known to be less fertile. Hormones essential to ovulation and menstruation are reduced, with resulting irregular menstrual bleeding. There have been further suggestions that superobese women are biologically less sexually active (Crisp, 1978).

THE HEALTHY OVERWEIGHT WOMAN. Research findings propose that obesity is a genuine threat to an individual's health and well-being. It substantially increases that person's risk of developing cardiovascular disease, gallbladder disease, and/or diabetes. In addition, the excessive body weight itself may damage weight-bearing joints and bones, which may be further aggravated by gout or arthritis. This imposed threat of chronic illness and debilitation must not be ignored by either health care providers or obese health care consumers. At the same time, both should acknowledge the fact that healthy overweight people do exist. A healthy overweight woman is one who maintains her excessive weight at a stable level for long periods of time, is neither gaining nor losing weight, and is functioning physically, emotionally, and socially at a level that is satisfactory to her.

Healthy overweight individuals are not immune to the health burdens of obesity. However, when the difficulty of curing obesity is considered and the fact that many scientists suggest that repetitive losing and regaining of weight may be more damaging to the cardiovascular system than the excess body mass itself, an alternative health plan to weight loss should be considered.

Using the model of a healthy overweight individual as the basis of health planning, the suggested self-health care program consists of three parts. In the first phase, the healthy overweight consumer and health care provider identify and evaluate her potential health and well-being risk factors and burdens. The second phase is the development of a program to help her alter her life-style in a way that will significantly reduce the probability of chronic disease, using factors more amenable to self-control than weight loss, such as changes in cigarette smoking, alcohol consumption, cholesterol and saturated fat consumption, salt and sugar intake, and supervised regular exercise. In developing this program, neither the health care provider nor the consumer should neglect the constant fact that the obese person functions in a society that is generally hostile and derogatory toward overweight. Therefore, the third phase is intended to provide general therapeutic support and the specific buttress essential to continual effective handling of an abusive culture during this period of life-style change.

The proposed treatment plan is not meant to deny the emotional, physical, and social hazards of obesity. Instead, it is suggested as an alternative to traditional programs that focus on weight loss. In addition, it is suggested only as an alternative for those overweight women who are dealing effectively with the burdens to well-being imposed by obesity.

DIETS. The traditional treatment for obesity

focuses on the reduction of weight; the cornerstone of this rational approach is a systematic combination of reduced caloric intake and increased energy expenditure through systematic exercise. There are, however, no shortcuts or magic formulae that will accelerate or reduce the difficulty of the weight loss process. Although fasting or extremely low caloric (starvation) diets produce rapid weight loss, both methods are fraught with danger. The dangers, including sudden death, can be attributed to abrupt changes in the gut, acid-base balance, body potassium levels, and/or loss of essential body proteins. A more rational approach to weight reduction is the reduction of caloric intake, while maintaining a generally well-balanced distribution of nutrient source. The dietary regimen that most closely resembles the typical health maintenance diet consumed in the United States is one with approximately 20 percent protein nutrients, 30 percent fat (10 percent of which is saturated fat), and 50 percent carbohydrate.

To reduce daily intake of cholesterol, an additional risk factor, the diet should contain few animal products. In fact, recent research reports that when soybean constitutes the prevalent protein source in the diet, the soybean protein lowers cholesterol levels in the majority of patients. At the same time, soybean is deficient in one essential protein source, methionine. Wheat will provide this essential protein, but is deficient in others. It should be apparent that the development of a diet that will be both calorie restrictive and health promotive requires professional planning.

It should be noted that middle-aged, postmenopausal women may be less responsive to the soybean/cholesterol effect (Sirtori et al., 1979). In addition, the exact amount of calorie reduction essential to weight loss is a highly individual phenomenon. A great deal of variation exists in the reported caloric requirement for weight gain or loss. It has been calculated that the amount of excess calories essential to gain a gram of tissue can range from 1.1 to 10 calories, or from 500 to 4,500 calories for a pound. This difference depends on the type of tissue being formed, the individual's adjustment to a different caloric intake, sex, age, and previous obesity. Thus, diets should be professionally planned and must be individualized to the person's nutrient and calorie reduction needs.

It seems to take considerably fewer calories to put on weight in the person who was obese than in the person who was not. This fact must be built into weight maintenance diets, once the dieting former-obese person has reached her desired weight goal. Thus, successful weight loss depends on individualized caloric requirements, which should be flexible because they need to be periodically altered as different weight loss phases occur, including the body's adjustment to dietary change, water loss, and the approach of the desired weight loss goal. A well-balanced diet is as essential to health maintenance as is the weight loss itself. A diet containing essential nutrients can be maintained while losing weight, even with many "fad" diets, but probably not with all.

A long-term restricted diet should be supervised by knowledgeable professionals. In choosing that professional—by interview or by referral from someone else—the obese woman should accept only the services of a health expert who acknowledges: (1) the metabolic uniqueness of each person, (2) the extreme differences between men and women in weight loss trends and body fat, (3) the health benefits of all nutrients, fats, and carbohydrates as well as proteins, (4) the disruptive effect of dieting on the person's life-style, and (5) the need for other experts to work with the multiple aspects of this complex phenomenon—obesity.

Although dieting is an essential element in any weight loss program, it is not the only important ingredient for success. Obesity is frequently defined as a disorder of the energy balance equation. It occurs when energy intake exceeds the energy requirements of the body for both physical activity and for growth. Thus, the equation can theoretically be balanced from either or both sides. Balancing can be aided by the obese woman through systematic daily increases in exercise.

Fat people can and should exercise (see chapter 11). Exercise does not actually lead to massive loses in poundage; it does however, in the presence of a reduced calorie diet, burn up the body's own fat in its effort to meet its increased energy needs. When dieting occurs without exercise, body proteins (lean body mass) are used as a fuel source, and only half as much fat tissue will be expended to meet energy requirements. Exercise inhibits the breakdown of body protein for energy use and speeds up weight loss during calorie reduction.

DIETING AND LIFE-STYLE. Dieting and exercise together comprise the traditional rational obesity treatment program; however, in all honesty it would appear that there is no current cure for obesity. Even when persons are able to lose weight, maintaining the weight loss is a difficult process. Despite these depressing facts, the treatment program that combines individualized diet and exercise plans and does not depend on that current "fad," either diet or exercise, provides the only real basis for hope in obesity treatment.

The loss of weight and weight loss mainten-ance demand more than calorie reduction and daily exercise; they mean a maximum change in life-style. Life-style reflects what people are and is, thus, very resistant to change. Dieting is hard work, and no "fad" diet has been found that reduces this workload while demonstrating positive long-term effects. One factor that has been used to reduce the chore of dieting is appetite-reducing (anorexigenic) drugs. Recent studies suggest, however, that these drugs are effective only for short periods of time. Most people develop tolerance to the majority of drugs within 12 weeks, although some have been effective for up to six months. Once the person develops resistance to the drug, it has no effect for prolonged periods of time.

Appetite-suppressive drugs provide only short-term support, and this aid must be weighed against the fact that these drugs can have profound effects on other parts of the brain. They can significantly increase the user's heart rate or blood pressure, and most are associated with insomnia, increased nervousness, and anxiety. Thus, anybody with heart or blood pressure problems or anxiety and nervousness should avoid appetite-suppressive drugs. They provide only short-term support and are at the same time actually dangerous and addictive.

Another supportive trend is the combination of behavior modification with dieting. Behavior modification is appropriate when there is a characteristic obese eating style and that style is both learned and alterable. However, as already mentioned, there is little evidence to support a single characteristic obesity eating style, although evidence suggests that individual eating styles contribute to obesity development. So, behavior modification techniques do support modest weight loss in some obese persons. In general, however, it has proven to be a great disappointment to most of its initial advocates and disciples.

Many techniques of behavior therapy— record-keeping, restriction of cues that signal eating, slowing the rate of eating, and rewarding of the foregoing behavior—are logical components of the comprehensive treatment program proposed here. These techniques can support necessary life-style changes, as can self-help groups—Weight Watchers, TOPS (take off pounds sensibly), and others—group therapy, psychotherapy, individual counseling, and family therapy. Of course, no one person would need or probably could afford all that support, but the emotional support that best meets the needs of the individual obese woman is an essential part of the extensive life-style changes important to obesity cure.

A comprehensive review of obesity is not complete without a comparison of this comprehensive, conservative treatment to the more radical methods of weight loss, as represented by intestinal bypass operations and jaw wiring. Intestinal bypass operations, recommended only for the massively obese, do promote greater consistent weight loss than any other current method of weight reduction. They are, at the same time, major surgical procedures with frequent complications, and, thus, are both expensive and dangerous. On the other hand, jaw wiring is cheaper and less dangerous, but it offers no better long-term effects than any current program. In fact, because jaw wiring does little or nothing to support long-term life-style changes, it probably has a lower probability of positive long-term effects than more conservative, comprehensive treatments.

As we struggle with the complexities of obesity and its treatment, it becomes apparent that the ultimate solution to the problem is prevention. Prevention of obesity in women demands that we all examine our current life-styles and alter those eating and exercise patterns that are inconsistent with maintaining ideal weight. Maybe even more importantly, we must each assume our responsibility to future generations by helping our children develop life-styles that are consistent with health maintenance.

other problems of overnutrition

Health problems of overnutrition are not limited to excessive calorie consumption. Immoderate ingestion of cholesterol and saturated fats is linked to atherosclerotic plaque formation on artery walls. It is currently believed that this relationship between overindulgence in foods with high cholesterol and elevated blood cholesterol levels may occur only in persons susceptible to this metabolic abnormality. A daily breakfast of bacon and eggs may not significantly affect the health potential of many American women. On the other hand, eating cholesterol is actually not necessary since it can be manufactured by most of the body's tissues from other substances. Therefore, reduced daily cholesterol intake is a rational act for those women whose history suggests susceptibility and for those who see it as a thoughtful alternative to routine blood cholesterol checks.

Finally, a discussion of food additives or supplements requires thoughtful consideration of the use of saccharine. Some laboratory studies suggest that saccharine is a weak carcinogenic agent. Much of the evidence is still contradictory and inconclusive. However, a health risk apparently exists with the consistent use of this food additive. This risk should be considered thoughtfully by pregnant women and mothers. On the other hand, most researchers still imply that the health risk of obesity far outweighs that imposed by the use of saccharine.

anorexia nervosa

Although undernourishment is, in general, an uncommon occurrence in the developed countries of the Western world, one phenomenon of self-imposed starvation is seen only in the same developed industrial societies where food deprivation is generally the exception. This phenomenon is anorexia nervosa.

Anorexia nervosa occurs primarily in women; only from 4 to 6 percent of diagnosed anorexic patients are men. Although in the general population it is quite rare, it may be as prevalent as one in every 200 females in the high-risk age groups (between 12 and 18).

The symptoms of this nutritional disorder usually occur between early and late adolescence, but they could begin before puberty or even as late as the early thirties. Most commonly, anorexia nervosa occurs as a single episode of self-starvation that is precipitated or associated with a stressful life situation. However, it is not uncommon to find women with anorexic episodes that fluctuate between periods of more normal eating patterns.

The essential features of this disorder are behaviors directed toward losing weight and an intense fear of gaining weight. Weight loss is accomplished by extreme reduction in the total amount of food eaten, with a disproportionate decrease in those foods that contain large amounts of carbohydrate and fat. Other methods may be self-induced vomiting or laxative and/or diuretic abuse. A consistent use of vomiting and/or purging as a means to compensate for a loss of control in caloric restriction is viewed as a poor sign in regard to successful treatment.

Anorexia is defined as a loss of appetite, but most anorexia nervosa patients do not experience a genuine loss of appetite for food until late in the illness. Thus, the term *anorexia* is a misnomer for this disorder. Instead, it is characterized by fear, fear of losing control, fear of becoming fat, and a preoccupation with food and calorie intake.

Some suggest that errors of metabolism or alterations in the brain could create this self-starvation abnormality. Others imply it is a disorder of psychosexual immaturity or a distortion of body image perception. Social theorists classify it as the result of family problems, and they suggest that a predisposing factor may be frustrated, overachiever parents and a childhood exemplified by a perfectionistic model child. As with obesity, there is not enough evidence to support any of the current theories.

In contrast to obesity, anorexia nervosa could be classified as a mental illness, based primarily on the patient's inability or unwillingness to see her gaunt, emaciated appearance as unusual or a sign of illness. Unlike obesity, this disease is not merely a health risk factor; it can and does actually lead to death in 20 percent of those persons diagnosed.

Any incidence of self-imposed starvation demands professional medical and psychological therapy. It is a unique and totally unnatural phenomenon, even in the United States where so much social support is given to the art of reducing natural body fat levels to the bare minimum. Thin may be beautiful, but is it ideal?

Although most adolescent women in the United States see themselves as fatter than they would like to be, true anorexia nervosa can be differentiated from the natural concerns of maintaining the socially required "body beautiful" by the following (Halmi, 1978):

1. Refusal to maintain body weight over a minimal normal weight loss of at least 25 percent of original body weight. (If less than 18 years of age, weight loss for original body weight plus projected weight gain expected on pediatric growth charts may be combined to make 25 percent.)

2. Disturbance of body image with an inability to accurately perceive body size.

3. Intense fear of becoming obese, a fear that does not diminish as weight loss progresses.

4. No known medical or psychiatric illness that would account for weight loss.

5. Amenorrhea (suppression of menstruation, not due to pregnancy or menopause).

Effective professional treatment may be more loosely related to the pretreatment characteristics of the individual anorexia nervosa patient than to the type of therapy itself (Halmi, Goldberg, Casper, Eckert, & Davis, 1979), suggesting that like obesity, this disorder may be a complex, but individual phenomenon. It may have multiple causes and reflect many types; similarity among patients may be restricted to similarity of symptoms.

True anorexia nervosa requires professional treatment. If a daughter or adolescent friend demonstrates any of the peculiarities listed above, she should be encouraged to find professional guidance that will focus on helping her deal with her fear.

Crisp, A. H. Some aspects of the relationship between body weight and sexual behavior with particular reference to massive obesity and anorexia nervosa. *International Journal of Obesity*, 1978, *2*, 17–32.

Faust, I., Johnson, P. R., & Hirsch, J. Adipose tissue regeneration following lipectomy. *Science*, July 1977, *197*, 391–393.

Gordon, T., & Kannel, W. B. The effects of overweight on cardiovascular diseases. *Geriatrics*, 1973, *28 (8)*, 80–88.

Halmi, K. Anorexia nervosa: Recent investigations. *Annual Review of Medicine*, 1978, *29*, 137–148.

Halmi, K., Goldberg, S., Casper, R., Eckert, E., & Davis, J. Pretreatment predictors of outcome in anorexia nervosa. *British Journal of Psychiatry*, 1979, *134*, 71–78.

Hytten, F. E. Nutrition in pregnancy. *Postgraduate Medical Journal*, May 1979, *55*, 295–302.

Kolata, G. B. Obesity: A growing problem. *Science*, December 1977, *198*, 905–906.

Sirtori, C. R. et al. Clinical experience with the soybean protein diet in the treatment of hypercholesterolemia. *The American Journal of Clinical Nutrition*. August 1979, *32*, 1645–1658.

Vermeulen, A., & Verdonck, L. Sex hormone concentrations in post-menopausal women. *Clinical Endocrinology*, 1978, *9(1)*, 59–66.

10

JEAN REESE R.N., M.N., and
LOUISE KRUSE, R.N., M.A.

women and smoking

Smoking is not like loving—
it's better not to at all.

An unmistakable increase in the incidence of diseases commonly associated with smoking is occurring in women. Concern about this increase became acute in the early 1970s when the death rate for lung cancer in women, according to the National Vital Statistics and Bureau of Census, had doubled since 1960. In addition, there was some evidence that the birth weight of babies born to smoking women averaged less than babies born to nonsmoking women.

The increase in the death rate of women with cancer of the lung reflects the number of women who started to smoke around the time of World War II. In 1930, only 2 percent of women over 18 smoked; men were smoking at a rate 30 times greater than women (Burbank, 1972). With the war years and resultant job opportunities came a habit indicative of the camaraderie in the war effort. Not only did Rosie the Riveter perform a man's job, she also "lit up" with her female coworkers. The tension of the war, stress of the job, and a new-found freedom undoubtedly contributed to more women acquiring the smoking habit.

Diseases related to smoking take 20 to 30 years to develop and usually have few symptoms along the way. By the time major symptoms appear, irreversible damage has occurred, causing illness. Statistics show that women between 44 and 54 years of age who have inhaled deeply for about 20 years have a mortality ratio of 1.78 as compared to 1.0 for women who do not smoke (Hammond, Garfinkel, Seidman & Lew, 1976b). Women who smoke like men are beginning to die like men. The ratio of male to female deaths due to lung cancer is decreasing, and it is not due to a reduction in male deaths (Schneiderman & Levin, 1972).

A conclusion reached in *Smoking and Health*, a report of the Surgeon General, in 1979 was that if the present trends continue, cancer of the lung will be the leading cause of cancer deaths in women in the 1980s. This sur-passes the relatively stable but high mortality death rate for breast cancer in women.

The silence in the development of smoke-related diseases in women has ended with a bang. The current trend in the incidence of these diseases is the basis for Meigs (1977) of the Connecticut Cancer Epidemiology Unit to label cigarette smoking as an "epidemic in women." The epidemic is the health problems resulting from cancer of the lung, cardiovascular disease, and respiratory ailments. The earlier notion that women are immune to such diseases has proven to be untrue.

profile of the woman smoker

In the years since World War II, the number of women who smoke has been steadily rising. Fewer social restrictions on woman's behavior, nurtured by the feminist movement and taking hold in a changing society, provided fertile ground for such industries as the tobacco companies to find new marketing areas. Not all of the smoking increase can be blamed on advertising, but, presently, a target population of tobacco advertising is the young, educated, career-minded woman.

Figures on smoking compiled by the National Center for Health Statistics in 1976 show that this group of women smoke more and at a rate greater than women who are older and/or work only in the home. For example, about 42 percent of the women in managerial positions are smokers. In contrast, 28 percent of women not in the paid work force smoke. Nearly one-half of the women employed as waitresses, buyers, or clerks are smokers; less than 20 percent of librarians and elementary school teachers are smokers. A high percentage (40 to 45) of real estate agents, hair dressers, and foremen are smokers. Almost 40 percent of the women who are editors, bookkeepers, or nurses are smokers (Sterling & Weinkam, 1976).

Age also determines extent of smoking. According to a 1970 survey sponsored by the National Center for Health Statistics, women at ages 35 to 44 have the highest percentage (39.3) of smokers. Next is the 25-to 34-year-old-group, at 38.7 percent. Smoking women in the 65 and over group taper off considerably to 11 percent, a figure that will probably increase because of the rising number of smoking women in the younger age brackets.

Of greatest concern is the rise of smoking in teen-age girls and young women. There seems to be a willingness on the part of young women to start smoking with low-nicotine cigarettes to avoid feelings of nausea. It has been suggested that if low-nicotine cigarettes were less available young females might choose not to smoke rather than experience the unpleasant effects of nicotine. (Silverstein, Feld, & Kozlowski, 1980).

In the 17-to 24-year-old age group, 31 percent are smokers. This has great implications for the children of these women, plus the increased likeliness of smoke-related diseases occurring earlier and more frequently in their lives. Clerical workers and waitresses have the greatest percentage of women who start smoking before the age of 20. Women who start smoking after age 20 are more likely to be in professional or managerial positions. It appears that social class, education, and occupational field may have a bearing on when women start to smoke (Sterling & Weinkam, 1976).

The young female smoker trend continues, even though voluntary and government health agencies have been issuing warnings since 1964 about the hazards of cigarettes. Taxation, advertising bans, and public smoking restrictions have all been used to deter smoking. In light of these efforts, the overall percentage of women over 21 who smoke does show a modest decline from 32 percent in 1964 to 29 percent in 1975, as reported in *The Smoking Digest*. However, enough women have now smoked long enough with resulting diseases to make an impact on the health status of women as a group.

smoking and disease

The association between smoking and specific diseases is unquestionable. But even with the continued accumulation of knowledge and conduction of better designed studies, the exact substance or mechanism of how smoking causes disease is unclear. We know the human lung was never intended to regularly and periodically exchange air that was hot and loaded with particulate matter. The lungs told anyone this the first time he or she inhaled cigarette smoke. But many people continue to expose their lungs to a concentration of smoke ranging from 1 billion to 5 billion particles per cubic centimeter. (A cubic centimeter is about the area of a fourth of a teaspoon.) The smoke that bypasses the nose is not filtered, and it deluges the lungs with tar, nicotine, and gases in amounts that the lung cannot return to the atmosphere. As a result, the excess substances remain in the lung tissue or are absorbed in the bloodstream.

smoking and cancer

Scientific studies show that most of the smoke (85 percent) is made up of nitrogen, oxygen, and carbon monoxide. Eight percent is particulate matter that makes the smoke visible. Tar is what remains of the particulate matter after the nicotine and moisture have been removed. It is in the tar where most of the cancer-causing substances, called carcinogens, have been found (Wynder & Hoffman 1967). (Women and cancer are discussed in chapter 22.)

Just how these carcinogens cause aberrations in the cells lining the respiratory tract is not fully understood. Normally, the upper respiratory tract and the lungs provide an efficient method for removing debris from the air we breathe, (Figure 10.1). The respiratory airways are lined with cells that have hairlike projections called cilia. These cilia have a coating of mucus produced by the goblet cells, which also line the respiratory airways. The mucus sheet traps minute debris, and the cilia, with wavelike motions, propel the mucus upward and out of the lungs. The continuous motion of the cilia actually "sweeps" the lungs clean. The mucus is then either swallowed or expectorated.

Another cell, called a macrophage, patrols the distensable sacs (alveoli) at the end of the airways where oxygen and carbon dioxide exchange from the air and blood. This macrophage literally eats debris that happens to reach the alveoli. Once a macrophage ingests a piece of debris, it either rides out of the lung on the mucus sheet or enters the lymph system, which disposes of it.

Smoking overwhelms these protective mechanisms. Smoke decreases the action of the cilia. For the lung to rid itself of the overload of particulate matter, it needs the coughing mechanism—hence, the smoker's hack. In addition, the goblet cells are stimulated to increase in number and produce more mucus, which results in a "loose" cough.

The ciliated cells can be destroyed by smoking. When this happens, the basal and squamous cells are exposed to the inhaled smoke and the various carcinogens in the tar. The irritation to these cells can be severe enough to produce a malignancy. The malignancy invariably associated with cigarette smoking is bronchogenic carcinoma. This is the type of cancer that accounts for about 90 percent of all malignancies affecting the lung.

The cells of other structures that repeatedly come in direct contact with cigarette smoke or tobacco can also develop abnormalities, for instance, the lips, mouth, gums, tongue, and pharynx. People who use tobacco have an increased incidence of malignancies at these sites when compared to nonusers. The mortality for women as a result of cancer in these sites is low when compared to men or to other common cancer sites. Women do not generally smoke pipes and cigars, or chew tobacco in enough numbers to produce any trends. However, cancer of the larynx is related to the amount of cigarette smoking and the type of cigarette smoked. When compared with men, women who smoke have less risk of cancer of the larynx because more women prefer filtered cigarettes than do men (Mushinski & Stellman, 1978).

smoking and chronic obstructive lung diseases

Changes in the cells of the respiratory tract can produce diseases other than cancer of the lung. Emphysema and bronchitis, which cause difficulty in breathing, are prime examples. The inhalation of smoke causes an immediate constriction of the airways. This in turn requires more effort to move air in and out of the lungs. As a person smokes year in and year out, the constriction of the airways traps air in the alveoli, which causes a decrease in the amount of air that can be exhaled. The alveoli lose the ability to recoil, and the smoker cannot exchange the air in her lungs as efficiently as before. This leads to a decrease in ventilation and shortness of breath. The overproduction of mucus and loss of cilia action aid bacterial growth. As a consequence, the smoker who develops emphysema (Figure 10.2) and chronic bronchitis has frequent bouts of respiratory infections.

It is not known exactly which substance or combination of substances in cigarette smoke

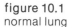

figure 10.1
normal lung

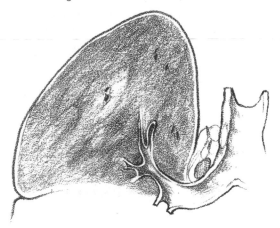

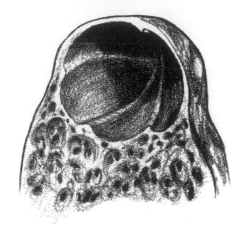

Figure 10.2
inner lining of lung showing emphysema

cause the airway constriction or the destruction of the alveoli. However, a similar mortality ratio is seen with bronchitis and emphysema as with cancer of the lung. All are associated with smoking. A 1975 report of a World Health Organization expert committee states that smokers of 20 or more cigarettes a day have a mortality rate due to bronchitis and emphysema that is about 15 times greater than nonsmokers.

smoking and cardiovascular disease

It is not only the tar in the cigarette smoke that may cause harm. Carbon monoxide and nicotine have been implicated in diseases of the heart and blood vessels.

Carbon monoxide, a gaseous vapor in cigarette smoke, displaces the oxygen that normally would be carried by the hemoglobin in the blood. The carbon monoxide also causes the walls of the arteries to become more porous so that cholesterol can be deposited within the walls, aiding the development of atherosclerosis. This process makes the arterial walls thicker and decreases the size of the vessel channel so that less blood reaches vital tissues such as the heart and brain. Added to this are the indirect effects of the nicotine, which causes constriction of the blood vessels and makes the heart beat faster. As a result, heart attacks can occur because of the narrowed or blocked arteries and blood being transported without its full complement of oxygen. The heart muscle is stimulated to beat faster and, in turn, to require more blood to function. With this imbalance of supply and demand, the heart muscle develops areas of ischemia (not enough blood to nourish the tissue) or infarction (actual death of tissue).

Women who smoke are now recognized as being as vulnerable to myocardial infarctions (heart attacks) as men. One study that supports this discovery was a review of the autopsy records of men and women who had died suddenly between 1967 and 1971 in a New York State county. A report in a major medical journal revealed that 62 percent of the women who died suddenly from coronary heart diseases were heavy cigarette smokers (more than 20 cigarettes per day) as compared to 28 percent of smoking women who died suddenly from other causes. The average age for the smoking women who died suddenly from coronary heart disease was 48 years, while the age of smoking women who died from other causes was 67 years. The ratio of male to female sudden deaths due to coronary heart disease changed in relation to amount of smoking. For the nonsmoking males and females, the death ratio was 11 to 1. In contrast, the death ratio was 3.5 to 1 when both males and females had smoked 20 or more cigarettes per day. These figures become even more impressive as the study excluded women who had diabetes mellitus or hypertension. These diseases are highly correlated with coronary artery disease (Spain, Siegel & Bradess, 1973).

Another medical report estimated that women under the age of 50 who smoke 35 or more cigarettes per day have 20 times the chance of developing a myocardial infarction as those women who have never smoked (Sloan, et al., 1978).

smoking and fetal development and perinatal mortality

Numerous studies report the effects of smoking on fetal development and perinatal (infant) mortality. Of particular interest is the large Ontario Perinatal Mortality study (1960–1961), which included over 51,000 women who gave birth in 10 Ontario hospitals. The data showed that women who smoked and had other risk factors—high number of previous births, low socioeconomic status, low hemoglobin levels (Meyer, Jonascia & Buck, 1974) had perinatal mortality rates of 70 to 100 percent more than those for nonsmokers. The nature of this interrelationship is obvious. The less than ideal nutritional habits and perinatal care of women in lower economic levels are known factors that obviously complicate the natural process of childbirth.

Smoking seems to have a hand in disruption of the natural process. If a mother has decreased hemoglobin and is a heavy smoker, the carbon monoxide will have a greater effect on the amount of oxygen that is in her blood. In other words, she has less oxygen-carrying power of the blood to begin with, and it is further decreased with the carbon monoxide from cigarette smoke. It is suspected that the nicotine indirectly causes constriction of the arteries leading to the placenta, which further reduces the blood flow to the fetus. This reduction in nourishment to the fetus can result in lower birth weights for children born of heavy smoking mothers.

For women who have been smoking for 20 years, it is a critical time. This is the beginning of the period when diseases associated with smoking begin to appear. As long as the smoking has not started an irreversible process, the cells of the respiratory airways can return to normal functioning. Once one stops smoking, the first two to three years show a decline in lung cancer mortality rates, but it takes 10 to 15 years before the rates are similar to those of nonsmokers (Rogot, 1974). Mortality rates for coronary artery disease also decline for people who become ex-smokers.

changing the habit

Smoking is interwoven into the fabric of society by its portrayal of people who smoke while experiencing important feelings—joy, pathos, love, loneliness, victory, defeat, fear, comradeship, boredom, relaxation, and so on. With such associations, many people will not or cannot reject the habit of smoking. It provides powerful and immediate physiological and psychosocial satisfactions, and the reasons why one starts to smoke and then

continues the habit are not always related (Christen & Cooper, 1979).

Smoking is primarily learned in adolescence, and studies reveal that if one is not a smoker by age 20, one is less likely to begin. The reasons for starting to smoke are psychosocial in nature, with the two major influences being smoking by one or more parent(s) and social-peer pressure. In the beginning, smoking is intermittent and tends to occur mainly in social situations. It is believed to be almost an entirely learned behavior mainly in response to a variety of social pressures. However, as the habit becomes ingrained into one's life-style and social maturity is realized, the psychosocial rewards for smoking weaken and fall away, leaving the rewards of nicotine to maintain the habit. After one has become habituated to nicotine, a new set of learned psychological and social needs requires fulfillment. Therefore, smokers who desire to quit have two problems to overcome—physiological and psychosocial (Russell, 1974).

The physiological addictive nature of nicotine is such that the smoker unconsciously modifies the puff rate until a "brain level" is reached. Addictive smokers need nicotine reinforcement to maintain nicotine brain levels every 20 to 30 minutes throughout waking hours. Maintaining a physiological level of nicotine is directly related to psychological status in that nicotine acts on various parts of the brain as a stimulant, depressant, or tranquilizer, depending on the dosage and type of smoker. Yet, smoking is generally viewed as a psychological habit since there is no innate or inborn need for nicotine (Russell, 1974).

According to the American Cancer Society (Saunders, 1971) there are six major psychological categories or types of reasons why smokers continue to smoke. These categories are crutch, craving, stimulation, relaxation, handling, and habit. Smokers fit roughly into one or more of the six types, depending on the development of individual habits. Thirty percent of the smokers smoke as a crutch, that is, for tension and stress reduction. The next largest category (25 percent) of smokers are those who crave cigarettes and, hence, are psychologically addicted. Ten percent smoke primarily for stimulation; 15 percent continue smoking for relaxation. Another 10 percent

enjoy manipulating the cigarette, matches, and ashes, while the 10 percent in the habit category smoke automatically and with little awareness of satisfaction.

A test developed by Dr. Daniel Horn of the National Clearinghouse for Smoking and Health can assist smokers in identifying the psychological factors involved in maintaining individual smoking habits. Understanding the psychological reasons why one continues to smoke can assist in developing a plan to quit by meeting the smoking-related needs through substitute or alternative methods. For example, if one smokes primarily as a crutch, other ways for handling tension and stress might be used (Figure 10.3).

the quitting process

Studies reveal that successful ex-smokers have usually tried to stop several times and are more likely to stop for health than for other reasons (Pederson and Lefcoe, 1976). Half of the people appear to quit in a graduated fashion over a long period of time, and the other half suddenly quit (Adams, 1973). Regardless of how one quits smoking, a "given" in the process will be physiological and psychological withdrawal symptoms. To stop smoking leaves an awkward emptiness since it is integrated into one's life-style (Christen & Cooper, 1979).

Physiological withdrawal involves excretion of the built-up nicotine from the bloodstream and body tissues through the kidneys. The bulk of this nicotine is eliminated in the first 3 to 4 days; hence, most individuals will experience the worst symptoms during this time. Frequently reported symptoms include nervousness, shortness of breath, heart palpitations, visual (cont. on page 126)

figure 10.3

Why Do You Smoke?

Take this short test, and you will understand some of the reasons why you smoke. Your answers to the test questions will help you choose the best way to quit.

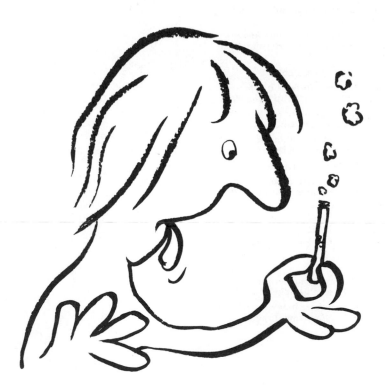

Why do you smoke?

Here are some statements made by people to describe what they get out of smoking cigarettes. How often do you feel this way when smoking?

Circle one number for each statement. Important: ANSWER EVERY QUESTION.

		always	fre-quently	occa-sionally	seldom	never
A.	I smoke cigarettes in order to keep myself from slowing down.	5	4	3	2	1
B.	Handling a cigarette is part of the enjoyment of smoking it.	5	4	3	2	1
C.	Smoking cigarettes is pleasant and relaxing.	5	4	3	2	1
D.	I light up a cigarette when I feel angry about something.	5	4	3	2	1
E.	When I have run out of cigarettes I find it almost unbearable until I can get them.	5	4	3	2	1
F.	I smoke cigarettes automatically without even being aware of it.	5	4	3	2	1
G.	I smoke cigarettes to stimulate me, to perk myself up.	5	4	3	2	1
H.	Part of the enjoyment of smoking a cigarette comes from the steps I take to light up.	5	4	3	2	1
I.	I find cigarettes pleasurable.	5	4	3	2	1
J.	When I feel uncomfortable or upset about something, I light up a cigarette.	5	4	3	2	1
K.	I am very much aware of the fact when I am not smoking a cigarette.	5	4	3	2	1
L.	I light up a cigarette without realizing I still have one burning in the ashtray.	5	4	3	2	1
M.	I smoke cigarettes to give me a "lift."	5	4	3	2	1
N.	When I smoke a cigarette, part of the enjoyment is watching the smoke as I exhale it.	5	4	3	2	1
O.	I want a cigarette most when I am comfortable and relaxed.	5	4	3	2	1
P.	When I feel "blue" or want to take my mind off cares and worries, I smoke cigarettes.	5	4	3	2	1
Q.	I get a real gnawing hunger for a cigarette when I haven't smoked for a while.	5	4	3	2	1
R.	I've found a cigarette in my mouth and didn't remember putting it there.	5	4	3	2	1

How to score

1. Enter the number you have circled for each question in the spaces below, putting the number you have circled to Question A over line A, to Question B over line B, etc.

2. Add the 3 scores on each line to get your totals. For example, the sum of your scores over lines A, G, and M gives you your score on Stimulation—lines B, H, and N give the score on Handling, etc.

Totals

_____ + _____ + _____ =
A   G   M   =   Stimulation

_____ + _____ + _____ =
B   H   N   =   Handling

_____ + _____ + _____ =
C   I   O   =   Pleasurable Relaxation

_____ + _____ + _____ =
D   J   P   =   Crutch: Tension Reduction

_____ + _____ + _____ =
E   K   Q   =   Craving: Psychological Addiction

_____ + _____ + _____
F   L   R   Habit

Scores can vary from 3 to 15. Any score 11 and above is high; any score 7 and below is low.

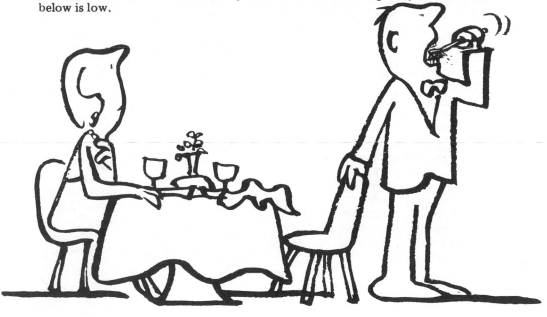

What kind of smoker are you? What do you get out of smoking? What does it do for you? This test is designed to provide you with a score on each of 6 factors which describe many people's smoking behavior. Your smoking may be characterized by only one of these factors, or by a combination of factors. In any event, this test will help you identify what you use smoking for and what kind of satisfaction you think you get from smoking.

The six factors measured by this test describe different ways of experiencing or managing certain kinds of feelings. Three of these feeling-states represent the positive feelings people get from smoking: a sense of increased energy or stimulation; the satisfaction of handling or manipulating things; and the enhancing of pleasurable feelings accompanying a state of well-being. The fourth is the decreasing of negative feelings by reducing a state of tension or feelings of anxiety, anger, shame, etc. The fifth is a complex pattern of increasing and decreasing "craving" for a cigarette, representing a psychological addiction to smoking. The sixth is habit smoking, which takes place in an absence of feeling — purely automatic smoking.

A score of 11 or above on any factor indicates that this factor is an important source of satisfaction for you. The higher your score (15 is the highest), the more important a particular factor is in your smoking and the more useful the discussion of that factor can be in your efforts to quit.

A few words of warning: when you give up smoking, you may have to learn to get along without the satisfaction that smoking gives you.

Either that, or you will have to find some more acceptable way of getting this satisfaction. In either case, you need to know just what it is you get out of smoking before you can decide whether to forego the satisfactions it gives you or to find another way to achieve them.

1. Stimulation

If you score high or fairly high on this factor, it means that you are one of those smokers who is stimulated by the cigarette — you feel that it helps wake you up, organize your energies, and keep you going. If you try to give up smoking, you may want a safe substitute: a brisk walk or moderate exercise, for example, whenever you feel the urge to smoke.

2. Handling

Handling things can be satisfying, but there are many ways to keep your hands busy without lighting up or playing with a cigarette. Why not toy with a pen or pencil? Or try doodling. Or play with a coin, a piece of jewelry, or some other harmless object.

There are plastic cigarettes to play with, or you might even use a real cigarette if you can trust yourself not to light it.

3. Accentuation of pleasure—pleasurable relaxation

It is not always easy to find out whether you use the cigarette to feel good, that is, to get real pleasure out of smoking (Factor 3) or to keep from feeling so bad (Factor 4). About two-thirds of smokers score high or fairly high on accentuation of pleasure, and about half of those also score as high or higher on reduction of negative feelings.

Those who do get real pleasure out of smoking often find that an honest consideration of the harmful effects of their habit is enough to help them quit. They substitute eating, drinking, social activities, and physical activities — within reasonable bounds — and find they do not seriously miss their cigarettes.

4. Reduction of negative feelings or "crutch"

Many smokers use the cigarette as a kind of crutch in moments of stress or discomfort, and on occasion it may work; the cigarette is sometimes used as a tranquilizer. But the heavy smoker, the person who tries to handle severe personal problems by smoking many times a day, is apt to discover that cigarettes do not help him deal with his problems effectively.

When it comes to quitting, this kind of smoker may find it easy to stop when everything is going well, but may be tempted to start again in a time of crisis. Again, physical exertion, eating, drinking, or social activity — in moderation — may serve as useful substitutes for cigarettes, even in times of tension. The choice of a substitute depends on what will achieve the same effects without having any appreciable risk.

5. "Craving" or psychological addiction

Quitting smoking is difficult for the person who scores high on the factor of psychological addiction. For him, the craving for the next cigarette begins to build up the moment he puts one out, so tapering off is not likely to work. He must go "cold turkey."

It may be helpful for him to smoke more than usual for a day or two, so that the taste for cigarettes is spoiled, and then isolate himself completely from cigarettes until the craving is gone. Giving up cigarettes may be so difficult and cause so much discomfort that once he does quit, he will find it easy to resist the temptation to go back to smoking. Otherwise, he knows that some day he will have to go through the same agony again.

6. Habit

This kind of smoker is no longer getting much satisfaction from his cigarettes. He just lights them frequently without even realizing he is doing so. He may find it easy to quit and stay off if he can break the habit patterns he has built up. Cutting down gradually may be quite effective if there is a change in the way the cigarettes are smoked and the conditions under which they are smoked. The key to success is becoming aware of each cigarette you smoke. This can be done by asking yourself, "Do I really want this cigarette?" You may be surprised at how many you do not want.

Source: Daniel Horn PhD., Director of National Clearing-house for Smoking & Health; U.S. Dept. of Health, Education & Welfare.

disturbances, sleepiness, headaches, fatigue, and short temper, along with an intense craving for tobacco (Saunders, 1971). Physiological withdrawal symptoms generally subside within a week, and symptoms occurring after this period are considered psychological in nature (Christen & Cooper, 1979).

The psychological element of withdrawal is much more complex and lasts a longer period of time. The first three months after stopping is a very critical period; within this block of time most relapses occur. After one year, 1 out of 5 ex-smokers resume the habit, and after two years, relapse rate decreases to 1 out of 20 (Fredrickson, McAlister, & Danaher, 1976). Therefore, if one can be a successful ex-smoker for at least three months, chances increase for continued success.

OBSTACLES TO CESSATION OF SMOKING. Women particularly identify with the obstacle of "anticipated or actual weight gain" and use this as an excuse for resumption of smoking. In a study of weight gain in 57,000 women who quit smoking, there was more weight gained by former two-pack-a-day smokers (up to 30 pounds) than for former one-half-pack-a-day smokers (5 pounds) (Blitzer, Rimm, & Giefer, 1977). It appears that another "given" in the quitting process is weight gain, with an average gain of 5 to 15 pounds. However, the equivalent health risk of one pack of cigarettes a day would be a gain of 50 to 75 pounds (Saunders, 1971). The person trying to stop smoking should not reduce calorie intake until a month of nonsmoking has passed.

Although long-term quitting is a complicated, lengthy process, which produces a great deal of constructive and painful inner conflict, close to 30 million smokers have successfully quit smoking (American Cancer Society, 1980).

METHODS AND APPROACHES TO QUITTING SMOKING. A number of approaches and methods are available to assist one to quit smoking. Approaches include group sessions, individual medical or psychological counseling, and self-help guides. Methods used include drugs, hypnosis, and behavior modification.

Studies reveal that drugs such as lobeline, a nicotine substitute found in over-the-counter drug aids to deter smoking, are not any more effective than are other methods. The usefulness of all drug agents in smoking treatment is considered unproven at this time (Danaher & Lichtenstein, 1978).

Evidence relating hypnosis to smoking control suggests that it does not eliminate the need for personal effort, and by itself may not be helpful to most people (Danaher & Lichtenstein, 1978). Although there are a large number of case reports on the effectiveness of hypnosis in smoking control, they are considered inadequate from a scientific viewpoint, and the conclusion is that "alone or in combination with other approaches, hypnosis has not been demonstrated to be effective" (Johnston & Donoghue, 1971).

Behavior modification methods for smoking control generally involve the use of one or a combination of two broad strategies referred to as "aversion" and "self-control." Aversion strategies aim at suppressing smoking behavior through laboratory sessions using such techniques as overexposure to smoke, rapid smoking, breath holding, and electric shock. For example, one technique has people smoke at a normal rate while a fan blows heated smoky air directly into their faces. The safety of this method is under question, and studies are being conducted to determine the worth of these potentially hazardous techniques (Fredrickson, McAlister & Danaher, 1976).

Self-control strategies emphasize more personal involvement in the quitting process.

This involvement includes homework assignments, self-analysis of one's own smoking styles, and active participation in a personal plan to quit smoking. The major focus is on self-control and on the application of specifically planned alternatives to smoking behavior in one's natural environment.

A number of smoking cessation programs using the group approach are being initiated by the American Cancer Society, the American Lung Association, and concerned religious organizations, such as the Seventh Day Adventists. In addition, profit-making organizations, such as the Schick Corporation clinics, SmokeEnders, and Smokewatchers, assist the smoker who is looking for a structured approach.

Most group sessions involve from 15 to several hundred persons and may meet daily or weekly for a specified period. Group programs usually include lectures, inspirational messages, films, and group interaction. Participants are generally urged to keep personal activity records, force fluids, stay in contact with buddies, and avoid tension-causing situations. Fees for noncommercial sponsored programs range from $3 to $10 as compared to commercial programs, which may charge as much as $450. Nevertheless, commercial programs are attracting smokers and are a resource for those who desire a structured group approach and can afford the fees.

Of the 29 million Americans who stopped smoking between 1964 and 1975, it is estimated that 95 percent of them quit on their own, with only 2 percent attending a structured group program (Smoking Digest, 1972). Because of this factor, a number of "do-it-yourself" materials have been developed and are available to assist smokers. Health agencies such as the American Cancer Society and the American Lung Association have available on request a number of self-help aids

at minimal or no cost for smokers desiring to quit on their own. Step-by-step books can be purchased or borrowed from public libraries.

Evaluation studies by experts on the topic of antismoking methods and approaches conclude that no specific technique or program achieves outstanding success. The crucial success factor of any program appears to be the motivation level of the participant. No matter what treatment methods are used, about 20 percent will be successful in quitting (Smoking Digest, 1977).

changing the cigarette

Since the smoking habit is extremely hard to change, scientists have investigated methods of changing the cigarette itself. The tar and nicotine contents of cigarettes have been significantly modified by agricultural methods, processing, and cigarette design. Although still denying any link between cigarette smoking and health hazards, the tobacco industry has moved swiftly to meet federal regulatory and consumer demands for cigarettes with low tar and nicotine contents. About 25 percent of all cigarette sales fall into the low tar-nicotine category, which places the amounts at less than 17.6 milligrams of tar and less than 1.2 milligrams of nicotine per cigarette (Holleb, 1978). Previously, the average of these amounts was as much as 39 milligrams and 2.5 milligrans respectively (Wakeham, 1976). The switch to low tar cigarettes since the 1960s has been worthwhile in that lower death rates from cancer of the lung have occurred in smokers using these cigarettes versus those who smoked unfiltered cigarettes (Hammond, Garfinkle, Seidman, & Lew, 1976a). However, even the death rates for lung cancer and coronary heart disease for smokers of low tar and nicotine cigarettes far exceed the death rates of people who had never smoked (Holleb, 1978).

It has been stated (Russell, 1976) that "people smoke for the nicotine but die of the tar." What will be an acceptable level of tar and nicotine per cigarette to smokers remains to be seen since these ingredients do affect the taste of the cigarette. The success of some new cigarette brands containing 2 to 8 milligrams of tar and .2 to .8 milligrams of nicotine indicates that lower limits are possible technologically, along with an acceptance by smokers of the new taste and flavor (Gori, 1976). There is concern that low tar-nicotine cigarettes may undo the slight potential benefit if they encourage people, especially the young who have never smoked, to begin smoking or if in the cigarette's production, tobacco companies add new untested ingredients that will ultimately prove harmful (Holleb, 1978). Other outcomes may be the increased number of cigarettes smoked and holding the smoke in the lungs longer in order to compensate for the reduced tar and nicotine content.

Switching from cigarettes to other forms of tobacco and controlling the amount of smoking are other methods to reduce the effects of smoking. All smoking-reduction methods are based on the principle of bringing less smoke in contact with lung tissue. However, there is currently no method of smoking without risk.

It is evident that if women continue to smoke at the present rate, we will constitute a major portion of the mortality rates of diseases associated with smoking. To achieve less tension or, perhaps, a liberated image, we seem ready to risk our health and that of our children. If we actually want to control our destiny, this may be the place to start—and with urgency. Our future health lies within ourselves.

Adams, E. An approach to patients who can't stop smoking. *Preventive Medicine*, 1973, *2*, 313–317.

American Cancer Society. *Cancer Facts & Figures 1980*.

Blitzer, P. H., Rimm, A. A., & Giefer, E. E. The effect of cessation of smoking on body weight in 57,032 women: Cross sectional and longitudinal analysis. *Journal of Chronic Diseases*, July 1977, *30(1)*, 415–429.

Burbank, F. U.S. lung cancer death rates beginning to rise proportionately more rapidly for females than for males: A dose-response effect? *Journal of Chronic Disorders*, 1972, *25*, 473–479.

Christen, A. G., & Cooper, K. H. Strategic withdrawal from cigarette smoking. *CA: A Cancer Journal for Clinicians*, March/April 1979, *29(2)*, 96–107.

Danaher, Brian & Lichtenstein, Edward. *Become An Ex-Smoker*. Prentice-Hall: Englewood Cliffs, N.J., 1978.

Frederiksen, L. W., Peterson, G. L., & Murphy, W. D. Controlled smoking: development and maintenance. *Addictive behaviors*, 1976, *1*, 193–196.

Fredrickson, D. T., McAlister, A., & Danaher, B. Giving up smoking: How the various programs work. *Medical World News*, Nov. 1, 1976, 52–57.

Gori, G. B. Low-risk cigarettes: A prescription. *Science*, 1976, *194*, 1243–1246.

Hammond, E. C., Garfinkel, L., Seidman, H., & Lew, E. A. Tar and nicotine content of cigarette smoke in relation to death rates. *Environmental Research*, December 1976, *12(3)*, 263–274. A.

Hammond, E. C., Garfinkel, L., Seidman, H., & Lew, E. A. Some recent findings concerning cigarette smoking. *World Smoking and Health*, 1976, *1*, 41–44. B.

Holleb, Arthur I. A safe cigarette? *CA: A Cancer Journal for Clinicians*, November/December 1978, *28(6)*, 375–376.

Johnston, E., & Donoghue, J. R. Hypnosis and smoking: A review of the literature. *American Journal of Clinical Hypnosis*, 1971, *13*, 265–272.

Meigs, J. W. Editorial—Epidemic lung cancer in women, *Journal of American Medical Association*, September 5, 1977, *238(10)*, 1055.

Meyer, M. B., Jonascia, J. A., & Buck, C. The interrelationship of maternal smoking and increased perinatal mortality with other factors. Furter analysis of the Ontario Perinatal Mortality Study, 1960–1961. *American Journal of Epidemilogy*, December, 1974, *100(6)*: 443–452.

Mushinski, M. H., & Stellman, S. D. Impact of new smoking trends on women's occupational health. *Preventive Medicine*, 1978, *7*, 349–365.

Pederson, L. L., Lefcoe, N. M., A psychological and behavioral comparison of ex-smokers and smokers. *Journal of Chronic Disorders*, 29(7), 431–434, July, 1976.

Rogot, E. Smoking and general mortality among U.S. veterans, 1954–1969. U.S. Department of Health, Education, and Welfare, Washington, D.C.: DHEW Publication No. (NIH) 74-544, 1974, 65 pp.

Russell, M. A. H. Low-tar medium-nicotine cigarettes: A new approach to safer smoking. *British Medical Journal*, 1976, *1*, 1430–1433.

Russell, M. A. H., The smoking habit and its classification, symposium on 'addiction'. *The Practitioner*, June 1974, *212*, 791–800.

Saunders, G. M. *Stop Smoking Program Guide.* California Division of American Cancer Society, 1971.

Schneiderman, M. A., & Levin, D. L. Trends in lung cancer: Mortality, incidence, diagnosis, treatment, smoking and urbanization. *Cancer*, 1972, *30*, 1320–1325.

The smoking digest: Progress report on a nation kicking the habit. Office of Cancer Communications, National Cancer Institute, U.S. Department of Health, Education and Welfare, Public Health Service, National Institutes of Health, October 1977.

Smoking and its effect on health. Report of a WHO Expert Committee, Technical Report Series 568, World Health Organization, Geneva, 1975.

Smoking and Health: A report of the surgeon general. DHEW Publication No. (PHS) 79-50066, 1979.

Silverstein, B., Feld, S., & Kozlowski, L. T. The availability of low-nicotine cigarettes as a cause of cigarette smoking among teenage females. *Journal of Health and Social Behavior*, 1980, *21*, 383–388.

Slone, D. et al. Relation of cigarette smoking to myocardial infarction in young women. *New England Journal of Medicine*, June 8, 1978, *298(23)*, 1273–1276.

Spain, D. M., Siegel, H., & Bradess, V. A. Women smokers and sudden death: The relationship of cigarette smoking to coronary disease. *Journal of American Medical Association*, 1973, *224(7)*, 1005–1007.

Sterling, T. D., & Weinkam, J. J. Smoking characteristics by type of employment. *Journal of Occupational Medicine*, 1976, *18*, 743–754.

Wakeham, H. Sales weighted average "tar" and nicotine deliveries of U.S. cigarettes from 1967 to present. In E. L. Wynder, S. S. Hecht (eds.), *Lung Cancer. A Series of Workshops on the Biology of Human Cancer.* Report No. 3. UICC Technical Report Series, Geneva, International Union Against Cancer, 1976, *25*, 151–152.

Wynder, E. L., & Hoffman, D. *Tobacco and tobacco smoke, studies in experimental carcinogenesis.* New York: Academic Press, 1967.

LINDA PETERS, R.N., M.N.

women and exercise

Since the mid-1960s, we have seen some of the most dramatic changes in society with regard to women and their roles and images. Emphasis, in particular, has been on rights, alternative life choices, and independence from restrictive beliefs and expectations. In the area of exercise and sports, thousands of women are learning that with changes in the mind come changes in the body, and vice versa; through appreciation and use of physical abilities, strength is gained and new identities closely follow.

Strengths and uses of the body that were once seen as "masculine" are becoming more and more acceptable challenges for women. As a consequence, what follows is a changing ideal of what the American woman is: her image of herself, her image of others, and her capabilities as a participant, companion, and competitor in sports. What was once inappropriate for a woman is now fashionable. "Being in shape" now means more than gentle stretching exercises that don't even cause perspiration. The word is spreading that it can feel good to breathe hard, and actually sweat, and that it is ridiculous to feel weak and dependent when one has just run two miles!

Slowly, the terms *woman* and *athlete* are becoming less of a contradiction. Increasing numbers of women are living proof that the athletic female can continue to be "feminine" and expand her own self-concept and appreciation through activities that once would have been labeled "masculine" or "macho."

130

In this chapter, we will study the effects of exercise on women by focusing on the case study of one woman. Through Sara, we can see how a previously inactive female was able to integrate exercise into her life—successfully.

family and exercise history

Sara was 28 years old when she became a client for exercise consultation. She is the mother of two children, ages eight and five years. In addition to homemaker responsibilities, Sara is a substitute grade-school teacher, which involves an average of two days per week of work. She wanted exercise consultation because she was concerned about being 20 pounds overweight and had noticed that her regular clothes size did not fit well even though she had maintained the same weight since the birth of her second child.

Sara's opening comment to the exercise consultant was: "I've been thinking for about five years that I should exercise more, but I never seem to get very far with it—I mostly just feel bad about the 'should.' " She sought assistance after having made a firm commitment to herself to make the necessary changes in her daily life that would allow her to include exercise regularly. Her decision to involve an exercise consultant was based on her recognition that any activity programs she had started in the past had all failed. She felt that outside support and guidance could give her what she had lacked from her own experience. She readily agreed to a six-month commitment that involved weekly visits with the exercise consultant.

The first visit consisted of completing a comprehensive exercise and health history and brief physical exam. The limited physical examination revealed these data:

Height: 5' 7"
Weight: 144 pounds

Pulse: 84
Blood pressure: 140/80

Sara's personal and family health history showed no cardiopulmonary problems, hypertension, diabetes, hyperlipemia, or significant obesity. The absence of these diseases, plus the fact that her age was under 35 years, negated the need for a more comprehensive exam (Elrick et al., 1978, p. 41; *Runner's World*, 1979, p. 48). Had she been over 35 or had any history of these diseases, she would have been referred for a complete physical examination, lab work, and cardiovascular stress testing to determine whether an increase in activity would be likely to precipitate an immediate health threat.

Sara was also asked to discuss her past exercise experience. She recalled being an active child who enjoyed outdoor play. In her first year of junior high, she participated in gymnastics. But because she "grew too fast" that year, the teacher encouraged her to attend regular physical education classes the following year. The classes, she recalled, were uninteresting because they were 40-minute calisthenic workouts, which she tended to skip whenever possible. In her third high school year, Sara convinced her father that she would "not break her leg" if he allowed her to try downhill skiing. She took ski lessons through the high school program for two seasons.

"I was pretty lousy at skiing. I mostly remember falling a lot, being cold, and looking forward to the bus ride home with my friends.

"During college there was so much to do, I don't remember thinking much about exercise for exercise's sake. Activities were usually associated with some social attraction." Sara also recalled feeling confident that she could eat "all she wanted" and never seemed to gain weight.

Soon after she was married, Sara became pregnant. She gained 35 pounds during the pregnancy, but easily lost the weight following the delivery. She remembered doing sporadic situps, but lost interest quickly as she didn't notice any difference.

Sara's husband, Jeff, is active on weekends and enjoys tennis and skiing. In the previous four months, he had been jogging during his noon hour at work. Some of his enthusiasm about how "much better" he was feeling had influenced Sara, but she reported feeling skeptical about how much time and effort it might take for her to enjoy similar feelings. Jeff had volunteered to jog in the morning or after work with Sara, but she was doubtful about how helpful his company would be. She remembered too many times of feeling "like a burden" when they had participated in other sports together.

deterrents to success with exercise

Sara was asked to identify what she saw as deterrents to her success with exercise. Her list was fairly long, but it showed what many women identify as blocks to regular exercise.

1. I was never encouraged in my family to be athletic or to learn physical skills.

Without a doubt, most young girls do not receive the encouragement, opportunity, and positive feedback that is necessary to reinforce them for living physically active lives. Furthermore, there are outright discouragements for women who may be naturally interested in sports. Consider for instance, these recurrent themes against physical exercise: threat to fertility, sagging breasts or breast injury, and bulging muscles. Through these kinds of messages comes the belief that women's biological destiny is best fulfilled through reproduction and that physical strength and expression are incompatible with that process. These beliefs about physical activity and women's functioning contribute to a female self-concept of inherent physical weakness and a consequent attitude of "substandard" with regard to physical achievements.

2. There simply don't seem to be enough hours in the day to include even 30 minutes of exercise.

For many women, the management of home, family, career, and/or education seems to leave no extra time for exercise. In the midst of going to work, running errands, carrying groceries, cleaning the house, and hurrying to classes, the perceived goal sometimes becomes to "conserve energy." Exercise is often seen as just another "thing to do" and it does not receive a high priority. Because of this experience, it is important for women who wish to increase their exercise to learn that time to rejuvenate themselves, release tension, and have fun is not a luxury; it is a necessity to good health and a source of increased energy with many benefits for other aspects of their lives (Elrick et al., 1978, p. 29).

3. Exercise has never been something I could rely on to be fun. As a matter of fact, I often just end up feeling worse about myself because I can't do any sport very well.

This lack of positive experience with exercise is common among many women. A feeling of inadequacy is not only nonreinforcing of repetition, but can make a strong case for avoidance!

4. I don't like the feeling of breathing hard and the sore muscles afterward.

The physical discomfort of stress to joints, muscles, and lungs is very unpleasant to many women. First, many women have been taught that these are the body's signs to stop whatever is causing the feelings. Second, for many women, activities are not repeated frequently enough to get beyond unconditioned bodies that truly do not tolerate exertion very well.

5. There isn't anyone else to exercise with who is at my level.

The idea of doing an exercise activity alone or with someone who is much more skilled is discouraging for many women. Their fear may be that "everyone" else is "better" at whatever activity is being considered. On an intellectual level, it may not be difficult to accept the fact that with practice and repetition an activity will get easier and even possibly rewarding, but in the beginning, when it is awkward and painful, the image of the long-term effects can be easily lost.

6. I am embarrassed to be seen exercising because I'm fat and slow—I know I jiggle when I move.

Another belief that many women hold is that exercise is for the already skillful, beautiful, and thin women. Overcoming the self-

concept of "jiggly, slow, and fat" can be a barrier to exercise.

changing old beliefs

The goal of completing the "deterrents" list was to allow Sara to examine for herself her own beliefs and ideas about exercise that could interfere with her attempt to make a life-style change. She was then asked to rewrite each of the six beliefs about herself, changing them to a more affirming, positive statement. Her new list looked like this:

1. I have the potential for being a strong, physically skilled woman; I can learn through my body.
2. I am worth at least 30 minutes a day for taking care of myself.
3. I accept myself as I am now and believe that I will grow physically and psychologically through my efforts.
4. Exploring the capabilities of my body is an exciting adventure.
5. A goal for my exercise program is to learn more about my body. I will compare my progress to where I am starting from.
6. Exercise is a route to becoming my ideal image of myself.

Sara was instructed by the exercise consultant to review these positive affirmations at least once a day during the first weeks of her increased activity plan. She was asked to read and write them to herself over and over to reinforce them in her mind.

choosing an exercise activity

During the second visit to the exercise consultant, Sara was instructed about some basic principles of exercise physiology. This background information is helpful in selecting an

activity that will provide maximum health benefits, as well as defining what are optimal and realistic exercise goals.

exercise for optimal health

When activity is viewed on a scale from a sedentary person to a competitive athlete, where is the point at which maximum health benefits are realized? It is important to evaluate how much is enough and not to assume, as do many people, that "more would always be better." For instance, it is known that the risk of musculoskeletal injury from running increases sharply when weekly mileage exceeds 30 miles (Osler, 1978, pp. 20–21), or perhaps much less mileage for those with the beginnings of degenerative joint disease or mild back problems. It has also been demonstrated that athletes who spend their lives involved with activity that pushes them to their physical limits, do not have longer lives than do less active people, and, in fact, such stresses do have liabilities that must be weighed against the benefits (Osler, 1978, p. 20). In evaluating health in general, it is typical but limiting to think in terms of what is "normal" rather than in terms of what is "optimal." "Normal" reflects averages rather than what is possible. One definition of "optimal" is "standards which encourage the highest reachable level in the physical, biochemical and physiological tests in general use" (Elrick et al., 1978, p. 6). Specifically, optimal health involves the highest levels of cardiovascular-pulmonary fitness, the lowest rates of cardiovascular and other degenerative diseases, and the longest life-span (Elrick et al., 1978, p. 6). The level of fitness or health is also associated with "quality" or zest for the good life (Elrick et al., 1978, p. 7).

As a woman considers what she can expect from herself physically, it is important not to limit oneself by the old myths that say women are weak and fragile. Instead, she may look to research done on children, which shows that the *development* of skill and strength is the most important variable, not any sexually inherent ability (Kaplan, 1979). Generally speaking, exercise begun early in life contributes to greater expected physical achievement. However, systematic use of proper conditioning methods will yield great improvements in health fitness, regardless of age, and that includes exercise classes in nursing homes or other homes for the elderly.

aerobic exercise

Aerobic means "in the presence of air." With regard to exercise, this translates to "promoting the supply and use of oxygen" (Cooper & Cooper, 1972, p. 19). Activity requires energy, which comes from a combination of food taken into the body and ignited into energy by oxygen. Through aerobic conditioning comes a "training effect," which means that the body can increase its efficiency in supplying the tissues with oxygen. An "endurance" or aerobic exercise is an activity that is vigorous enough to produce and maintain a heart rate of between 120 and 160 beats per minute, depending on age, conditioning, and other health factors. The training effect from such exercise begins about five minutes after the exercise starts and lasts as long as the heart rate remains between 120 and 160 beats per minute. Activities that achieve and sustain this heart rate are running or jogging, swimming, bicycling, and cross-country skiing, to name some familiar sports. Activities such as tennis, downhill skiing, basketball, and racquet ball, although vigorous, do not sustain the heart rate even though they will intermittently raise the rate to training levels. Consequently, these activities will require longer periods of participation to achieve improved fitness (Elrick et al., 1978, p. 25). In their book, *Aerobics for Women*, Cooper and

Cooper (1972) compare various activities of aerobic benefit and outline the amounts and regimens for improved fitness.

SELECTING AN AEROBIC ACTIVITY. By this point in the exercise consultation, a lot of information is available about Sara's past experience with exercise and her skills. These data are helpful in identifying an activity most likely to be successfully integrated into an active life-style. The following criteria for an aerobic activity are associated with a consistent pattern of exercises:

1. Little preparation time.
2. Little or no equipment (or equipment that is easily maintained).
3. Something about which a person feels some sense of skill (although that skill may be regarded as minimal).
4. Associated with some degree of fun or specific rewards recognized that contribute to a sense of pleasure.

Based on these criteria, her past experience, and present skills, Sara decided to begin her fitness program with running. She felt that running would fit into her life most easily due to time and equipment considerations. She also felt supported in this choice by several friends who were running. An additional advantage of running for Sara was that it could be done in most all kinds of weather and she lived in a location with a variable climate.

EQUIPMENT CONSIDERATIONS. Sara was encouraged by the exercise consultant to be generous with herself regarding equipment. Basically, the guidelines for equipment purchases were:

1. Purchase whatever equipment is needed to make an activity as easy, safe, and hassle-free as possible. The beginner should reinforce an intellectual commitment with finan-

cial support. This attitude also helps eliminate deterrents to success with exercise that are based on equipment failure.
2. Become an informed shopper and learn as much as possible about the specifications of the equipment to be used and how it will be affected by female weight and size. Most sports equipment is available for women, but sometimes special ordering or shopping is required.
3. Choice of the clothing that will best serve the demands of the activity will pay off in the long run. For instance, for running choose nonrestricting, sweat-absorbing, comfortable clothing. Choose clothing that will look the part of the sport; it is easier to develop a self-concept of an active person by appearing as such.

During the equipment discussion, Sara raised the question of whether a special "athletic" bra was a necessity. The answer was that what is necessary with regard to breast protection is good support and comfort. "Athletic" bras are generally expensive, and most women find that the bra they wear during nonactive time is also adequate for activity periods. Women who do not usually wear a bra may find that they are more comfortable with some added support during exercise, especially if they have large breasts (*Runner's World*, 1979, p. 11).

assessing fitness and making a conditioning plan

The third visit to the exercise consultant marked the real beginning of a structured activity program for Sara. She came prepared with running clothes and good, supportive shoes, ready to see just where she was "aerobically" at that time. The session began with instruction by the exercise consultant in a warm-up and stretching routine that took about 7 to 10 minutes. (Stretching and warm-up routines are found in Anderson, 1979, and Couch, 1979.) The importance of this preparation was stressed for its value in injury prevention (Cooper & Cooper, 1972, p. 61).

Accompanied by the exercise consultant, Sara then began to jog along a level, regular surface *at her own pace (Runner's World,* 1979, p. 13). She was encouraged to continue talking with the exercise consultant as she jogged; the ability to continue talking is a helpful indication that the heart rate is within the range of aerobic training. Sara found that talking was difficult so she was instructed after about four minutes of jogging to walk for two minutes. This jog-walk pattern was continued for 10 minutes during the first session. At the end of the 10 minutes, Sara was feeling like her body was "ready" to stop, even though she was also feeling enthusiastic about trying to do more. She was encouraged to "listen to her body" and look forward to the next day (Elrick et al., 1978, pp. 68–72; *Runner's World,* 1979, pp. 13, 177). The stretching part of the warm-up routine was repeated at the end of the session (Anderson, 1979; Couch, 1979; Elrick et al., 1978, p. 78).

This method of assessing present ability is simple and easy to use. There are, however, more specific methods that may be preferable for some women, especially if health problems are involved. Two references for such assessment techniques are *Aerobics for Women* by Cooper and Cooper (1977) and *Living Longer and Better* by Harold Elrick et al. (1978, pp. 41–47).

Having established a baseline, Sara was given written guidelines on frequency, duration, and intensity of exercise sessions to reinforce the verbal instructions. She would also continue to see the exercise consultant on a weekly basis to evaluate her progress, discuss her feelings about her exercise program, and set goals. At each visit, the exercise consultant

would be jogging with Sara to give her support and encouragement; she would also receive instruction on jogging form and style. The written guidelines were:

1. Plan to do your chosen activity at least three times per week (preferably four times), with no more than two days between exercise sessions. This will assure that the exercise will have a building effect and that fitness will be improving. More than two days between exercising will cause the conditioning effects to be lost (Cooper & Cooper, 1972, p. 39; *Runner's World,* 1979, p. 17; Sevene, 1979).

2. A reasonable goal for exercise duration is 10 to 20 continuous minutes per workout in the first eight weeks of the program. This range is based on a starting level of zero activity and should be greater if the beginning level of fitness is somewhat developed (*Runner's World,* 1979, p. 17; Sevene, 1979).

3. Identify the time of day when it is most convenient and comfortable for exercise activity. This may seem self-evident, but women who have not previously been involved in an activity plan may not realize that there are body rhythms that play a big part in one's motivation toward exercise. For example, some women will find that to get out of bed at 6:00 a.m. to run is a perfect way to begin the day. Other women find that exercising at the end of the day is a good way to release tension, and it gives them added energy for the rest of the evening. For others this seems to be the last time in the day when there is energy for physical activity. Some experimentation will identify the time of day in which there is maximum motivation toward exercise and minimal disruption of other daily routines.

4. Following the first eight weeks, activity should be increased by 10 percent each week. This may be accomplished either by adding time to each workout or adding an additional exercise session or day (Sevene, 1979).

5. Within six months of beginning an exercise program, most women can expect to be active from 30 to 40 continuous minutes from 4 to 5 times per week and consequently realizing "optimal" cardiac/pulmonary health benefits (*Runner's World,* 1979, p. 19).

6. It is valuable to appreciate from the beginning of a fitness plan that progress will be characterized

by periods of acceleration followed by leveling off or periods of plateau performance. And, in general, as an individual nears optimal fitness, the rate of improvement will tend to slow. Being aware of these normal variations will help to avoid discouragement.

7. Exercise sessions will not necessarily always be fun or easy, especially in the beginning. Don't expect immediate "euphoria," but believe that the rewards will come and be ready to enjoy them. Sara was encouraged to take it slowly and at her own pace. She was assured that if she gave running a "fair" try and persisted through the first three months of the program, she would very likely continue running on a regular basis (*Runner's World*, 1979, p. 11).

8. Avoid responding too much to advice from outsiders about how fast one can or should progress—personal assessment of progress generally proves to be most trustworthy. Accepting the integration of any life-style change as a slow, gradual process will increase its chances of success (Ullyot, 1976, p. 19).

9. In a similar vein to making an exercise program slow and comfortable is the idea of learning to "listen to your body." Even when following what seems to be a reasonable plan, at times flexibility will have more benefit for long-term goals than simply "sticking" to the goals. For instance, anyone who is a consistently active person has experienced days of feeling overwhelmed and of dreading anticipated exercise with a generally tired and lethargic body. There may be no explainable cause for these feelings, or there may be clearly identifiable sources of external stress such as extra work, lack of sleep, emotional problems, or worry. All of these factors take energy even though not through physical exertion. Allowing for decreasing or skipping a planned activity session is usually followed by an increase in energy and motivation for continuing with a routine. In low-energy or low-motivation periods, it is worth weighing the immediate benefits against the long-term drain that an accumulation of negative experiences can bring. Most women who exercise regularly will begin to recognize a pattern in their internal motivation and will learn to anticipate and plan for unscheduled "days off."

rewards and reinforcements

During the beginning weeks for her exercise program, Sara was encouraged to build in rewards and reinforcements for her achievements. This is an especially important component of success for a newly active woman or one who is beginning at a relatively low level of fitness and skill. Ultimately, most active women will find that activity is its own reward, but for many women the beginning is simply hard work, which demands a high degree of motivation and determination. In such circumstances, it is important to build in outside incentives.

Sara found in the beginning of her exercise program that she was rewarding herself with extra or special foods. She believed that her increased activity warranted an increase in calories. It was helpful for her to acknowledge that her 10-to15-minute exercise sessions really did not make her more hungry and, in fact, she often felt less hungry after running. (For women of ideal weight who are exercising 30 minutes or more, the result will be a recognizable increased calorie demand.) Sara found that she needed to remind herself consciously that food would not be a reward for exercising.

Following is a list of ways devised by Sara and the exercise consultant to reinforce her new activity pattern:

1. For Sara (and for many women), keeping a log or chart of exercise is very reinforcing. Adding up miles, minutes, hours, or "aerobic" points at the end of the week, month, and year can give a tremendous sense of accomplishment. This record also sets up a competitive situation with oneself to

see if activity can be maintained or increased. Recording in the exercise journal is most reinforcing when done as soon as possible after the exercise session is completed.

2. If the motivation for exercise is to lose weight, look better, or improve cardiovascular fitness, use appropriate measurements as indicators of progress. Check your pulse, your weight, and changes in your body girth at regular intervals. Record them as they happen. It is reasonable to expect to begin seeing these changes as early as 4 weeks, and by 6 to 8 weeks, measures of physical fitness will improve appreciably (Elrick et al., 1978, p. 67).

3. Set short-term goals that will ultimately progress to the ideal level of fitness. Short-term goals should be set frequently and with flexibility with regard to alterations necessary to accommodate any unforeseen problems or accelerations in progress. Frequent short-term goal-setting is a mechanism for positive reinforcement and a perspective of growth.

4. Sara found that exercising with another woman or with a group of women was a real motivator. She was cautioned, however, to recognize negative feelings that might be generated in an environment where comparisons will be made. Unless there is an attitude of competence or an experience of support, others may not contribute to enjoyment. This may be especially true regarding participation with men in exercise. Obviously, this is a variable issue based on the man or men involved and the woman's competence, but there may be pitfalls in trying to keep up with or participate in sports with men. Most men will be physically stronger right from the beginning and almost always progress more quickly toward physical fitness (Ullyot, 1976, p. 19). This is primarily due to men's past development and some inherent ability. Regardless of reason, it is usually not encouraging to be compared to a higher standard that seems to have been so easily attained (*Runner's World*, 1979, pp. 13, 16).

5. Sara found that setting up a competitive situation with herself or a friend was a good motivator for her. Recognition and acceptance of a competitive nature is one of the ways that mind and body work together in women's realization of their potential. For many women, exercise can also become an outlet for the expression of aggression, hostility, and anger (*Runner's World*, 1979, p. 212). One woman described this benefit: "I find that I can cope much better with the frustrations and demands of getting three kids to school, soccer practice, music lessons and all the rest, if I've taken 30 minutes to run—there is something very relaxing about breathing like that."

6. Exercise "time out" from the routine pressures and stimulation of external stress is considered essential rejuvenation by women who have learned to use it in this way. One of the ways to develop this positive effect is to be aware of the thoughts and ideas that come to one's mind during exercise; this is an opportunity to build one's self-concept and self-esteem. Self-suggested messages such as "I do this for myself," "I am in control of my life," "I experience myself as a capable and strong woman through exercise" all contribute to expanding the psychological value of exercise.

7. Sara was encouraged to avoid becoming bored with running by planning for variety in route or scenery. For some women, variety may mean having several routes over which to run or ride, several friends to exercise with, or even more than one form of exercise. For example, perhaps to plan for seasonal changes based on weather-dependent sports like skiing or skating will contribute to an attitude of enthusiasm and positive anticipation.

positive effects of aerobic exercise

A follow-up interview was completed with Sara 12 months after the initial visit to the exercise consultant. The purpose of the interview was to discuss her progress and determine what she felt were the results of her running program. At the time of the interview, Sara was running for 40 minutes, six times a week. She had been at this level for four months and felt satisfied with the schedule.

The following list of changes summarizes what Sara identified as her payoffs for her more active life-style:

1. At the time of the follow-up interview, Sara's blood pressure was 110/60 (from 140/80 at the initial visit). Her pulse was 60 beats per minute (as opposed to 84 beats per minute).

This drop in blood pressure is commonly seen in people who move from a sedentary to a more active life-style. This change is indicative of a decrease in stress to the cardiovascular system (although the initial reading of 140/80 is considered in the normal range). The blood pressure reflects the internal tension in the heart and blood vessels, and above normal readings are associated with coronary artery disease, heart failure, and cerebral vascular disease. The heart rate reflects the work demands of the heart and the duration of the resting phase of the cycle.

In the past, the risk of cardiovascular disease has essentially been considered a threat to men and not significantly to women. Presumably this was because men were involved in highly stressful and demanding careers, which contributes to cardiovascular disease. As women move into similar situations, will their incidence of cardiovascular disease also increase? Many researchers are predicting such increases, especially in postmenopausal women where protective estrogen levels are lower. Exercise physiologists have shown that sedentary women who become active on a regular basis will achieve a decrease in blood pressure and heart rate even if neither was elevated before exercise began. It is logical to anticipate that this reduced stress on the cardiovascular system will have preventative effects (Elrick et al., 1978, pp. 25–27; Wood, 1979).

Although Sara's blood fat levels were not measured at the initial visit, since she had no history of disease, people who are involved with regular aerobic exercise do have lower blood fat levels than nonexercisers. The implications are that lowering of blood fat levels will reduce the risk of cardiovascular disease, although research continues in this area (Wood, 1979).

2. From her original 144 pounds, Sara weighed 124 pounds one year later. She was also aware of her improved muscle tone simply by her appearance.

Consistent exercise will produce a decrease in body fat relative to the muscle weight of the body. In other words, not only should a woman expect to lose excess weight, but fat will be exchanged for muscle tissue. Benefits of this redistribution include an improvement in muscle tone, strength, and appearance. It is this type of change that accounts for an improvement in the way a woman's clothes fit her rather than what she may see on the scale. Twenty to 25 percent of the weight of the average American woman consists of fat tissue; with consistent exercise that percentage can be expected to lower to 10 to 15 percent, which is considered ideal (Elrick et al., 1978, pp. 9, 11–14).

3. Sara reported improved sleep patterns; she now falls asleep more quickly and is less likely to wake up during the night. This improved sleep pattern is an important common difference between active and inactive people (Elrick et al., 1978, p. 28).

4. Another benefit of running for Sara was alleviation of an intermittent problem with constipation.

Digestion is improved with exercise due to the increase in circulation and stimulation, which increases the contractions of the intestine. Constipation is uncommon in consistent exercisers (Elrick et al., 1978, p. 27).

5. For Sara, as for many women, exercise alleviates or reduces problems associated with menstruation. Probably one of the best ways to relieve the bloated feeling that many women have, which is due to increased fluid in the body, is to perspire. Significant amounts of fluid are lost from the skin and through respiration during sustained, aerobic exercise. Dysmenorrhea, or painful menstrual cramps, is frequently alleviated or reduced with activity. The mechanism involved in this benefit probably comes from the improved circulation and relaxation that follows a somewhat stenuous effort (Cooper & Cooper, 1972, p. 30; Kaplan, 1979, p. 20; Runner's World, 1979, pp. 20, 134).

6. Sara also reported a generally more energetic feeling most of the time since increasing her physical activity.

Active people enjoy higher levels of energy than do inactive people. Physiological and psychological factors account for this change. Physiologically speaking, metabolism is accelerated, and conditioning results in improved function of the heart, lungs, blood vessels, and muscles, with the subsequent ability to work harder, play harder, and endure stress better (Elrick et al., 1978, p. 26).

7. Sara also reported generally feeling more relaxed and better able to "cope."

Many women learn that a relaxed mind accompanies a relaxed body and that the most consistently effective route to that relaxation is through exercise. This effect is a consequence of the "fight-flight" response of the body. As people are exposed to stress, their internal coping mechanisms provide the chemicals essential for a "fight" or "flight" response. However, because neither of these alternatives are usually appropriate in the situation, the accumulation of these chemicals probably accounts for the tense, irritable way the "stressed" person feels. Through exercise, these chemicals are used or eliminated, which results in the subsequent feeling of relaxation (Elrick et al., 1978, p. 28).

8. Another benefit associated with use of bones and muscles comes in a preventative form by reducing degenerative bone changes that frequently follow the menopause. As bones are used, the demand for mineral deposits to strengthen their structure increases. With aging, and especially with a decrease in estrogen, osteoporosis (demineralization of bone with consequent increased fragility) can account for easy fracturing. Exercise that stimulates an increase in mineral storage is probably the best insurance against this problem (Cooper & Cooper, 1972, p. 34; Kaplan; 1979, p. 40).

9. The psychological benefits experienced by Sara were as powerful and positive as the physical changes that accompanied her increase in activity. The changes in self-concept, self-esteem, and sense of control are dramatic for many women (*Runner's World*, 1979, p. 21). The belief that "I can do this" transfers into other aspects of interaction. The ability to be self-accepting is nurtured through positive achievements.

Anderson, B. The runner's guide to stretching. *The Runner,* September 1979, *1(12),* 24.

Cooper, K. *The aerobics way.* New York: Bantam Books, 1977.

Cooper, M., & Cooper, K. *Aerobics for women.* New York: Bantam Books, 1972.

Couch, J. The perfect post-run stretching routine. *Runner's World,* April 1979, *14(4),* 84.

Elrick, H. et al. *Living longer and better, a guide to optimal health.* Mountain View, Calif.: World Publications, 1978.

Kaplan, J. *Women and sports.* New York: Viking, 1979.

Osler, T. *Serious runners handbook.* Mountain View, Calif.: World Publications, 1978.

Runner's World (eds.). *The complete woman runner.* Mountain View, Calif.: World Publications, 1979.

Sevene, B. How to begin running. *Runner's World,* June 1979, *14(6),* p. 48.

Ullyot, J. *Women's running.* Mountain View, Calif.: World Publications, 1976.

Wood, P. Does running help prevent heart attacks? *Runner's World,* December 1979, *14(6),* 68, 86–88.

NADA J. ESTES, R.N., M.S.

women and alcohol

Until recently, researchers studying the effects of alcohol on human behavior have concentrated primarily on the male drinker. It has been assumed that whatever was learned about male alcoholics could be generalized to women with similar problems. This assumption is currently being challenged, and there is increasing concentration, both in research and treatment efforts, on women with alcoholism.

Given the history of this sexual imbalance in alcoholism studies, there still remain many unanswered questions about alcoholism in women, and current findings are sometimes conflicting and not thoroughly substantiated. Nevertheless, some findings are becoming clearer and these will be the emphasis of this chapter.

prevalence

Women today are more likely to drink than ever before in history, and the increase is especially true for young age groups. In addition, female drinkers are developing heavier drinking patterns than in the past, similar to the drinking patterns of men (Carrigan, 1978).

It is a large step from drinking to alcoholism, but the number of women with alco-

141

holism is also increasing. Conservative estimates range from 1.5 to 2.25 million, or 15 to 22½ percent of the total alcoholic population in the United States (sec. of HEW, 1978). The number of men alcoholics continues to outnumber women alcoholics, but the gap is closing.

Reasons for the increase in alcohol use and alcoholism in women are not entirely clear, but changing life-styles and mores have most likely had an effect, especially because they have led to a redefining of roles for many women. The women's liberation movement has been identified as a factor in the increase, in that liberation for some women brings mixed blessings. Women are less bound to the traditional wife-mother role, but as they enter the work world outside the home, they are more exposed to the stresses typically experienced by men, which induce heavier alcoholism rates and early mortality (Alcoholism and Women, 1974).

There is some evidence, too, that society's attitudes toward alcoholism in women are gradually becoming less negative and punitive. As women feel less guilty about drinking, the need to conceal it diminishes. This has led to more accurate identification of numbers of women affected by alcoholism, and subsequently to increased research and treatment efforts directed solely at women. It is a very hopeful sign for alcoholic women that their problems are finally reaching the attention of workers in the field.

classification of alcoholic women

Just as there is no typical alcoholic man, there is no typical alcoholic woman. Alcoholic women come from all segments of society, and their drinking varies not only with the stage of alcoholism, but with age, social class, living conditions, and cultural background. Assigning them into general categories, however, is helpful in bringing increased recognition to the variations that exist in the total population of women alcoholics. One classification includes "lace curtain" women, single career women, and Skid Row women (Fraser, 1976, pp. 45–56).

The "lace curtain" women include the secretly imbibing housewife. She has been described so often in movies and novels that she has almost assumed the role of the prototype alcoholic woman in the minds of many. She is typically in her mid thirties to forties. While her children were growing, she failed to formulate worthwhile goals for herself and used her energies to focus on her children's needs and furthering her husband's career. In her middle years, she no longer feels worthwhile or needed. She easily learns that alcohol temporarily removes the ugly feelings of loneliness and depression, and therefore she drinks (Fraser, 1976, pp. 45–56).

The second category includes the single professional or career woman. She differs considerably from the lace curtain drinker, and she may have more in common with her male counterpart. Often she has never married or is divorced or widowed. She may have an interesting, fulfilling job. The problem begins when she returns home at the end of the day and the excitement of the work world is ended. The career woman may have neglected her social life in favor of her business life, and she only knows how to fill the void during the evening and on weekends with alcohol (Fraser, 1976, pp. 45–56).

The homeless alcoholic woman has been described as possibly the most socially isolated and disaffiliated member of Skid Row (Garrett & Bahr, 1973). Although Skid Row is the name for a society featuring a great deal of social interaction for the men who live there, for a female inhabitant, it is a solitary life. The Skid Row woman is far less likely to drink in public places, such as bars or taverns, and even when seen in bars she has limited interactions with others, especially other women. Her contacts with male patrons may be limited to attempts to use sex as a means to continue alcohol consumption. Rooming-house relationships are often short term, but it is easy to find another man and room—at

least until she has completely lost her youthful appearance, which happens at a rather young age for a Skid Row woman, largely as a result of her alcohol abuse and life-style (Garrett & Bahr, 1973).

These categories obviously do not include all females who have alcohol problems, most notably the teen-ager, women of ethnic minorities, or lesbian women. But the categories do provide a broad overview of the variations, indicating the need to respond to alcoholic women in an individual way.

special findings

attitudes toward drunkenness

Alcoholism still caries a greater stigma for women than for men. Although there seems to be a more permissive attitude in American society about social drinking in women, many people continue to view female intoxication with disgust and scorn. Drunkenness in men, on the other hand, is often looked upon with indifference, amusement, or pity (Gomberg, 1974, pp. 169–190).

The rejection of female intoxication involves at least two aspects, one relating to the division of labor between the sexes and the other to the loss of customary sexual inhibitions and restraints (Knupfer, 1964). In the woman's traditional housework role, high levels of skill are not generally required and moderate degrees of intoxication are not particularly incapacitating. The aspect of life that may be impaired by alcohol intake is the woman's sensitivity to the needs of others in her roles as wife, mother, daughter, sister, or caretaker. For example, a drunken mother is incapable of being consistently responsive to the needs of a young child. This factor alone makes drunkenness in women more threaten-

ing than in men. The second issue relates to the historical position noted in the Bible and in Roman law that a woman's drinking and sexual irregularities are linked. Although the popular image persists of the drunken woman and loose sexual morals, promiscuity seems to be involved with only 5 percent of all women alcoholics. Most of the other 95 percent complain of diminished interest in sex (Schuckit, 1972b).

Disapproval of female drunkenness may be a constraint against heavy drinking, thereby providing some cultural protection against alcoholism in some women. At the same time, it has no doubt contributed to the fact that many women with alcohol-related problems drink in secret and delay seeking treatment until the alcoholism is far advanced.

depression

Family history data reveal that depressive disorders and alcoholism are closely related illnesses, and this association is most marked in women alcoholics. When compared with the backgrounds of male alcoholics, women alcoholics have more close female relatives who suffer from depression, as well as a higher incidence of alcoholism in all close relatives. At the same time, women alcoholics themselves are more likely to suffer from depression, while alcoholic men are more likely to be sociopathic (Schuckit, 1972a). The reasons for these differences are unclear, but they may be a result of the contrasting ways in which females and males function in our society. Females are likely to learn that it is acceptable to express feelings through crying, and they may receive extra attention when they are sad. Males are more likely to be taught aggressive responses and be rewarded for fighting when frustrated.

Several similarities between alcoholism and depression are readily seen. With both conditions, the person displays a dysphoric mood, complains of sadness and of feelings of worthlessness, hopelessness, and helplessness. The risk of suicide is high in both alcoholism and depression, and especially so for women alcoholics. The rate of completed suicides among female alcoholics is 23 times the rate for females in the general population; among males it is 22 times the population rate (Carrigan, 1978).

In appraising women alcoholics, it is of particular importance to determine if the alcoholism is a primary condition or secondary to some other problem, most notably depression. Are the depressed effects, feelings of hopelessness, and suicidal ideations, seen so often in women alcoholics, the cause of or the result of the drinking problem? In many instances, an accurate diagnosis of primary depression cannot be made until the woman is free of alcohol for some period of time. Clearly, the adequacy of subsequent care will be determined on the basis of correct diagnosis.

precipitating factors

The onset of alcoholism and heavy drinking in women has been repeatedly linked to psychological stress and to some specific precipitating circumstances. Social, environmental, and gynecological factors, such as death of a parent or spouse, divorce, hysterectomy, or menopause, are thought to play a special role in the origin of alcoholism in women (Curlee, 1969; Lisansky, 1957). One study found that twice as many women as men cited a specific past experience as the point when they started drinking (Lisansky, 1957). However, a more recent study done on a heterogeneous sample of 191 women seen at a detoxification center did not agree with these findings (Morrissey & Schuckit, 1978). An evaluation of the time relationship between a number of life stresses and the onset of alcoholism did *not* support the supposed tendency of female alcoholics to begin drinking in response to stressful situations. In this study, women were asked about their history of alcohol problems and their gynecological and family histories in separate sections of the interview so that the relationship between the problems would be less likely due to the women's reconstruction of events. Since excessive drinking produces a guilt complex for many women, they greatly need an acceptable reason for drinking. Earlier researchers may have made it easy for subjects to state a reason by the sequencing of questions. Whether, in fact, women are more likely than men to develop alcoholism in response to stress needs further investigation in which men and women alcoholics are compared along similar dimensions.

Once heavy drinking begins to be a problem for a woman, the course into alcoholism tends to be severe and rapid. This generally shortened developmental period of alcoholism in women has been referred to as "telescoped" effect (Curlee, 1970), and, as a result, alcoholism in women has been viewed as a more virulent process than alcoholism in men.

polydrug use

Women, in general, exceed men in their consumption of psychotropic drugs (Cooperstock, 1976, pp. 83–111). The excessive use of prescription drugs by women in the United States would appear to be related to several factors. Women engage in help-seeking behavior more readily than men, and they tend to describe their symptoms in emotional or psychological terms. They report feeling worried, tense, or having insomnia, whereas men are more likely to seek help for physical pain. Therefore, when women bring their complaints to their physicians, they are more likely than men to receive prescriptions for minor tranquilizers such as Valium and Librium. Women accept these prescriptions, many of them believing the cultural stereotype that they need psychoactive medications for relief of emotional discomfort associated with certain aspects of womanhood, such as menstruation, pregnancy, and menopause.

An additional factor that sometimes leads to excessive use of prescription drugs by women has to do with the myths and misconceptions regarding the female that are still endemic in much of medical education (Howell, 1974) where the majority of educators are male. For example, it is often taught in medical schools that patients with psychogenic problems are likely to be women. Compounding this is the fact that pharmaceutical advertisements and literature, readily available to medical practitioners, often convey negative attitudes toward female patients (Prather & Fidell, 1975) and promote the use

of psychoactive drugs to treat symptoms common to women. With such influences, male physicians may find it difficult to be objective in their approach to female patients.

Women alcoholics use drugs other than alcohol more than do men alcoholics, and as a result multiple dependencies on alcohol and other drugs (predominantly those legally prescribed by physicians) is increasing for women. A major concern, as yet little known by professional workers and the general public, has to do with how alcohol interacts with other drugs. When taken in conjunction with other psychoactive drugs, alcohol has an additive effect, so it is possible to take a low dose of alcohol and a low dose of Librium, for example, and get the combined effect of taking a large dose. The combination of intoxication, common to alcoholic women, and the ingestion of a psychoactive drug can lead to unintentional overdose, resulting in coma or death.

Also important for women with polydrug addictions is the fact that they require a longer time to detoxify. It may take up to two weeks of detoxification to achieve a drug-free state before referral to a structured rehabilitation program can be made (Fraser, 1976, pp. 45–56).

The increasing problem of polydrug addictions among women must be confronted on several levels. Educational programs should inform consumers and prescribers of drugs about the dangers involved in mixing alcohol and other drugs. Women especially must become knowledgeable about drug interactions and take special note of their help-seeking behavior with the goal of learning to expect and accept remedies other than drugs for their symptoms. Physicians need to alter their beliefs and understandings about women, and pharmaceutical agencies should make certain that their advertisements are unbiased toward women. Finally, a variety of treatment options must be provided to all women seeking relief of symptoms.

biological factors

A larger proportion of women than men suffer from cirrhosis of the liver associated with heavy drinking, and women alcoholic patients, on the average, die at an earlier age— 48.6 years vs. 56.3 years for men (Spain, 1945). Women also appear to develop cirrhosis at a lower level of alcohol intake (Pequignot et al., 1974) and following a shorter duration of excessive drinking (Lelbach, 1974).

Another biological factor of importance to women alcoholics is that the same dose of alcohol, corrected for body weight, apparently produces higher blood alcohol levels in women than in men (Carrigan, 1978). Additionally, blood alcohol level varies at different times during the menstrual cycle. The relationship between hormonal balance, menstrual cycle, and alcoholism in women needs further clarification.

psychosocial factors

Alcoholic persons may have poor self-image and low self-esteem (Wood & Duffy, 1966), a tendency that is more pronounced in women then in men. It appears that being alcoholic and a woman constitutes a double jeopardy for females in American society. Related to this sense of inadequacy is the difficulty many alcoholic women experience with regard to feminine role identity. It has been shown that although women alcoholics may wish to be feminine, their unconscious sex-role confusion causes them to feel somehow inadequate as women (Wilsnack, 1973). The doubts of the

woman alcoholic may be increased by acute threats to her sense of feminine adequacy as a result of such experiences as marital problems, hysterectomy, or children leaving home. Alcohol is used to gain feelings of womanliness, but the typical consequences of heavy drinking—neglect of appearance, disapproval by family—eventually make her feel less of a woman, and thus the proverbial vicious circle is set in motion.

In regard to psychosocial aspects of family life, alcoholic women marry to the same extent, but they have higher divorce rates than the general population (Gomberg, 1974, pp. 169–190). Alcoholic women are far more likely than alcoholic men to have an alcoholic spouse. The man married to the alcoholic woman is a relatively unknown entity. He has not been the subject of much research, in contrast to his female counterpart, and has received more sympathy than censure (Lindbeck, 1972). Wives of alcoholic men, on the other hand, have been studied extensively and often have been cast in a negative light. Clinical impressions in the literature indicate that the husband of the alcoholic woman reacts to her drinking in several ways. He may deny her illness, attempt to control her drinking, or abandon her by such actions as divorce (Estes & Baker, 1977, 186-193). Male spouses, in particular, need help in comprehending and dealing constructively with alcohol problems in their wives. A useful book for assisting in this process is available (Curlee-Salisbury, 1978). Women married to alcoholic men are less likely to divorce their husbands and will often struggle for long periods to make their marriage work.

Women alcoholics, as a rule, have experienced more traumatic and disruptive events in their early lives than the normal population and to a greater extent than male alcoholics (Gomberg, 1974, pp. 169–190). The events include having an alcoholic parent, losing a parent through divorce, death, or abandonment, and psychiatric illness in the family of origin. The deprivations of childhood may contribute to the alcoholic woman's intense search for love and reassurance through marriage and motherhood. When her relationships with people significant to her falter, she is especially vulnerable to the ravages of excessive drinking.

the alcoholic mother

The deleterious effects of an alcoholic mother on her children are undoubtedly manifold. One effect, difficult to measure, has to do with the kind and degree of social, physical, and emotional deprivation that children with alcoholic mothers experience. Alcoholic mothers are apt to abuse their children through neglect due to preoccupation with alcohol intake and its effects, including intoxication and hangovers.

The children of chronic alcoholic women risk developing fetal alcohol syndrome (FAS), caused by the effects of alcohol on the developing fetus. The severity of FAS is related to dosage, timing, and individual fetal response. The damage, severe or mild, is irreversible.

Children with full-blown FAS exhibit four main abnormalities: (1) central nervous system dysfunctions, resulting in varying degrees of mental deficiency or development delay, (2) growth deficiencies exhibited by smaller than normal heads, and smaller heights and weights, both prenatal and postnatal, (3) characteristic cluster of facial anomalies such as short eye slits, thinned upper lip, absence or near absence of the vertical ridges between the nose and upper lip and epicanthal (eyelid) folds, and (4) malformations such as heart defects, minor abnormalities of the joints, and external anomalies (Clarren & Smith, 1978).

Although FAS is more often associated with alcoholism, the effects of moderate levels of alcohol intake during pregnancy are still being investigated. The Department of Health, Education, and Welfare issued a health caution statement to the general public in mid-1977, describing the potential effects on the fetus of heavy use of alcohol during pregnancy. The statement said that safe levels of drinking for pregnant women are unknown, but it appears that a risk is established with more than 3 ounces (89 ml) of absolute alcohol, or 6 drinks per day. For intakes of 1 and 3 ounces per day (30–89 ml), there is still uncertainty, but caution is advised.

Given the questions regarding safe levels of alcohol during pregnancy, the wisest decision for a woman anticipating pregnancy is to refrain from all alcohol intake prior to conception through delivery. The danger of becoming pregnant and not knowing it for a period of several weeks makes the cessation of alcohol important prior to conception. The anguish of giving birth to a child with FAS is difficult to comprehend. Raising a child with this syndrome presents an almost overwhelming challenge to the healthiest of parents. Such an event only compounds the already problem-laden life of the alcoholic woman, promotes the waste of human life, and must be prevented whenever possible. If prevention efforts fail, the option of terminating a pregnancy may have to be considered.

Alcoholism and Women. *Alcohol Health and Research World*, experimental issue; Summer 1974, 2–7.

Carrigan, Z. H. Research issues: Women and alcohol

abuse. *Alcohol Health and Research World* 1978, *3*, 2–9.

Clarren, S. K., & Smith, D. W. The fetal alcohol syndrome experience with 65 patients and a review of the world literature. *New England Journal of Medicine* 1978, *19*, 1063–1067.

Cooperstock, R. Women and psychotropic drugs. In A. MacLennan (Ed.), *Women: Their use of alcohol and other legal drugs.* Toronto: Addiction Research Foundation of Ontario, 1976.

Curlee, J. Alcoholism and the "empty nest." *Bulletin of the Menninger Clinic*, 1969, *33*, 165–171.

Curlee, J. A comparison of male and female patients at an alcoholism treatment center. *Journal of Psychology*, 1970, *74*, 239–247.

Curlee-Salisbury, Joan. *When the woman you love is an alcoholic.* St. Meinrad, Indiana: Abbey Press, 1978, p. 278

Estes, N. J., & Baker, J. Spouses of alcoholic women. In N.J. Estes, & M. E. Heinemann (Eds.), *Alcoholism development, consequences and interventions.* St. Louis: C. V. Mosby, 1977.

Fraser, W. The alcoholic woman: Attitudes and perspectives. In A. MacLennan (Ed.), *Women: their use of alcohol and other legal drugs.* Toronto: Addiction Research Foundation of Ontario, 1976.

Garrett, G. R., & Bahr, H. M. Women on Skid Row. *Quarterly Journal of Studies on Alcohol*, 1973, *34*, 1228–1243.

Gomberg, E. Women and alcoholism. In V. Franks and B. Vansanti (Eds.), *Women in therapy—new psychotherapies for a changing society.* New York: Brunner/Mazel, 1974.

Howell, M. C. What medical schools teach about women. *The New England Journal of Medicine*, August 8, 1974, *291*, 304–307.

Knupfer, G. Female drinking patterns. Paper presented at the Fifteenth Annual Meeting of the North American Association of Alcoholism Programs, Washington, D.C., September 1964.

Lelbach, W. K. Organic pathology related to volume and patterns of alcohol use. In R. J. Gibbins et al. (Eds.), *Research Advances in Alcohol and Drug Problems.* New York, Wiley, 1974.

Lindbeck, L. J. The Woman alcoholic; A review of the literature. *International Journal of Addiction*, 1972, *7*, 567–580.

Lisansky, E. Alcoholism in women: Social and psychological concomitants I. Social History Data, *Quarterly Journal of Studies on Alcohol*, 1957, *18*, 588–623.

Morrissey, E. A., & Schuckit, M. Stressful life events and alcohol problems among women seen at a detoxification center. *Journal of Studies on Alcohol*, 1978, *39*, 1559–1576.

Pequignot, G. et al. Increasing risk of liver cirrhosis with intake of alcohol, *LaRevue De L'Alcolisme* 1974, *20*, 191.

Prather, J., & Fidell, L. S. Sex differences in the content and style of medical advertisements. *Social Science and Medicine*, January 1975, *9*, 23–26.

Schuckit, M. The alcoholic woman: A literature review. *Psychiatry in Medicine*, 1972a, *3*, 37–43.

Schuckit, M. Sexual disturbance in the woman alcoholic. *Medical Aspects of Human Sexuality*, 1976, *6*, 44–45, 48–49, 53, 57, 60–61, 65.

Secretary of Health Education and Welfare. Third special report to the U.S. Congress on *Alcohol and Health.* Washington, D.C.: U.S. Government Printing Office, 1978.

Spain, D. M. Portal cirrhosis of the liver: A review of 250 necropsies with reference to sex differences. *Am. J. Clin. P.*, 1945, *15*, 215.

Wilsnack, S. Femininity by the bottle. *Addictions*, 1973, *20*, 3–19.

Wood, H. P., & Duffy, E. L. Psychological factors in alcoholic women. *American Journal of Psychiatry*, 1966, *123*, 341–345.

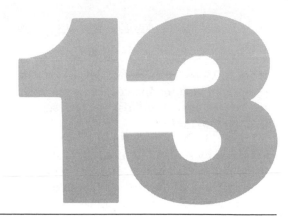

PAMELA MITCHELL R.N., M.S.

physiologic responses of women to stress

Everywhere one sees hints on managing stress, detecting stress, thriving on stress, avoiding stress. The popularity of the concept as an explanation for many of the ills besetting humankind can be traced to the work of Hans Selye, a specialist in the study of endocrine function. Although his work was concerned with the body's nonspecific response to a variety of physical stimuli, his speculations regarding emotional stimuli as a stressor formed the basis for the concept of "stress" as the mediator of interactions between people and their environments. Many diseases and problems in managing living came to be viewed as "stress-related." In other words, the way in which one deals with the wear and tear of living seems to be a factor in whether one stays well or becomes ill; it also becomes a factor in the zest with which one lives life in the "well" state.

Women account for a larger percentage of visits to health care professionals than do men. Is this a sign that women are under more stress than men? Does it indicate that women react to the stress of living by becoming ill more often than men? Or does it indicate that women are more willing to take on the sick role, to identify themselves as not well more frequently than men? Some illnesses in which stress is often identified as a contributing factor have a different distribution between men and women. For example, the rate of myocardial infarction (heart attack) is greater among men than among women, prior to the menopause. Is this due to differences in response to stress, to hormonal differences, or to some combination thereof? Or is the difference related to a third risk factor, such as cigarette smoking?

The incidence of ulcers and hypertension, considered by some to be affected by stress, is higher in men than in women. Are women exposed to fewer of the stresses that predispose men to these disorders (sometimes thought of as "executive diseases"); do women respond in a different manner than men? Women have a higher rate of psychiatric diagnoses, in particular neurosis and depression. Are these manifestations of the way women deal with stress; are they related to the biology of women; are they related to the particular demands of living on women in contrast to men? Or is the description of mood and affect (upon which the making of these diagnoses is partially dependent) more socially acceptable for women than for men?

These observations raise intriguing questions regarding the degree to which such problems and diseases are the results of stress in men and women, or due to differences in the manner of expressing problems with living among groups of men and women. When health status is being considered, the assumption is that men and women react to the problems of living differently. Women have been characterized as expressive, using words and communication to deal with problems; men are often typed as instrumental, using action and movement. Although such differences may not characterize individual men and women, observations of large numbers of people have, indeed, suggested such differences. If so, are they based on differences in the way men and women are raised and treated in a society? Are they inherently biological, or do the biological differences interact with the socialization processes? Are there physiologic differences in the responses of men and women to stress that can account for all these contrasts? If so, can an individual man or woman use the knowledge of these differences to deal most effectively with the demands of daily situations on him or her?

perspectives on stress and physiologic responses

Before turning to the processes that the human body uses in interacting with changes in the environment, we must deal with the problem of defining the term *stress*. The definition is elusive even though it is used by many people, all of whom assume they share a common meaning. Selye (1965) uses it quite specifically to mean the nonspecific *response* of the body to a variety of stimuli. Regardless of stimulus (heat, cold, pain, chemical), he found a characteristic general response of the body. He calls the provoking stimulus a *stressor*. However, many investigators use stress to mean that which is "out there" and which provokes the Selye-type responses. Others use it to mean the interaction between the provoking stimulus and the response; still others use it to mean the whole process of being stimulated, appraising the stimulus as threatening, and responding. Many state or imply that the term applies to those situations that are deemed *threatening*. Although this notion of threatening or negative situations as stressful is common, it is not consistent with scientific definitions, which attempt to use the bodily response as the key variable.

When scientists measure some of the biochemicals thought to reflect the stress response, situations with both negative and positive content produced similar changes.

For example, Levi (1972), noted for his work with the sympathetic nervous system and adrenal gland medulla (center) found that catecholamines (chemicals that indirectly measure emotional arousal) are elevated when people view either fearful or funny movies, but change little during emotionally neutral scenes (such as nature documentaries). Thus, in Levi's view, both negative and positive emotionally arousing situations serve as stimuli to the stress response.

adaptive response

In all definitions of stress, a key point is that a *change from the ongoing* state has occurred. When such change occurs, a number of psychophysiologic responses deal with it. Many of the responses are relatively nonspecific; they occur whenever there is change, regardless of its nature, provided that the change is seen as emotionally arousing. There is considerable scientific evidence to suggest that psychosocial arousal (fear, happiness, anger, for example) is the key to Selye's nonspecific stress response.

Changes may occur in either the external or internal environment. For example, changes in environmental temperature, interpersonal activity, or the quality of the air are all external to the person. Both psychological and physical processes occur in the internal environment. For example, fears about an examination, joy at the thought of a lover, or infection of the lung from a microorganism are changes in the internal environment. In addition, the physiological response to these changes constitutes yet another change in the internal environment and can act as feedback to the whole system.

Consequently, in this chapter the initial focus is on determining and describing the physiologic means by which humans and animals respond to perceived changes in the equilibrium of the external and internal environments. These mechanisms are called *adaptive responses.* Second, the known differences in physiologic adaptive responses of men and women are discussed for the few areas in which they have been studied. Questions are raised regarding the origins of these differences, and, last, the implications of the known differences for women's health are discussed.

major physiologic response systems

Most of the experimental work regarding physiologic response systems has been in the context of physiologic responses to emotionally arousing situations and to physical stressors such as heat, cold, and exercise. A great deal of the work involved animals in laboratory situations. Studies of humans have generally been limited to indirect measures of the responses of the various systems because of the difficulties involved in direct measures. For example, changes to the skin are often used as an indirect measure of arousal, rather than the more specific measure of plasma catecholamines, which involves taking blood (itself a stressful experience) and sophisticated laboratory analysis techniques. Finally, physiologic measures of humans in real-life situations are very few, primarily because it is difficult to collect appropriate specimens during the course of daily activity. Although there are few real-life studies of women as well as men, there are even fewer that collect physiologic as well as psychologic data. Consequently, the reader must be aware that the generalizations here are gained primarily from laboratory settings, and the data are primarily from male human and nonhuman primates and male rodents.

Stimuli arising from within or without the organism are appraised by central processing mechanisms, which in some manner signal physiologic response systems: autonomic nervous system, endocrine systems, and musculoskeletal system. Some responses are highly specific to the stimuli, for example, increased heat production in cold environments, heat-losing mechanisms in hot ones. Others seem to be general and nonspecific to a number of stimuli when elements of novelty, challenge, or threat are present.

These systems do not operate independently, but interact with one another. For example, the increased heart rate associated with a frightening stimulus may serve as a further stimulus of alarm and increased muscle tension. The increased tension may create pain, which further serves as a signal of alarm, thus increasing the experiences of anxiety.

Neural connections exist between the neocortex (thinking brain), limbic cortex (feeling brain), and brain stem (vegetative brain) and the sensory systems by which we have contact with external and internal environments. These connections form a circuit by which our thoughts, feelings, and behavior can influence the functioning of body systems, and the feedback loops by which our perception of body functioning can influence thoughts and feelings.

When the neural systems become aware of any change in the environment that requires response, a number of physiologic systems come into play. The German neurophysiologist, Walter Hess, described two balanced, integrated systems consisting of components of autonomic nervous system and musculo-skeletal responses. Gellhorn (1965) expanded the concept to include endocrine and immunologic patterns of response. These scientists called the emergency preparedness response system *ergotropic* (from the Greek, meaning to turn toward work) and the return to normal response *trophotropic* (turning toward nourishment).

Still others (for example, Henry, 1976) have suggested that individual animals develop a primary physiologic pattern of response depending on their social status in the colony. In colonies of mice, dominant animals develop a high activity response, whereas subordinate animals manifest a predominantly withdrawal, low-activity response. Although Henry does not use Hess's terms at all, the patterns of behavior suggest similar integrated systems (action-oriented and withdrawal-oriented). The fact that all the animals are in the same social situation (establishing social dominance in the colony) is a strong argument against looking *only* at the external environment in defining stress. It could be argued that the animals are genetically predisposed to be either dominant or subordinate, that they have an inherent "prewired" response pattern. However, this argument does not hold up when one takes a dominant animal from one colony and puts it in a colony that has already established its dominance patterns. The once-dominant animal changes to the withdrawal pattern of the subordinates.

Although one must be cautious about inferring human reactions from animal responses, particularly when the animals are not primates, differing methods of response to life situations are evident in human experience, and within given individuals as well. Responses to environmental stimuli may be broadly categorized into two modes: (1) active-aggressive defense reaction, and (2) withdrawal-conservation reaction. Any given organism may respond with elements of both sides or at one or the other extreme from defense to withdrawal.

active–aggressive defense reaction

In studies of emergency situations and strong arousal (positive or negative), many physiologic systems are involved. These include the autonomic nervous system, neuroendocrine and immunologic systems, musculoskeletal system, and cognitive (thinking) processes.

AUTONOMIC. The sympathetic nervous system increases activity, which results in the release of the neurotransmitter hormones norepinephrine and epinephrine (also called noradrenaline and adrenaline). While norepinephrine is always circulating in the body, epinephrine is secreted only by the adrenal medulla and only in highly arousing situations. The effect of these hormones is to increase heart rate and blood pressure, aid in increasing glucose metabolism, and facilitate the function of other endocrine hormones that are catabolic (energy-using). In short, the sympathetic system assists the body to meet the emergency by the classic fight or flight mechanisms.

NEUROENDOCRINE. The anterior pituitary gland initiates secretion of various hormones that increase energy production and utilization of nutrients. These include increased production of thyroid, testosterone, and glucocorticoids. Simultaneously, hormones that normally act to store and maintain energy are suppressed. This is reflected in decreased production of growth hormone and insulin. The immune system gears itself to fight any invaders by increasing platelets and lymphocytes.

MUSCULOSKELETAL. In keeping with the general emergency readiness of the rest of the body system, the musculoskeletal system responds by increasing muscle tension in preparation for vigorous activity. This increase can be initiated locally, for example, in response to injury. It can also be stimulated centrally in the brain and probably uses connections between limbic brain and hypothalamus.

COGNITIVE PROCESSES. The cognitive interpretation and accompanying mood depend on both the conscious appraisal of the situation and the conscious or unconscious awareness of the sensations that accompany the physical processes. The bodily sensations that most often accompany the emergency reaction primarily reflect muscle tension and increased epinephrine—tense muscles, pounding heart, cold and clammy hands, dry mouth, shortness of breath. The mood (or the name given to the emotion that is associated with these sensations) varies with the meaning of the situation that provoked them. For example, one interprets the pounding heart and flushed face as joy if they happen at the approach of a loved one, and as fear if a wild animal shows up. In a classic experiment, Schachter and Singer (1962) injected adrenaline (epinephrine) into volunteer subjects. Only some of the subjects knew the actual symptoms to expect. Others were told not to expect any body sensations, and still others were told incorrect sensations to expect. In addition, some members of the investigating team, in the guise of subjects, pretended to be angry or euphoric while the real subjects were experiencing the effects of the injection. The subjects who knew what to expect did not report any emotion attached to the experience; those who had been told incorrect information tended to report emotions that corresponded to the behavior shown by the "false" subjects. In other words, when these people felt body symptoms they could not explain, they took their cues from the social environment to explain these symptoms to themselves and to others.

withdrawal-conservation reaction

The "playing dead," or withdrawal, reaction is characterized by behavioral inhibition and activation of the pituitary-adrenal-cortical system. Its purpose is anabolic (energy-storing) rather than catabolic (energy-using). Gluconeogenesis (formation of new glucose stores) occurs, stimulated by adrenocortiotrophic hormone (ACTH). ACTH and subsequent corticosteroid responses are increased. There is increased activity of the parasympathetic nervous system, characterized by decreased heart rate, increased pepsin (stomach secretion), decrease in reticuloendothelial cells (immune system activity). Muscle tension is decreased and there is less movement than normal.

Aspects of this reaction are seen when subjects are recovering from emotional stimuli produced in the laboratory (Mason, 1968) and following stimulation of the ergotrophic (emergency preparing) system (Gellhorn, 1965). However, Henry's work suggests that the withdrawal reaction may be a main response pattern in itself in naturally occurring social situations. The similarity of the behavioral and biochemical sides of the withdrawal-conservation response to those seen in human depression is striking.

defense and withdrawal as opposite poles

The stress response described by Selye (1965) appears to contain components of both defense and withdrawal. Although he did not measure sympathoadrenomedullary function (the interaction between adrenal gland and the sympathetic nervous system), he assumed it to be present, based on Cannon's (1939) early work. Strong pituitary-adrenocortical response was evident by the classic findings in Selye's animals—enlarged adrenals, stomach ulcers, and shrunken thymus. These organ changes reflected increased adrenocortical activity, changes in stomach secretion, and impaired immune system. In all of Selye's experiments, the animals were restrained and essentially helpless to control the situation. Hence, his findings may show the epitome of the "playing dead" reaction. The response is an adaptive mechanism in conserving energy, but fails to preserve the organism if the environmental situation, and possibly fear, are too strong. In situations in which animals can influence the timing of the stimulus, more elements of the defensive response are seen. The withdrawal response becomes more evident when the animal's perception of the ability to control is altered or the actual ability to control is impaired. In such cases, some animals just give up and die.

In real-life situations, both human and animal, it is likely that these two patterns represent opposite poles and that individual responses are combinations of the two. Human situations that might represent extreme stimuli are such events as severe physical trauma (accidents with trauma to many systems, or severe burns). Studies of metabolic function in such persons support the idea that both defensive and withdrawal patterns function simultaneously. Such combinations appear in animal studies in which the animal has no control over the situation of extreme fear or arousal. For example, a tree shrew, when exposed to the sight of an animal it has fought, initially has a strong sympathetic reaction—its hair stands on end. If the inescapable exposure continues, the animal may die (literally of fright) and exhibits the classic triad—enlarged adrenals, stomach ulcers, shrunken thymus. Animals that can exert control over the experimental stimulus show more of a defensive reaction (Henry, 1976).

Thus, the key elements that determine the

kind and degree of response to psychosocial stimuli appear to be: (1) appraisal of control over the situation, (2) predictability of stimulus, and (3) severity of stimulus (Levine, Weinberg, & Ursin, 1978; Weiss, 1968). The idea of appraisal as a prime factor in determining the response to stimuli comes from the work of Richard Lazarus (1975, pp. 47–67).

sex-related differences in physiologic response to stress

Very little of the research defining adaptive response of physiologic systems to physical and emotional stimuli has been done with women or female animals, still less comparing the responses of male and female to the same stimuli. Nevertheless, even with so little data, some consistent differences in physiologic adaptive response do emerge. The areas studied most frequently are physiologic responses to exercise, heat and cold, and emotion and mental tasks.

exercise

Muscular exercise is commonly classed as stress by physiologists because consistent adaptive responses are evoked in a number of physiologic systems. Heart rate and cardiac output increase to meet the increased blood flow need of muscles. Muscles increase their requirement for and use of cell nutrients— oxygen and glucose. At the same time, rate of breathing increases to supply more oxygen to cells. Breakdown and utilization of glucose increases (glycogenolysis); manufacture and storage of glucose for future needs (gluconeogenesis) decreases, as do other energy-conserving processes. Catecholamines (epinephrine and norepinephrine) are released and serve to increase cardiac output and utilization of glucose.

Most research describing physiologic response to exercise was conducted with well-trained male athletes. In most cases, comparison data of male and female response was derived from studies of nonathletically trained women and men with different degrees of skill. In addition, many studies did not take into account differences in weight between male and female subjects in reporting variables in which weight is a factor. Measures of cardiac output, oxygen utilization, and catecholamines are examples in which body mass affects the numerical value of the data.

In studies in which body weight and level of athletic training are not held constant or taken into account, women after puberty consistently have lower oxygen consumption, lower oxygen utilization, higher pulse rate, but lower cardiac output than men with a given degree of exercise stimulus. Prior to puberty, there are no significant differences in male-female response to exercise (Astrand & Astrand, 1978). The most common stimulus is stationary bicycle pedaling or running in place on a treadmill with a given slope and speed.

When both men and women in a study are given specific conditioning exercise and when lean weight is taken into account (by expressing values in units/kilogram), the differences in cardiac output and maximal oxygen uptake are smaller, but women continue to show about 20 percent smaller oxygen uptake than do men. Heart rates are higher on the average during maximal exercise. There is some evidence that, in endurance exercise, such as marathon running, women utilize glucose more efficiently than men. It is interesting to note that, although laboratory measurements of exercise variables show an average 20 percent difference between women and men—suggesting a physiologic disadvantage to women in athletic contests—actual differences in competitive times in swimming and running are considerably smaller (Astrand & Astrand, 1978). Similarly, the times for women to complete such endurance events as marathon running have been decreasing at a far more rapid rate than for men (Weissman, 1980). These observations support the contention that in real-life situations relative lack of physical training, rather than absolute limitations in physiological response capacities, have accounted for most of the observed differences in competitive athletic performance.

heat and cold

Change in environmental temperature has been used as a "physiologic" stressor for many years. Selye's (1965) work suggested that both heat and cold acted to produce the nonspecific stress response. In other words, the corticosteroid, immunologic, and gastric changes that occurred in addition to the sweating and shivering were not specific to the heat or cold stimulus itself.

Mason (1975) points out, however, that the nonspecific responses (Selye's "general adaptation" syndrome) were more likely related to psychological distress regarding the manner in which the primary stimuli were applied. In all of Selye's experiments, the animals were handled, restrained, or removed from contact with human keepers. Such factors likely provoke intense emotional arousal, which then acts as the nonspecific stressor. If the environmental temperature is changed in such a manner that emotional arousal is not added as a variable, physiologic response to heat and cold are quite different (Mason, 1975). The primary goal of physiologic response systems

with environmental temperature changes is to maintain the core temperature (around the heart, brain, and vital organs).

In general, heat acts as a stimulus to the energy-dissipating systems: catecholamine production decreases, thyroid hormone decreases, surface vessels dilate, and perspiration occurs to lose heat from the body. Cold has the opposite effect. Energy is produced in an attempt to make heat and thus conserve the core temperature of the body. Catecholamines are released and stimulate increased heart rate, increased force of cardiac contraction, and a general increase in metabolism. Surface blood vessels constrict to prevent heat loss to the environment. Visceral vessels dilate to provide more blood to core organs. Eventually, shivering occurs and the increased muscular metabolism involved produces more heat. Glycogenolyis (glucose breakdown) occurs to produce more fuel for energy; thyroid hormone is released to increase metabolism. In summary, the response to cold is similar to the defensive stress response described earlier, and the response to heat is similar to the withdrawal response.

It is a common assumption that men perspire more readily and more profusely than do women in hot environments and that women tolerate cold better than men due to their relatively greater insulating fat layer. There is little research directed toward validating these assumptions. Concern with protection of the health of industrial workers in the late 1960s promoted some studies of male and female responses to heat and exercise. In men and women who were not conditioned for the physical task (bicycle pedaling), there was a distinct difference in response, with women's responses to exercise being similar to sedentary men (Nunnelly, 1978).

When men and women in the same study have both had physical conditioning, the men have a greater maximum oxygen uptake than women in both cold and hot environments. This difference stems from difference in lean body weight. In several studies of conditioned men and women who exercised in hot environments, the men began to perspire sooner and had a greater volume of sweat. The rectal temperature of the women returned to normal at a much faster rate than did that of the men (Hori, Mayuzuni, Tanaka, & Tsujita, 1978; Nadel, Roberts, & Wagner, 1978, pp. 391–52; Nunnelly, 1978). These results suggest that, despite greater heat-losing mechanism in men, women's bodies are more efficient in returning body temperature to normal. Core temperature in both groups rose to about 39°C (102°F) during the peak of exercise (Fox et al., 1969). Exercise in hot laboratory environments has been described as comparable to physical labor in a hot factory. Both men and women performed equally well physically. Nor were there any sex-related differences in maximum tolerable temperature (Nadel et al., 1978, pp. 29–38; Paolone, Wells, & Kelly, 1978). It is important to repeat that these findings are from a relatively small number of people, with highly specialized testing conditions. The responses of individual men and women to everyday extremes of heat and cold will be highly variable.

There is almost no controlled data regarding male-female response to environmental cold. Nunnelly (1978) reviewed the available studies and concluded no evidence that metabolic response (energy production) differs between men and women in cold air. Women consistently had lower skin temperatures than men, related to the greater subcutaneous fat layer of women. This insulating layer may account for the disproportionate number of women who are successful in distance swimming in cold water (such as across the English Channel).

emotional arousal and mental tasks

The majority of stress research in recent years has focused on stimuli that carry emotional connotations, perhaps in recognition of the key role of psychological factors in the "nonspecific" stress response. Unfortunately, the majority of studies, particularly in humans, have measured either the pituitary adrenocortical axis (hormone-pituitary response) *or* sympathoadrenomedullary axis (adrenal-sympathetic nervous system chemical response), but not both. While early stress theory supported the idea that corticosteroid measures were good indicators of generalized stress and emotional arousal, current work demonstrates that many measures of arousal are necessary (Mason, 1975). If there is more than one mode of "nonspecific" physiologic response to the same stimulus, and if the pattern is consistent with such factors as social position, magnitude of the stimulus, sex, or other factors, it is imperative that researchers incorporate multiple neuroendocrine measures and evaluate individual patterns as well as group response.

Here, we consider emotional arousal and mental tasks together. In most persons, the accomplishment of a mental task (such as arithmetic, color matching, word recognition) in a laboratory or real-life setting can be presumed to carry some degree of emotional arousal. Such elements as time limit and internal or external pressure to do well can be expected to contribute to a view of the situation as emotionally arousing. Levi (1972) has shown that even those situations viewed as pleasurable create sufficient arousal to activate the sympathetic nervous system. Almost the entire literature supporting generalizations regarding activation of the sympathoadrenomedullary and pituitary adrenocortical systems in emotional arousal stem from male volunteers in laboratory or real-life situations. Such groups as armed forces recruits in navy pilot training and combat situations have furnished rich data regarding neuroendocrine responses (Bourne, 1969). Only Ursin, Baade, and Levine (1979), however, have furnished long-term data for multiple systems, and only in men.

Two laboratory studies showed a decrease in plasma corticosteroid metabolites (which indirectly measure pituitary adrenal activation) during hypnosis in both males and females. Interestingly, when anxiety was induced during the trance, only the women showed an increase in plasma corticosteroids (Grosz, 1961; Persky et al., 1959). A more recent study by Frankenhauser and her colleagues evaluated cortisol (hormone) levels in the urine of men and women during entrance examinations and during laboratory cognitive-conflict tasks. In both cases, urinary cortisol increased in both sexes, but most markedly in men (Collins & Frankenhauser, 1978; Frankenhauser et al., 1978). These findings are in direct opposition to those of the earlier hypnotists.

Levi and Frankenhauser have done extensive work with catecholomine responses of humans to laboratory and real-life psychological stressors. Their early work was primarily with men or with women only in a work situation. The unexpected absence of the "typical" epinephrine response in women in studies in the 1970s led Frankenhauser to begin comparing the catecholamine response of men and women to both laboratory and real-life mental and emotional stimuli. Her work, although with small samples, has consistently shown, on the average, a considerably smaller epinephrine response in women than in men to a variety of emotional stimuli. It must be remembered, however, that individual men

and women will be quite variable from the average. Any given woman may have a considerably greater or smaller epinephrine response than may a given man.

Norepinephrine is released at nerve endings of the sympathetic nervous system and is always found in the plasma portion of circulatory blood. Epinephrine is secreted primarily by the adrenal medulla (central portion of the adrenal gland) and only when there is a stimulus requiring a defensive response. Both epinephrine and norepinephrine increase in such circumstances, with epinephrine to a much greater degree.

One of the first studies to suggest a sex-related catecholamines response to emotionally arousing stimuli was conducted by Levi (1972). He had previously found (in a male population) that both funny and frightening movies produced a rise in urinary epinephrine and norepinephrine, while a neutral (nature scenes) movie created little change. He then investigated the effects of an erotic film on males and females. The men, as a group, showed the expected effect of emotional arousal; both epinephrine and norepinephrine increased significantly from baseline. The values for women, however, were not significantly different from baseline. For both men and women, some individuals had little change and some had marked change; however, as a group, the differential response was evident.

At that time it was assumed that male and female catecholamine responses to emotional arousal were similar; thus, Levi concluded that these women were not as emotionally aroused by the films. Indeed, the self-reports supported this idea, although many women did report arousal. If this study is viewed in the light of Frankenhauser's more recent work, one must conclude that the women's physiologic response to the erotic film differed from men's more than did the ability of the film to serve as an arousing stimulus.

Frankenhauser and her colleagues have conducted a series of studies investigating the effects of mental tasks, cognitive conflict, venipuncture (fear), and college entrance examinations in male and female children and adults (Collins & Frankenhauser, 1978; Frankenhauser, Dunne, & Lundberg, 1976; Frankenhauser & Johansson, 1975, pp. 118–126; Frankenhauser et al., 1978). All values for urinary catecholamines were equalized for differences in weight between male and female.

The studies together showed remarkable consistency in the following features:

As a group, women had significantly less rise in epinephrine and cortisol during emotional arousal than did men; norepinephrine values were similar for both.

Real-life testing (entrance exam) provoked greater epinephrine rises in both men and women, but as a group, women's levels were significantly lower.

Children by age 12 had the same patterns as adults.

Mental tasks and venipuncture (fear) provoked the same pattern of response with the same male-female difference.

Women reported more feelings of psychic distress than men with each situation.

In women, those who felt most successful had low adrenaline and cortisol response. Actual success or performance was greatest in those who experienced high to medium discomfort.

In men, those who felt good about their performance tended to have higher adrenaline and to actually do well; women who felt bad about their performance actually did best.

Differences in adrenaline and cortisol excretion between men and women had no relationship to differences in performance. Men and women did equally well in both laboratory and real-life situations.

An earlier Levi (1972) study of 12 women alternately paid by piecework versus salary showed some increase in epinephrine and sense of distress during piecework days (assumed to be higher stress). The reported levels, if corrected for an "average weight," are similar to those reported by Frankenhauser for laboratory situations in women; that is, lower than men's in studies of real-life, time-pressured situations.

Although Frankenhauser's data are not reported for individuals, she noted marked individual differences among the women, and also in pilot data for a woman coworker. Wondering if women who choose more traditionally "masculine" work might have catecholamine patterns more similar to men, she and coworkers studied male and female engineering students with a laboratory mental test. This was the first of such studies to compare men and women on both catecholamines and pituitary adrenocortical measures. The women in this small sample did increase epinephrine significantly from baseline, but they were still significantly lower as a group than the men. There were no sex-related differences in norephinephrine. Interestingly, the increase in urinary cortisol was evident for both sexes, but not significantly greater than baseline in women. The increase in cortisol was greater than that seen in the female high school students during the matriculation examination (Frankenhauser et al., 1978). Pierce, Kupprat, and Harry (1976) reported that women athletes preparing for competition excreted significantly more epinephrine and norepinephrine than did their female teammates in training. They interpreted this increase as reflecting the "mental stress" of anticipated competition as additive to exercise alone. Unfortunately, it is impossible to compare their data to those of Frankenhauser because of the differences in the way the units of the biochemicals are reported.

The physiological mechanisms underlying

this apparent difference between men and women in epinephrine responses are not known at this time. Estrogen and epinephrine share enzymes at one point in their metabolic pathways (Paul & Axelrod, 1977; Yen, 1978). Thus, it may be that circulating estrogen is a factor in the lower response of women. No variations in epinephrine response have been found during the menstrual cycle (Patkai, Johansson, & Post, 1974), and there are no data available from postmenopausal women to shed light on this theory.

Small numbers of comparative studies suggest quantitative differences in corticosteroid response between healthy men and women. The higher incidence of depression in women and the related disturbance in diurnal rhythm of corticosteroid indicate the need for more comparative study in this area.

These works represent a wide variety of environmental and emotional stimuli. A few consistent differences in response of men and women have emerged: decreased female oxygen capacity in exercise, increased rate of return to normal body temperature after heat stress in women, and decreased epinephrine and corticosteroid response to emotional stimuli in women. These differences are important in evaluating any data that would apply to people when the source of the data is only male people.

origins of differences
in response

The consistent differences between men and women in physiological response to the adaptive stimuli raises the age-old "nature versus nurture" questions. Are these differences inherent in the obvious differences in physical build of men and women, or are they learned as we learn other sex roles? Do some of the socially assigned sex roles arise because of inherent physiologic differences, for example, to work, heat, aggressive defensive response to threat? Or does the assumption of sex roles suppress certain physiologic responses? For example, do women who assume the traditional female nurturing role suppress epinephrine response in the face of emotional arousal, or is the decrease in epinephrine a factor in promoting a withdrawal response to threat? The poor correlation between subjective sense of distress and epinephrine levels in women suggest that epinephrine may not play a significant role in subjective sense of comfort in women related to emotional arousal. Although male aggressive behavior has been linked to greater levels of testosterone, the relationship of testosterone to epinephrine is not clear.

One might speculate that the heightened catecholamine defensive response to psychosocial stimuli in men is a factor in the higher incidence of cardiovascular disease. There is direct evidence in animals, but not in humans, that prolonged stimulation of the brain areas influencing sympathetic response results in arteriosclerosis, hypertension, and heart disease. The incidence of such disease is lower in premenopausal women and is often attributed to the antiatherogenic effect of estrogens. Perhaps the decreased catecholamine response in women interacts with estrogen in a protective fashion.

Depressive illnesses have been linked in both animals and humans with decreased brain and circulatory norepinephrine, and with altered diurnal cycles of corticosteroids. In animal studies, situational variables such as loss of control, lack of predictability of aversive stimuli, and extreme fear without an avenue of escape have all produced physiologic changes characteristic of the withdrawal mode—depleted catecholamine, gastric ulcers, increased corticosteroids, altered immune mechanisms. There is insufficient data to even speculate regarding male-female differences in these responses.

Frankenhauser (1978) sums up implications of sex-related differences in catecholamine response as: " . . . the physiologic cost involved in coping with the situation seems to have been lower for females than for males. In psychological terms . . . the results suggest that the cost was higher for females. More intense sense of discomfort and lack of a sense of satisfaction with performance characterized women more than men" (p. 334).

It is impossible to define succinctly the implications of sex-related physiologic differences in response to stress for one's personal guidance. Although groups of men and women differed from each other, given individuals did not necessarily conform to the group pattern. Thus, an individual woman may have higher epinephrine, oxygen-carrying capacity or earlier sweat level than an individual man, and vice versa.

Any individual, seeking to understand his or her own patterns of response to environmental or psychosocial stimuli (stressors), will do best to become aware of the signals given by our own bodies in these situations—in other words, "get in touch with one's own body."

Patterns of defensive-aggressive reaction are shown by musculoskeletal responses—tight muscles, clenched fist, "nervous fidgeting"; automatic sympathetic nervous system responses—dry mouth, dilated pupils, increased heart rate or pounding heart, perspiring palms and underarms, and in some situations sensations of skin tightening or "crawling."

The felt perceptions of withdrawal response are not so closely correlated with physiologic systems, but may be evident in decreased movement, psychomotor apathy,

"blue" or depressed feelings, awareness of stomach and intestinal movement. Once aware of one's own typical pattern of response, analysis of its appropriateness to the stimulus is necessary. Responses that are prolonged or continual (too much, too long, too often) are signals that a change in patterns may be in order. Even if a particular pattern of response is more common to males than females, it can be changed if it is leading to ill health.

Astrand, I., & Astrand, P. Aerobic work performance: a review. In F. J. Folinsbee (Ed.), *Environmental stress*. New York: Academic Press, 1978.

Bourne, P. (Ed.). *The Physiology and psychology of stress* (wtih special reference to studies of the Viet Nam War). New York: Academic Press, 1969.

Cannon, W. B. *The wisdom of the body*. New York: Norton, 1963 (reprint of 1939 edition).

Collins, A., & Frankenhauser, M. Stress responses in male and female engineering students. *Journal of Human Stress*, June 1978, *4(2)*, 43–48.

Fox, R. H. et al. Comparison of thermoregulatory function in men and women. *Journal of Applied Physiology*, 1969, *26*, 444–453.

Frankenhauser, M., Dunne, E., & Lundberg, U. Sex differences in sympathetic-adrenal medullary reactions induced by different stressors. *Psychopharmacology*, May 5, 1976, *47*, 1–5.

Frankenhauser, M., & Johansson, G. Behavior and catecholamines in children. In L. Levi (Ed.), *Society, stress and disease*, Vol. 2, *Childhood and adolescence*. London: Oxford University Press, 1975.

Frankenhauser, M. et al Sex differences in psychoneuroendocrine reactions to examination stress. *Psychosomatic Medicine*, June 1978, *40*, 334–343.

Gellhorn, E. The neurophysiological basis of anxiety: A (sic) hypothesis. *Perspectives in Biology and Medicine*, 1965, *8(4)*, 488–515.

Grosz, H. J. The relation of serum ascorbic acid level to adrenocortical secretion during experimentally induced emotional stress in human subjects. *Journal of Psychosomatic Research*, 1961, *5*, 253.

Henry, J. P. Mechanisms of psychosomatic disease in animals. *Advances in Veterinary Science*, 1976, *20*, 115–145.

Hori, S., Mayuzuni, M., Tanaka, N., & Tsujita, J. Oxygen uptake of men and women during exercise and recovery in a hot environment and a comfortable environment. In F. J. Folinsbee (Ed.), *Environmental stress.* New York: Academic Press, 1978.

Johansson, G. Sex differences in catecholamine output of children. *Acta Physiologica Scandanavia,* 1972, *85,* 569–572.

Lazarus, R. *Psychological stress and the coping process.* New York: McGraw-Hill, 1966.

Lazarus, R. Self-regulation of emotion. In L. Levi (Ed.), *Emotions: Their parameters and measurements.* New York: Raven Press, 1975.

Levi, L. Stress and distress in response to psychosocial stimuli. *International Series of Monographs in Experimental Psychology,* 1972, *17.*

Levine, S., Weinberg J., & Ursin, H. Definition of the coping process and statement of the problem. In H. Ursin, E. Baade, and S. Levine (Eds.), *The psychobiology of stress: A study of coping men.* New York: Academic Press, 1978.

Mason, J. W. Organization of the multiple endocrine responses to avoidance in the monkey. *Psychosomatic Medicine,* September-October 1968, *30(5),* 774–79;, suppl.

Mason, J. W. A historical view of the stress field, part 2. *Journal of Human Stress,* June 1975, *1(2),* 22–36.

Nadel, E. R., Roberts, M. F., & Wagner, C. B. Thermoregulatory adaptations to heat and exercise: Comparative responses of men and women. In F. J. Folinsbee (Ed.), *Environmental stress.* New York: Academic Press, 1978.

Nunnelly, S. A. Physiological responses of women to thermal stress: A review. *Medicine and Science in Sports,* 1978, *10,* 250–255.

Paolone, A. M., Wells, C. L., & Kelly, G. T. Sexual variations in thermoregulation during heat stress. *Aviation, Space and Environmental Medicine,* May 1978, *49, 715–719.*

Patkai, P., Johannson, G., Post, B. Mood, alertness and sympatheticadrenal medullary activity during the menstrual cycle. *Psychosomatic Medicine,* November-December 1974, *36,* 503–512.

Paul, S. M., & Axelrod, J. Catechol-estrogens: Presence in brain and endocrine tissues. *Science,* August 12, 1977, *197,* 657–659.

Persky, H. et al. Effect of hypnotically-induced anxiety on plasma hydrocortisone level of normal subjects. *Journal of Clinical Endocrinology,* 1959, *19,* 700.

Pierce, D., Kupprat, I., and Harry, D. Urinary Epinephrine and norepinephrine levels in women athletes during training and competition. *European Journal of Applied Physiology,* 1976, *36,* 1–6.

Schachter, S., & Singer, S. E. Cognitive, social and physiological determinants of emotional state. *Psychological Review,* 1962, *69,* 379–399.

Selye, H. *The stress of life.* New York: McGraw-Hill, 1965.

Ursin, H., Baade, E., & Levine, S. *The psychobiology of stress: A study of coping men.* New York: Academic Press, 1979.

Weiss, J. Effects of coping response on stress. *Journal of Comparative and Physiological Psychology,* 1968, *65,* 251–260.

Weissman, G. Guilty With an explanation: Reflections on the marathon. *Hospital Practice.* February 1980, *17(2),* 121–126.

Yen, S. S. C. The human menstrual cycle. In S. S. C. Yen and R. B. Jaffee (Eds.). *Reproductive endocrinology: physiology, pathophysiology and clinical management.* Philadelphia: Saunders, 1978.

14

KAREN VANDUSEN, M.S.P.H.

the effect of the environment on women's health

Personal health is intricately and intimately linked with the health and values of the community in which one resides. It may even be said that in creating its way of life, a society simultaneously creates its way of death (Eckholm, 1977). This can be seen by observing the impact on health that results from a community's beliefs, values, and decisions regarding basic environmental issues. In the lesser developed countries, the environment's contribution to disease transmission or cause is a poorly understood or rejected concept. It is not uncommon for low-income rural mothers to watch helplessly as any number of their children die from chronic diarrhea, unaware that sanitary water supplies and waste disposal would largely eradicate this infec-

tious killer. For contrast, in countries with advanced technologies, such as the United States, the cause of death is more likely to come from chronic illnesses such as cancer and diseases of the heart. The evidence is mounting that the environment plays a major and complex role in these deaths and diseases. Some estimate that 60 to 90 percent of cancer cases can be attributed to personal, voluntary environmental exposures, for example, smoking and life-style, or involuntary community environmental exposures (Warren, 1978). The involuntary exposures may reflect the changes characteristic of modern society, such as urbanization, increase and use of motor vehicles, discovery and use of several energy forms such as nuclear energy, and the spectac-

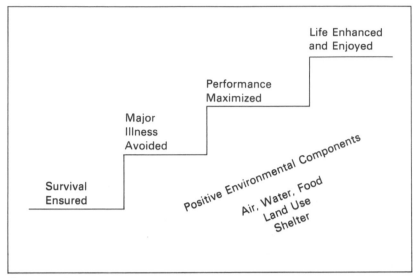

figure 14.1
environmental components and human health

ular rise of the synthetic chemical industry.

Almost any environmental factor can, and probably does, impact on the quality of a person's life. Some of the interactions are positive, and some are distinctly negative. While individuals constantly modify the environment in an effort to optimize living conditions, there is plentiful evidence that poorly planned modifications may actually lead to hazardous environments. Environmental factors influence survival, cause acute and chronic disease, interfere with or enhance the full use and enjoyment of lives or lands, and when well managed can maximize performance, enjoyment, and quality of life. They can be considered the foundation upon which individuals and communities can build and progress (see Figure 14.1).

Potentially hazardous environmental exposures can occur wherever a person is—whether at home or at work. With the emergence of a newer freedom for women in recent years and better opportunities for occupational fulfillment, women must analyze the potential that their roles and settings have for environmental exposures that may be detrimental to health. The following sections will examine some of the general environmental factors in the home and on the job that may be of particular concern to women.

the home

Few words project more emotionalism than the word *home*. For most Americans, it represents far more than basic shelter, but encompasses a host of hopes, memories, endeavors, and financial commitments. Although the average American spends about 55 percent of his or her time in a household environment, for many women—particularly those who may be pregnant, and for infants and young children—the indoor environment of the home determines a large part of their total environmental exposure (Fritsch, 1978; Kane, 1976).

While any shelter should provide for basic psychological and physiological needs, at least four types of potentially hazardous environmental agents may impact housing quality: agents arising outside the home; agents "built in" the structures; agents "brought-in" the home; and agents generated by the inhabitants themselves (Radford, 1976). Examples of some of these agents and other health impacts of housing follow.

environmental agents outside the home

The problems of multiple land use in communities and the juxtaposition of residential and industrial zones can significantly affect housing quality and health. As an example, in December 1971, the City-County Health Department in El Paso, Texas, discovered that an ore smelter was discharging large quantities of lead and other metallic wastes into the air ("Human Lead Absorption," 1973). From community surveys it was estimated that undue lead absorption affected persons across all of southern and western El Paso to a distance of at least four miles from the smelter. The resulting control measures involved the relocation to more distant public housing of approximately 500 persons who had lived close to smelter property.

In early 1980, two miles east of Globe, Arizona, approximately 120 residents in a 44-home mobile housing subdivision were found to be excessively exposed to asbestos ("Asbestos Exposure," 1980). The subdivision was built on the property of an inactive

asbestos mill, where mill tailings were used as landfill during the initial grading of the site. In addition, the active operating mill was situated 1,000 feet upwind of the mobile homes. Indoor air samples during household activities such as vacuuming revealed concentrations of asbestos fibers in excess of the occupational exposure standards recommended by the National Institute for Occupational Safety and Health (NIOSH). These standards, incidentally, were not designed for the population at large, who may be exposed to asbestos up to 24 hours per day, but for an occupational exposure based on only an eight-hour work day.

These serve as examples of air pollutants arising outside the home that clearly affect the quality of the home environment. However, effects on health from air pollutants, although strongly suspect, have been extremely difficult to document because of the multiple exposures people receive, the lag time typical of the chronic diseases that are suspected of being linked with air pollutants, and the many factors that govern exposure time and body reaction.

People with pre-existing health problems, such as asthma, bronchitis, emphysema, or related cardio-pulmonary problems, seem to be the most susceptible to the hazards of air pollutants. Most specific health links with air pollutants, such as sulfur dioxide and ozone, have been documented among such previously stressed individuals. However, for carbon monoxide (CO), evidence of both acute and chronic health effects has been documented for some time. Perhaps most disconcerting in this regard is a study conducted during the 1970s in New York City. Surprising results followed the monitoring of the air in an apartment building straddling an expressway and in an older 20-story office building located in mid-Manhattan. At ground level there were no significant differences between CO concentrations inside and outside the buildings. Although CO decreased with elevation, during the heating season CO standards established by the federal government were exceeded nearly 20 percent of the time even on the 32nd floor of the apartment building. On the third floor of the office building, CO standards were exceeded nearly 50 percent of the time ("26 Health Departments," 1973). In this instance, there was no escaping air pollution!

Particularly with the effort to insulate and tighten homes due to energy conservation, those women at home need to be aware that concentrations of their daily air pollutants may not be as readily diluted by air flow in and out of the home as in the past. The hazards and impacts they face may actually increase in the future.

Recognizing the limitations of little specific toxicology information and no firm concrete evidence, there is concern about community efforts in vector control through pesticide application. For example, in the spring of 1978, the U.S. Forest Service sprayed an Oregon valley with two herbicides. Within two weeks, 5 of 7 pregnant women in the area miscarried, and eventually about 50 households in the area reported new health problems. Coincidence or correlation? It is not known, but a few years before the same valley had been sprayed with the herbicide 2-4-5-T; a rash of miscarriages occurred and the herbicide was banned, at least temporarily ("Herbicides," 1979). The principle concern may not be whether the spraying caused the problems, but the fact that households were unknowingly exposed to a potentially toxic chemical. These examples clearly demonstrate how important agents arising *outside* the home may be to the health status of the home environment.

environmental agents built in

There are a number of "built-in" potential environmental problems in the home. Women who may in some way avoid major exposure to community-based air pollutants are still exposed to products derived from heating, cooking, and dust and lint from fabrics. Oxides of nitrogen, carbon monoxide, sulfur dioxide, and particulates generated by indoor activities may exceed outdoor concentrations of these primary air pollutants (Kane, 1976; Radford, 1976). Improperly vented gas stoves can contribute heavy nitrogen oxide concentration—even 20 times the federal air quality standards (Kane, 1976). The cozy fireplace and/or wood stove can be a major source of respirable air particulates ("Wood Burning," 1979).

Another built-in factor receiving much attention is formaldehyde. Widely used in the manufacturing industry and found in such items as pressboard, household paneling, cosmetics, deodorants, urea-formaldehyde spray-foam insulation, and in a permanent-press finish, formaldehyde has been shown to cause allergic reactions and subsequent dermatitis among some women in the textile and clothing industries (*Occupational Diseases*, 1977; Stellman, 1977). Recent evidence is pointing to the home as a significant site for formaldehyde exposures and subsequent eye and upper respiratory irritation. The growing number of consumer complaints and documented problems, particularly in mobile homes, marks this as a potentially widespread health problem in need of careful study (Breysse, 1979).

One of the major categories of death in all age groups is accidents, and built-in factors in housing contribute to their occurrence. Excluding motor vehicles, falls constitute the major category of injury-related deaths in the United States. Approximately 15,000 people are killed and 14 million are injured each year by falls. The majority of these falls occur in the home (*Healthy People*, 1979; Tate, 1979). Women are a particularly high-risk group for fall injury. Elderly females have a relative risk of death due to falling that is 660 times that of young boys and two times that of elderly men ("Injuries Due to Falls," 1978; Neutra, 1972). The sites typically associated with home injuries with respect to falls are stairways and bathrooms (*Design Guide*, 1972).

Drowning is another major cause of injury deaths. Surprisingly, it is not in the public swimming areas where drownings are likely to occur, but in one's own backyard. The estimated 4 million pool-owning families are increasing annually, and while only 7 percent of all drownings nationally occur in swimming pools, about half of these occur in residential home pools, with motels, hotels, apartments, and condominiums accounting for another 20 percent (VanDusen & Fraser, 1977). Unintentially falling into water accounts for nearly half of all drownings, particularly among young persons, but a variety of other contributing factors, including alcohol, are also important factors.

Deaths attributable to fires and burns are another major injury category. About 5,000 deaths result from fires each year—predominantly house fires—and about two-thirds of the burn injuries resulting in hospitalization occur in the home (Tate, 1979). Many deaths and injuries could be prevented with good fire and smoke detection, less flammable furnishings and structural materials, and buildings designed for ease of escape. A number of investigations have shown that the greatest hazard to individuals in a fire is exposure to combustion products; an estimated 55 to 75 percent of all fire victims die from inhalation of toxic combustion products (Schumacher & Breysse, 1976). The effort to make materials fire-retardant may actually be increasing the life hazard, since incomplete combustion of these products results in heavy smoke and toxic gases ("Fire," 1973).

Another built-in factor that is seldom viewed as a potential health problem is modern plumbing. Although probably infrequent, a plumbing cross-connection—an actual link between the water and waste water systems—is one example of such a potential health hazard. Residential premises are not immune from cross-connection hazards. For example, if the hose and nozzle used to rinse dishes in the kitchen sink are inadvertently left in the water that fills the sink, polluted sink water can easily be pulled through the hose into the supply lines should a vacuum develop. In New England, a termite-control operator pushed a garden hose to the bottom of a drum containing three gallons of a pesticide concentrate, unaware that simultaneously a water main flushing in the vicinity was causing a momentary negative pressure. This caused back-siphonage of the pesticide into the water lines and necessitated isolating and draining the water supply to 500 homes (Ruskin, 1968).

Corrosion of plumbing lines, particularly in areas of soft water, may be another problem. Improved heavy metal-detection techniques and increased consumer advocacy make it possible to question the potential health effects of corrosion products, such as lead, cadmium, and copper, which may be ingested with drinking water. Reports from a Boston study indicated that the lead contamination of drinking water in many Boston, Summerville, and Cambridge homes substantially exceeded minimum federal safety standards. Nearly 60 percent of the households had some lead in either the service line and/or plumbing ("Water Corrosion," 1976). There is good evidence that water, in contact with lead pipes, solder, or galvanized pipe, may cause excessive exposure and an increase in total body burden of lead. This is particularly true in water that has stood in house plumbing for an indeterminate period. For the "average" consumer, the chronic health impact of continuous ingestion of minute amounts of heavy metals from several environmental sources, including water, is unknown.

agents brought in

Other concerns in the home environment are those factors that may be brought in. For example, one of the newer cooking techniques finding its way into today's busy homes is the microwave oven. Slashing energy needs, cooking time, as well as clean-up time, it is touted as a redeemer for women working outside the home. However, it also introduces an energy form about which few consumers know a great deal. Basically, microwaves for cooking are an outgrowth of microwave technology employed in radar development. They are a form of nonionizing radiation. When absorbed, their primary effect is heating—the basic principle of microwave kitchen cooking. The interaction of microwaves and materials in their path depends on the conductivity of the material. A nearly perfect conductor, such as any metal, reflects microwave energy; a perfect insulator, such as glass, provides no absorption and hence transmits the energy. Biological tissue interacts in an intermediate way, showing some reflection, absorption, and transmission. The major impacts on humans have centered on the effects of heating in certain sensitive and critical organs, namely the eye and testicles. In the United States, the evidence of injury has been confined to cataracts and lens opacities, linked with high-powered occupational exposures. To date the safety standards set by the Food and Drug Administration seem to provide a good margin of safety for home microwave ovens. As long as operating procedures are followed, interlocks and safety devices not damaged, and door seals kept clean, home microwave ovens can be safely used (Chanlett, 1979).

A major portion of every family budget is marked for the groceries brought into the home. Yet, this food can be a real health concern. Anyone who has ever suffered from food poisoning a few hours after a delicious meal topped by a custard pie does not need elaboration on the realities of foodborne illness. Food serves as a medium in which bacteria and viruses flourish and can be transmitted to humans. Food also serves as a mode of transmission for chemicals that may be hazardous to health. It is for the latter reason that using cookware containing cadmium is not allowed; pottery glazed with lead-containing pigments should never be used with acid foods; and any food product consumed should be from an approved source. Ignorance of such basic requirements was a major factor behind the tragedy that occurred in Japan between 1953 and 1960. Fishermen along Minamata Bay noted that fish swam erratically and when caught often appeared sick. With typical commercial acumen, they sold the best and took the sickest-looking fish home to their families. An epidemic of congenital defects among babies, disabling neurological symptoms among ill persons, and 43 deaths resulted (Waldbott, 1978). It was found later that the waterway, and hence the fish, had been contaminated by waste methylmercury from a factory that made vinyl plastic.

Although spectacular, such incidences are probably small in number compared to the thousands of persons who suffer ill health because of food that is inadequately cooked, contaminated after or during preparation, or kept at improper temperatures—all factors

table 14.1
common foodborne disease

FOODBORNE DISEASE	SYMPTOMS	INCUBATION PERIOD	TYPICAL SOURCE
Botulism	dizziness, double vision, swallowing difficulty, respiration difficulty	2 hours to 6 days (avg: 12–36 hrs)	improperly processed canned food as green beans, corn, chili peppers, asparagus, mushrooms, tuna
Staphylococcal Food Poisoning	nausea, vomiting, diarrhea, cramps, acute prostration	1–7 hours (avg: 2–4 hrs)	improperly prepared custards, cream-filled pastries, dairy products, warmed-over foods
Clostridium perfringens	acute abdominal pain and diarrhea	8–24 hours	meat inadequately cooked or allowed to cool slowly and served next day
Salmonellosis	abdominal pain, diarrhea, chills, fever, vomiting, prostration	5–72 hours, (avg: 12–24 hrs)	meat, meat products, poultry, egg custards, and other protein food
Paralytic Shellfish Poisoning	tingling or burning and numbness around lips and fingertips, giddiness, staggering, drowsiness, rash, incoherent speech	1 hour	mussels, clams, soft-shell clams, scallops, butter clams, shell-fish (contaminated by plankton causing "red tide")
Trichinosis	swollen eyelids, eye problems, diarrhea, muscle soreness, sweating, chills, weakness, fever	2–28 days	raw or insufficiently cooked animal flesh, particularly pork or "beef products"

Source: Abram S. Berenson, ed. *Control of Communicable Diseases in Man,* 12th ed. (Washington, D.C.: Public Health Assn., 1975) and Ben Freedman, *Sanitarian's Handbook,* 4th ed. (New Orleans, Peerless, 1977).

that allow pathogenic organisms to thrive. It is estimated that 2 million people are stricken by foodborne illness each year in the United States (Bradley & Sundberg, 1975). The number of these outbreaks attributed to "home cooking" is uncomfortably high.

It is difficult to document foodborne illness, as its symptoms are generally of short duration and characteristic of the flu—nausea, vomiting, abdominal cramping, and/or diarrhea. Table 14.1 indicates a few of the common illnesses, their symptoms, and typical associated foods.

Even though foodborne illness is so common, seldom does a homemaker wonder if the leftovers are safe. Unfortunately, the typical forms of spoilage or infection rarely show up through discrepancies in odor, taste, or appearance. Much of the problem, at least in the home, could be eliminated with improved personal hygiene when handling food, using only clean work surfaces and utensils, and taking simple precautions in storing, preparing, and cooking food. For example, pet turtles and the Easter baby chicks are terrific sources of Salmonella and should never be left in kitchens. Any surface that raw meat encounters should be thoroughly cleaned and sanitized prior to using with fresh products such as fruit. Better still is the maintenance of separate cutting boards for such items. Thawing under refrigeration rather than at room temperature; refrigerating leftovers immediately to a temperature less than 40°F (4.5°C); keeping foods to be served warm at a temperature of 140° (60°C); and using a ready and abundant supply of cleaning water are all basic to safe food handling.

Unfortunately, much of what is considered intolerable in a restaurant is common in the home. Public food sources and preparation are relatively closely regulated and monitored. Perhaps if more homes were, too, there would be fewer foodborne illnesses—including the dread botulism, which in the United States is most frequently associated with home-processed, low-acid foods.

Inhabitants themselves can bring a variety of contaminants such as viruses, bacteria, and chemicals into the home. In February 1977, a 25-year-old woman and her year-old son were hospitalized and treated for lead poisoning. The woman had worked for eight months at a battery factory in Raleigh, North Carolina, and apparently lead dust carried home on work clothes contaminated the household

("Lead Poisoning," 1977). Subsequent studies and other episodes indicate that exposure to contaminants brought home from the occupational setting is not rare. More than one young woman has learned of an impending death from malignant mesothelioma, a rare cancer found in asbestos workers. Why? Perhaps because as a daughter she laundered the clothes of a family member who was a worker in an asbestos insulation factory (Hricko & Marrett, 1975). A study of women with this rare cancer, attempting to measure risk attributable to *indirect* asbestos exposure, showed a greater number of fathers and husbands of the cases than of the controls had worked in asbestos-related industries (Vianna & Polan, 1978). Asbestos has many uses and is found in many products. Once known primarily as the cause of one of the chronic lung diseases, asbestosis, concern more recently has focused on its links with cancer. Concern is severe enough, in fact, that when in 1979 certain hair dryers widely used in homes were found to contain asbestos as an insulating material, the federal Consumer Product Safety Commission began a massive public education and recall effort to eliminate such dryers from homes and the marketplace.

In summary, the environmental agents found within and without the homes in which we reside appear to have subtle, but real and significant physical and mental health effects on our health.

the occupational setting

Increasing numbers of women work outside the home. In 1920, only 20 percent of the nation's work force was composed of women; in 1976, the number rose to 40 percent of the

labor force, and it is still rising (Hricko, 1976; Kuntz, 1976).

Women are still concentrated in occupations that reflect the domesticity of the conventional female role (Oakley, 1974). Clerical work is the major area of employment for women workers (Stellman, 1977). Among the 20 leading occupations of employed women are the following: secretaries; sales clerks, retail trade; bookkeepers; elementary schoolteachers; typists; waitresses; sewers and stitchers; registered nurses; cashiers; private household cleaners and servants; hairdressers and cosmetologists (Hricko, 1976). Female workers are disproportionately represented in assembly-line jobs, and despite publicity regarding female expansion in male-dominated fields, only about 8 percent of the female work force are employed in skilled crafts or management (Stellman, 1978).

One of the first problems encountered by women working outside the home is that they now hold two jobs. The International Labor Office has actually calculated that women throughout the world work approximately 80 hours per week, in comparison to husbands who work 50 hours (Stellman, 1978). This excessive work load may well be one source of stress for females in such a situation. The complex relationship between disease and stress has already been discussed. Job stress and demands, particularly when juggled with family responsibilities, can lead to increases in disease risk factors such as increased cholesterol levels and hypertension or to mental suffering and ill health—hefty impacts for women entering the job market (Stellman, 1977).

Historically, men have dominated the occupational settings outside the home, and the few early studies and concerns about occupational health consequently focused on men. However, in the late 1800s women workers were employed to make matches using phosphorus (lucifer matches). The phosphorus caused their jaws to erode, a condition both painful and disfiguring. This so-called phossy

jaws is the only occupational disease to have been completely eliminated; it resulted in stopping the manufacture of phosphorus matches (Stellman, 1977). In the 1920s came the highly publicized account of women who painted the numbers of watch dials with radium-containing paint so the watches would glow. Radium emits ionizing radiation, and these workers were later shown to have excess cases of severe anemia, degeneration of bone tissue, and cancer. Although such early tragedies made people more aware that occupational exposures could be hazardous, if that exposure were the only way to bring home economic support, few were willing to challenge the safety inadequacies that employers might maintain. In the United States, it took until the 1970s and the intervention of the federal government, through the Occupational Safety and Health Administration, to provide the focus, study, and continual pressure needed to ensure improved working environments. Many of the health hazards encountered in the workplace still need to be recognized, identified, quantified, and controlled or eliminated. Whether women have special susceptibilities to certain types of occupational exposures is a topic likely to be addressed only minimally. The regulatory efforts currently underway are aimed at reducing hazardous occupational exposures for *all* workers. Until such time that more specific research clarifies any particular problems, there will be a lack of baseline data on specific occupational health impacts on women. Presently, it appears that there are no significant physiological differences between male and female, on the average, that inherently make occupational settings more hazardous for women (Hricko, 1976). Only in the areas of strength and red blood cell counts (lower for women) are there differences that may be of concern, and even in the area of strength there is considerable individual variation, not an entire gender characteristic (Hricko, 1976).

Occupationally induced diseases are often hard to diagnose and identify. It is difficult to isolate occupational exposures from the myriad exposures to many toxic substances that individuals receive throughout a lifetime. Part of the problem reflects the often intermittent and hence ignored symptoms that occupational diseases may present. Some of these symptoms, such as cough, increased fatigue, loss of appetite, pain, and indigestion, are characteristic of many nonoccupational problems (Stellman & Daum, 1973). Also, although acute occupational problems, such as an injury due to poor safety practices or maintenance, are very evident, several of the occupational diseases that will affect many workers are chronic in nature, with evidence of a health hazard being felt 20 to 30 years after exposure. Current concerns with exposures to asbestos, benzene, and radiation reflect this awareness of a long-term effect.

Effects may also be local or systemic, depending somewhat on organ susceptibility as well as mode of entry of the contaminant to the body. Most commonly, skin absorption or inhalation provides entry pathways for hazardous agents. Some agents penetrate without being felt, enter the bloodstream, and are carried throughout the body. Carbon tetrachloride, a common ingredient in cleaning solvents, is one such chemical. It is extremely toxic to the liver and kidneys, and recent animal research links it with potential fetal damage and cancer (Hricko, 1976). Most of the poisons affecting the internal organs enter the body by inhalation (Stellman & Daum, 1973). Soluble substances, such as carbon monoxide, can then be absorbed from the lungs and travel via the blood to susceptible organs. Others, such as asbestos, may remain in the lung and cause serious local reactions.

Another complicating factor is that hazards may be encountered in physical, chemical, or biological form. In summary, for male *or* female, the number of potential occupational hazards and exposures is astounding.

physical hazards

The physical environmental hazards one may encounter in the work setting include noise and vibration, heat and cold, pressure differences, microwaves, radiation, illumination, general structural, and ergonometric factors. Some of these hazards are discussed in this section.

Exposure to noise has received much focus in occupational health programs. Noise, defined as unwanted sound, can be a matter of judgment, since sounds that one person appreciates are definitely noise to another. Excessive exposure to noise can result in physical or mental distress of either an acute or chronic nature. Although stress has a variety of causes, noise is certainly one of them, as the body stress reaction is continuous in the presence of noise (Stellman & Daum, 1973). Workers exposed to noise have complained of irritability and sleeping disturbances. Foreign studies report increased cardiovascular ailments in workers exposed to high levels of industrial noise (Lenihan & Fletcher, 1976). Chronic physical distress may be experienced when exposure to high levels of noise (over 80dBA) are encountered. The decibel (dB), a term used to measure sound, is a logarithmic scale based on sound-pressure levels. An arbitrary scale, the A scale (dBA), reflects the human ear's response to various pressure levels and frequency ranges.

Initial symptoms of hearing damage may include discomfort and headache, but permanent damage can develop if extensive exposure to noise continues over a period of years. A temporary threshold shift—temporary hearing loss after exposure to excessive sound—is not uncommon. Once away from the source of noise and given enough time, the ear usually recovers. But repeated exposures before complete recovery gradually erode hearing acuity. Levels of 85dBA and less are considered to be of negligible risk, although federal standards allow 90dBA exposure for an eight-hour day. Obviously, the length of exposure affects the possibility of hearing damage. Higher sound can be tolerated for shorter time periods.

Visible light is one form of electromagnetic energy, but it represents a very small band of the full electromagnetic spectrum, which includes such variable energy forms as microwaves, radar, AM-FM broadcasting, lasers, and X-rays. Ionizing radiation, which has enough energy to break atoms, cause electric charges, and thus produce "ions," is the portion of the spectrum people fear most. Numerous studies on groups of people with considerable exposure to ionizing radiation point out its hazards (Chanlett, 1979; Hricko, 1976; Waldbott, 1978). Among the evidence of health risk are the increased incidence of leukemia among radiologists and patients treated with X-rays for arthritis of the back; increased thyroid cancer among adults who as children were irradiated for enlarged thymus glands; a twofold increase in cancer among plutonium workers; and, depending on the gestation time for exposure, defects and increased risk for cancers among children whose mothers were exposed to radiation during pregnancy. It is well established that any woman, and particularly women workers who are pregnant, should avoid radiation exposure.

Although possibly considered a benign occupational setting, office work has many safety hazards, too. In this setting, the most common source of accidents is falls, followed by disabling injuries from lifting office equip-ment or working with office machines. One estimate records 40,000 disabling injuries and over 200 deaths among office workers annually (Warren, 1978).

chemical hazards

Even more impressive than the physical factors in occupational health are the incredible variety of chemicals to which workers are exposed. Chemicals can affect several different organs, cause a variety of diseases, and are common in many occupations. Typical chemicals found in occupational settings are arsenic, chromium, asbestos, free silica, vinyl chloride, lead, mercury, chlorine, carbon monoxide, hydrogen fluorides, and nitrous fumes. One or more affect the skin, lungs, liver, bone marrow, kidney, and blood (Corn, 1978).

Asbestos seems particularly ubiquitous, and while no longer simply an occupational problem, it was in that setting that its hazard was documented. Asbestos is a fibrous mineral composed of such fine fibers that they can be seen only with an electron microscope. Like cotton, it can be made into thread and cloth, and yet is extremely strong; it is nearly indestructible, heat- and fire-proof, and resistant to chemicals. It is found in thousands of products, such as potholders, welding rods, and insulation; hence, the industrial and commercial exposure is widespread (Stellman & Daum, 1973). The very fine fibers composing asbestos can float in the air much like water vapor, refusing to settle out. The fibers can also easily enter the lung, where they are as indestructible as outside the body. As many as 20 to 30 years after exposure to asbestos, the body cells can turn cancerous; the cells of the membrane lining the chest or abdomen seem particularly susceptible, producing the rare and fatal form of cancer known as mesothelioma. This can present a hazard to the worker, but also to family members, as discussed earlier.

Probably one of the most common occupational problems is contact dermatitis. Substances not normally irritating can cause dermatitis of the skin when an allergic reaction between the chemical and the skin immune system develops. Once the skin has become sensitized to a chemical, even years later minute quantities of the substance, and even at times similar substances, can cause a reaction. This complicated reaction, often termed hypersensitivity, is commonly seen around poison oak or poison ivy. In industrial settings, there are several common groups of chemicals causing contact dermatitis, such as plastics (as epoxy resins), germicidal agents (certain soaps and cleaners), nickel compounds (the nickel allergy is also common to many earring wearers), and a variety of organic and inorganic mercury compounds (Stellman & Daum, 1973).

Lead, produced in larger quantities than any other poisonous heavy metal, is widely used in industry and found in such products as paints, pesticides, gasoline, pipes, and solder (Hricko, 1976; Waldbott, 1978). It has been known as an occupational health hazard since ancient times. Lead is harmful to everyone, but especially to children. It affects the body's ability to produce red blood cells, can damage the nervous system, and has been related to kidney disease and high blood pressure (Stellman, 1977). As with asbestos, lead dust can and often does contaminate clothing, allowing occupational lead exposure to be inadvertently transferred home. There is some biological evidence that indicates women are more susceptible than men to the toxic effects of lead, and as early as the nineteeth century lead was known to have a damaging effect on fertility (male and female), fetal development, and

pregnancy (Rom, 1976). One theory holds that pregnancy produces a body stress that may mobilize lead from skeletal storage sites. Since both iron and calcium deficiencies, common during pregnancy and postpartum periods, increase susceptibility to lead toxicity, the particular risk that lead exposure may present to women cannot be ignored.

Hairdressers are occupationally and presumably extensively exposed to hair dyes, and recent studies link those products with increased risk of lung cancer. Hair dyes have also been found to be mutagenic (capable of causing mutations). Unfortunately, smoking habits among this occupational group may compound these problems (Menck, Pike, Henderson, & Jeng, 1977).

According to the industry, about 98 percent of the country's meat-wrappers are women. Normally, a polyvinyl-chloride (PVC) film is used to package meats. When the PVC film is cut with a hot wire during the wrapping process, over eight different chemicals and gases are released (Hricko, 1976). The resultant fumes have caused respiratory symptoms of shortness of breath, wheezing, and coughing while at work. At times, symptoms can be severe enough to force workers to quit their jobs. The specific agent càusing the "meat-wrapper's asthma" is unknown, but there are widespread accounts of the problem.

Table 14.2 shows some other occupational areas where women predominate and the hazards they potentially encounter. Improvements in occupational health are sometimes costly, but generally possible. However, it takes the awareness of the workers to avoid hazardous exposures and their cooperation to provide the data bases and control programs that enable the eight working hours to be not only productive, but environmentally enjoyable and safe.

table 14.2
potential health hazards in selected (female-dominated) occupations

OCCUPATION	ESTIMATED # OF WOMEN EMPLOYED	EXAMPLES OF POTENTIAL HEALTH HAZARDS	
Artists and Craftspeople (Professional)	250,000	lacquer and paint thinners paint and varnish removers lead, cadmium, and other metallic dust and fumes cleaning solvents	asbestos resins plastics
Clothing and Textile Workers (i.e., sewers, stitchers, textile operatives, ironers, pressers)	1,186,198	formaldehyde noise vibration cotton dust	flame-retardants solvents carbon disulfide benzidine-type dyes
Hairdressers and Cosmetologists	424,873	bleaches diethanolanine hair dyes nail varnishes (e.g., acetone, toluene, xylene, plasticizers)	heat noise ultraviolet light vibrating machines dermatitis
Health Care Professions (e.g., registered nurses, nursing aides, orderlies, attendants)	1,416,381	infection disinfectants and sterilizing agents (e.g., ozone, ethylene oxide, ultraviolet light) anesthetic gases	ionizing radiation mercury vapor back injuries puncture wounds and lacerations phenolic compounds
Household Workers	1,330,000	dermatitis (cleaning compounds) falls noise pesticides	formaldehyde solvents noise disinfectants
Laundry and Dry Cleaners	105,146	heat noise vibration back injuries solvents falls and sprains	infection contaminant dusts (e.g., asbestos) electrical shock
Meat Wrappers		decomposition fumes of wrapping film (PVC) (e.g., hydrogen chloride, carbon monoxide, phosgene) cold humidity infections from raw meat (e.g., Salmonellosis)	
Secretarial	5,396,061	falls and sprains back injuries	tenosynovitis
Waitresses, cleaners, cooks	2,075,129	falls and sprains back injuries burns	

Source: Michael McCann, The Impact of Hazards in Art on Female Workers," *Preventive Medicine*, 7, 1978, 338–48; Vilma R. Hunt, *Occupational Health Problems of Pregnant Women* (Washington, D.C. USDHEW, 1975); Carl J. Johnson and Herbert W. Anderson, "Meat-Wrappers Asthma: A Case Study," *Journal of Occupational Medicine*, 18(2), February, 1976, 102–4; Jeanne M. Stellman, "Occupational Hazards of Women: An Overview," in Forum: Women's Occupational Health: Medical, Social, and Legal Implications, *Preventive Medicine*, 7, 1978, 281–93; and A. J. Fritsch, ed., *The Household Pollutants Guide* (New York: Anchor Books, 1978).

childbearing

Regardless of their other interests, activities, and careers, women are indisputably potential childbearers. This unique role presents women with not only a variety of physiological, emotional, and life-style changes and challenges, but also a profound responsibility for a healthy newborn. Although the response to pregnancy varies from woman to woman, in most cases pregnancy interferes very little, if at all, with a woman's normal routine. This routine involves working outside the home for a significant proportion of women in the childbearing ages (Kuntz, 1976). In the United States, it is estimated that over a million babies each year are "at work" before being born and are potentially exposed to the same conditions as working mothers (NIOSH, *Guidelines*, 1977).

Pregnancy may be the event that causes a working woman to seriously examine and question her potential exposure to hazardous materials in the workplace. Although at one time the placenta was thought to be a protective barrier for the developing embryo and fetus, it is now known that almost all substances in the maternal bloodstream can pass through the placental membranes (Stellman, 1977).

There are thousands of chemicals in industrial and home use today, but very few have been tested for toxic effects on growth and development. The evaluation of the environmental impact on the growing human organism presents a real challenge. Exposure to a hazardous agent may produce abortion, malformation, or a neoplasia (tumor), depending upon the stage of development of the organism when exposure occurred. The glaring example of cancers resulting from chemical exposures in the prenatal period was the treatment of pregnant women with stilbestrol,

which has been linked to the development of vaginal cancer in their daughters (Fraumeni, 1974). Unfortunately, since the vast marjority of birth defects are from unknown causes, the impact of the environment on this tragedy is not clear. It is probably greater, however, than current estimates indicate. From the limited number of studies available, it is evident that a sizable number of women at work do encounter workplace hazards potentially harmful to a developing embryo or fetus. Table 14.3 is a partial list of such known or suspected hazards.

Although the leading cause of postnatal mortality in the United States is attributable to congenital malformations, 70 percent of these are presently of unknown etiology (Hunt, 1975). Up to 6 percent can be attributed to known environmental exposures (*Human Health*, 1976). Nonetheless, the acceptable occupational exposures set for most workplace hazards do not reflect that a chemical may cross the placenta, cause birth defects, be present in breast milk, or that it may cause genetic damage. The current occupa-

table 14.3
examples of substances known or suspect for adverse impacts on the embryo or fetus

Alcohol	Ionizing Radiation
Anesthetic Gases	Lead
Aniline	Methyl Mercury
Arsenic	Nicotine
Benzene	Nitrates, Nitrites
Cadmium	Pesticides
Carbon Disulfide	Phenol
Carbon Monoxide	Polychlorinated Biphenyls
Carbon Tetrachloride	Turpentine
Infectious Agents	Vinyl Chloride

Source: Velma P. Hunt, *Occupational Health Problems of Pregnant Women* (Washington, D.C.: USDHEW, 1975); Jeanne Stellman, *Women's Work, Women's Health, Myths, and Realities* (New York: Pantheon, 1977); and William D. Kuntz, "The Pregnant Woman in Industry," *American Industrial Hygiene Association Journal*, 37(7), July 1976.

tional "protection" afforded workers—men or women—does not insure workers protection against such reproductive effects (Hricko, 1976).

Although the pregnant woman is concerned for the safety and health of the newborn, the pregnancy also causes obvious biological changes to the mother, which need to be considered with respect to potential occupational hazards. The circulatory and respiratory systems are modified during pregnancy. Modifications in the respiration rate and reserve air in the lung may be hazardous if a woman is working with toxic substances. During pregnancy there is also a decrease in the relative percentages of iron in the blood, bringing it below levels of the nonpregnant state. The concentration of the red cells, and hence of hemoglobin, falls because of an increase in plasma volume (Hunt, 1975). For women exposed to lead, benzene, X-irradiation, and other factors that are known or suspected to interfere with the body's ability to produce red blood cells, this decreased percent of hemoglobin may be relevant to the health status of the woman, as well as to the fetus (Stellman, 1977). Detoxification mechanisms are also altered, including the ability of the liver to make substances "nonpoisonous" (Hricko, 1976). Thus, the physiological changes of pregnancy may make the female more sensitive to health hazards encountered at home, in the community, and particularly in the occupational setting.

conclusion

The environmental conditions that surround women at home, in the community, and on the job must be continually assessed for their health impacts. Some environmental conditions present obvious hazards. For others the verdict is not yet in, and more data are needed. Yet, of the many factors affecting health in this century, environmental degradation is one element that can be controlled and/or eliminated—if people are willing to pay the price. Women can influence and form the values, decisions, and activities in their communities and occupational settings that determine the level of environmental health considered acceptable. Life's quality, its quantity, and its characteristics rest on those decisions. There is every reason to view the environment as a supportive network with which we can positively interact and which can not only sustain, but enhance health conditions. To ignore this fact is to remove a major preventive technique from the health care system.

Asbestos exposure—Globe, Arizona. *Morbidity and Mortality Weekly Report*, USHEW, PHS, CDC, January 18, 1980, *29(2)*.

Bradley, H. & Sundberg, C. *Keeping food safe*. New York: Doubleday, 1975.

Breysse, P. A. Formaldehyde exposure in mobile homes and conventional homes. In Proceedings of the 43rd Annual Educational Conference of the National Environmental Health Association, Charleston, S. C., June 23–28, 1979.

Chanlett, E. *Environmental protection* (2nd ed.). New York: McGraw-Hill, 1979.

Corn, M. Factors affecting health. In Proceedings of National Conference on the Environment and Health Care Costs, Washington, D.C., August 15, 1978.

A design guide for home safety. U.S. Department of Housing and Urban Development, Office of Research and Technology, Washington, D.C., January 1972.

Eckholm, E. P. *The picture of health*. New York: Norton, 1977, (a) p. 25, (b) p. 19.

Fire and the built environment. *America Burning*. Report of the National Commission on Fire Prevention and Control, Library of Congress 73-600022, Washington, D.C., May 4, 1973.

Fraumeni, J. F. Chemicals in human teratogenesis and transplacental carcinogenesis. *Pediatrics*, part II, May 1974, *53(5)*, 807–812.

Fritsch, A. J. (Ed.). *The household pollutants guide.* New York: Anchor, 1978.

Healthy people: The Surgeon General's report on health promotion and disease prevention. U.S. Department of Health, Education, and Welfare, Public Health Service, Office of Assistant Secretary for Health and Surgeon General, Washington, D.C., 1979.

Herbicides: Risking too much. *The Washington Post,* Washington, D.C., August 17, 1979.

Hricko, A. *Working for your life: A woman's guide to job health hazards.* Berkeley: University of California, Institute of Industrial Relations, Center for Labor Research and Education, Public Citizen's Health Research Group, 1976.

Hricko, A. M., & Marrett, C. B. Women's occupational health: The rise and fall of a research issue. Paper presented at American Association for Advancement of Science Meetings, New York, N.Y., January 28, 1975.

Human health and the environment—Some research needs. Report of the Second Task Force for Research Planning in Environmental Health Science, U.S. Department of Health, Education, and Welfare, Public Health Service, National Institute of Environmental Health Sciences, 1976.

Human lead absorption—Texas. *Morbidity and Mortality Weekly Report,* U.S. Department of Health, Education, and Welfare, Public Health Service, Communicable Disease Center, December 8, 1973, *22(49).*

Hunt, V. R. Occupational health problems of pregnant women. Washington, D.C.: Department of Health, Education, and Welfare, 1975.

Injuries due to falls—Washington, *Morbidity and Mortality Weekly Report,* U.S. Department of Health, Education, and Welfare, Public Health Service, Communicable Disease Center, June 9, 1978.

Johnson, C., & Anderson, H. W. Meat-wrappers asthma: A case study. *Journal of Occupational Medicine,* February 1976, *18(2),* 102–4.

Kane, D. N. Bad air for children. *Environment,* November 1976, *18(9),* 26–34.

Kuntz, W. D. The pregnant woman in industry. *American Industrial Hygiene Association Journal,* July 1976, *37(7),* 423.

Lead poisoning in children of battery plant employees—North Carolina. *Morbidity and Mortality Weekly Report,* U.S. Department of Health, Education, and Welfare; Public Health Service, CDC, September 30, 1977, *26(39).*

Lenihan, J., & Fletcher, W. W. *Health and the environment* (Vol. 3). New York: Academic Press. 1976.

McCann, M. The impact of hazards in art on female workers. *Preventive Medicine,* 1978, *7,* 338–348.

Menck, H. R., Pike, M. C., Henderson, B. E., & Jeng, J. S. Lung cancer risk among beauticians and other female workers: Brief communication. *Journal of National Cancer Institute,* November 1977, *59(5),* 1423–1425.

Neutra, R. Accident epidemiology and the design of the residential environment. *Human Factors,* October 1972, *14(5),* 405–420.

Oakley, A. *Woman's work, The housewife, past and present.* New York: Pantheon, 1974.

Occupational diseases: A guide to their recognition (rev. ed.). U.S. Department of Health, Education, and Welfare, Public Health Service, CDC, National Institute for Occupational Safety and Health, June 1977.

Radford, E. P. Health aspects of housing. *Journal of Occupational Medicine,* February 1976, *18(2),* 105–108.

Rom, W. N. Effects of lead on the female and reproduction: A review. *The Mt. Sinai Journal of Medicine,* September/October 1976, *43(5),* 542–552.

Ruskin, J. H. A public health approach to plumbing defects. *Journal of Environmental Health,* January/February 1968, *30(4),* 370–378.

Schumacher, R. L., & Breysse, D. A. Combustion and pyrolysis products from synthetic textiles. *Journal of Combustion Toxicology,* November 1976, *3,* 393–424.

Stellman, J. M. *Women's work, women's health, myths and realities.* New York: Pantheon, 1977.

Stellman, J. M. Occupational health hazards of women: An overview. In Forum: Women's occupational health: Medical, social, and legal implications, *Preventive Medicine,* 1978, *7,* 281–293.

Stellman, J. M., & Daum, S. M. *Work is dangerous to your health.* New York: Pantheon, 1973.

Tate, C. L. Housing and health. In Proceedings of the 43rd Annual Educational Conference of the National Environmental Health Association, Chalreston, S.C., June 23–28, 1979.

26 health departments cooperate in carbon monoxide survey in dwellings. *Environmental Health Letter,* March 1, 1973, p. 5.

VanDusen, K. A., & Fraser, G. Swimming pool program study. Washington State Department of Social and Health Services, Office of Environmental Health Programs, October 1977.

Vianna, N. J., & Polan, A. K. Non-occupational exposure to asbestos and malignant mesothelioma in females. *The Lancet,* May 20, 1978, pp. 1061–1063.

Waldbott, G. L. *Health effects of environmental pollutants.* (2nd ed.). Saint Louis: C. V. Mosby, 1978.

Warren, C. Current knowledge on the environment. In Proceedings from the National Conference on the Environment and Health Care Costs, held in Washington, D.C., August 15, 1978. U.S. House of Representatives National Technical Information Service, U.S. Department of Commerce, Springfield. Va.

Water corrosion and health effects in Washington State—A status report. Publication No. 76-3, Washington State Department of Social and Health Services, Office of Environment Health Programs, October 1976.

Wood burning may be a hazard. *Journal of Environmental Health*, November/December 1979, *92(3)*, 155.

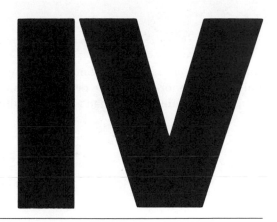

RUTH McCORKLE, R.N., Ph. D.

HEALTH SITUATIONS

There are a number of situations that can affect a woman's health. These situations can bring about changes that interfere with a woman's ability to carry out her normal day-to-day activities. Their occurrence can become sources of stress for a woman and rekindle unresolved feelings about previous experiences. Some situations give women more control than others in their willingness to participate. For example, a woman can plan to become pregnant and have a child, or she may choose not to become pregnant. In the event that she does become pregnant with an unwanted fetus, she may choose the option of having an abortion. In chapter 16 we learn of a unique problem related to the effects of the maternal hormone "guilt" and how this

feeling of shame has plagued some women for years. The costs and benefits of choosing the role of motherhood, work, a combination of both, or neither are carefully thought out. A choice for one role over another is not necessarily a decision that cannot be changed at a later time.

A number of other major health situations are discussed in this section. They are not meant to be exhaustive, but rather representative of health situations that are particularly troublesome to women when they do occur. Women become especially stressed in situations caused by violence from others, such as rape or the death of a loved one in an automobile accident. Also, situations that progressively occur or persist over long periods of

181

time, such as a diagnosis of cancer, low back pain, or osteoporosis, can be devastating and can affect not only the woman with the health problem, but the people with whom she comes in contact as well.

LYDIA KOTCHEK, R.N., Ph. D.

motherhood:
hazardous to your health?

Hormones are body secretions which clearly affect physiological functions. Their effect on social behavior is much less clear, although women's emotions and behaviors have all too often been glibly labeled as the result of female hormones. This causation is suggested by the word hormone itself, which is based on a Greek etymon meaning literally "an outflowing of emotion" or "to excite." During a menstrual cycle or a pregnancy a woman will have marked alterations in hormone levels. However, the "excitement" that can be associated with these changes is not inevitably caused by these physiological secretions. Rather, this "outflowing" may be based on a common female reaction to motherhood, the unhormonal—but nearly ubiquitous—emotion of guilt.

In the United States, a woman can deal with being a mother in several ways: by rejecting the role, accepting it, combining it with an occupation, being with a partner, or being alone. In all these choices—made for whatever reasons, optional or obligatory—guilt can be a part. She will fail standards held by some portion of the culture; she will not satisfy everyone. Those who believe that motherhood is the primary female role will censure a woman who is not a mother or who divides her time between work and children. Conversely, advocates of "find yourself" and

183

"do your own thing" may judge that a woman with children has denied herself true self-actualization.

Women, thus, are in the proverbial double bind—damned if you do and damned if you don't. Is this some fate peculiar to women, or is it a quirk of the American culture? No, the bind is not restricted to women or to this culture. The source of the bind lies in what are the unresolvable dilemmas of human life, ambiguities that affect both women and men and for which each culture proposes ideal resolutions.

Women, however, are more often trapped in these dilemmas; that is, women may find resolutions less easily than do men. This chapter will discuss these dilemmas and the paradox of resolving something that seems unresolvable. Then we will describe some cultural forces or pressures that affect parenting, a major part of life in which these dilemmas occur. And then we will suggest how women might deal with these pressures and their potential for engendering the maternal hormone of guilt.

unresolvable dilemmas

Each individual throughout her or his life needs to find a point of equilibrium between the poles of change and stability, closeness and distance, dependence and independence. There are advantages and disadvantages in moving toward either end. With closeness to others, comforting interpersonal contacts are developed. According to some theories of socialization, an individual learns who she or he is by seeing a reflection in the responses of others, since, alone, a clear view of the self is impossible. A human gains characteristics of being human (language and, as a consequence, the ability to abstract and to predict) only from contact with other humans. Yet, some distance from others is necessary to avoid a loss of identity. Although some religions idealize this loss as the ultimate possible achievement, in secular life a separate identity is valued. In some cultures, an individual's own name has a special, separate meaning. After death, this name is not spoken for fear that the person's afterlife repose will be disturbed and that the spirit will return to trouble the living.

With too much distance, on the other hand, a person can become isolated, which is a potentially morbid physiological state. Young children need close contact. Infants who are tended with detachment do not thrive as well as do infants given loving attention. Statistics indicate that for adults, too, isolation can be debilitating (Lynch, 1978). Possibly, all cultures have developed patterns of obligatory relationships because, although these are difficult to maintain (there are benefits in distance), they can be life-sustaining.

Dependence, related to closeness, could be similarly described. If we are close physically and emotionally to others, we may depend upon them and they upon us. From such dependence or, rather, interdependence can arise cooperative patterns with survival benefits. However, groups also need independent members, the expert who can lead the hunt, conduct the decision making, and discover new possibilities.

With stability, mutually predictable patterns can develop. Too much stability, however, can lead to dullness and inertia. Total stability can be a coma. In experiments of sensory deprivation, subjects who were cut off from stimuli that gave them information about change eventually began to fantasize changes—indicating that perception of some change is necessary. Fewer studies have been made of sensory overload, but the human mind is apparently limited in the amounts of random data it can manage at any one time. If change is excessive, if predictability is decreased, if information cannot be interpreted according to stable patterns from the past, the world becomes a confusion of randomness.

Finding optimal points of equilibrium between closeness and distance, change and stability, independence and dependence are unresolvable dilemmas. They are dilemmas because the search involves a continuous process of balancing the advantages and disadvantages of both ends of these poles. They are unresolvable because the optimal points for any individual may change as his or her environment changes; but inevitably the point of equilibrum will shift with age. As an individual grows older, she or he must deal with changing physiology and resources, with changing expectations, and yet with maintaining relative stability. Infants are dependent; adults must be sufficiently independent to provide for themselves and for others. No one can relate equally well to all others, in part because of limited time and resources. Numbers of kin increase and decrease from marriages, births, deaths, and migration. Managing such changes and yet retaining stable kinship ties involves processes of both closeness and distance.

In any culture, patterns exist that push toward both ends of these poles. Anthropologists have analyzed cultures, particularly non-Western, in terms of their patterns of traditional stability, of close and dependent kinship systems, of change within the culture as a result of contact with another culture. Less attention has been given to patterns of change, distance, and independence within the culture. But such patterns coexist with those of closeness, dependence, and stability (Gregor, 1969). Cultures vary in the relative emphasis placed on these patterns and in the idealized balance points. Samoans, for example, value the dependent, close family member more than they do the rugged individualist. They speak more highly of *Fa'aSamoa*, traditional Samoan customs, than of Western ways. American cultural values, in contrast, are weighted strongly toward the poles of independence, distance, and change. The cultural hero who most embodies these characteristics is a male, epitomized by the unencumbered (from entangling close relationships), inexpressive (detached) cowboy who moves farther west when he feels that he is too crowded by stable settlers. One could also cite the example of the playboy who moves on to other conquests when he feels that his independence is threatened by a current relationship.

The American frontier is now settled; the present frontiers for the restless male are those of work at which he strives, competes, achieves—actions that involve change, independence, and distance. Home and family are a separate world that provides him with the rest and relaxation he needs for renewed efforts at work. It has been the culturally idealized female role to maintain the stable home, to develop close family relationships, to produce the next generation (cowboys and playboys do not spring out of the dust by spontaneous birth), and to be dependent upon this sometimes undependable male.

mothering: hazards and dilemmas

The female role has been a cultural ideal in the United States as industrialization and mechanization have separated the areas of work from the home and have required a relatively smaller labor force. In the 1950s, a woman's most obvious choice was to marry (and, therefore, to become a mother) or to have a career (and, by implication, not to marry and become a parent). Times have changed. By the 1980s, the pressures toward both ends of the dilemmas increased—especially for women. Now they wonder: should I be a mother, should I work, could I or must I do both or neither? Whatever decision she makes will involve costs, guilt perhaps, as well as other physical and social consequences.

THE MOTHERHOOD CHOICE. If she chooses to be a mother and not to work for pay, she risks the accusation that she is a parasite (unwilling to face the harsh work world and earn her keep), that she has betrayed (by taking the lesser, traditional path) the sisterhood that has struggled to gain women's rights, and that she is selfish (contributing to overpopulation by her indulgence). Socially, she will be a member of a minority group. The numbers of mothers who now work outside of the home outnumber those who do not (Binstock & Shanas, 1976, p. 230). Physically, the risks of childbearing are minimal when compared with those of 100 years ago. Then, a woman risked a 5 percent chance of death related to childbearing. Now, only 1 mother in 8,000 dies from childbirth in the United States.

Physically, child-rearing is arduous. Combined with housekeeping, these activities can absorb more than 80 hours of labor a week, labor without pay, pension, vacation, and sick-time benefits. Such a mother could, because many other mothers work, be more involved in the extracurricular activities of parenting, car pools, school meetings, and children's organizations. Socially she is today—regardless of current commentary that men wish and need to be more involved as fathers—primarily responsible for child-rearing, both physically and emotionally. A mother is committed to her children's care, in sickness and in health (hers or her children's) 24 hours a day.

The best way to raise a child is still being debated. Current advice variously argues that a mother should form a close emotional bond with her child and yet keep her distance, dare to discipline and guide firmly, but also to encourage the child's natural independence and development—again, those troublesome dilemmas. Whomever she heeds, she will draw some disapproval from those she disregards. Included within the conflicting advice, however, is one firm consistency. All advisors agree that a woman's tenure as a mother is limited. On this point, the cultural pressure for independence is very evident. Her children must learn to function without her or she is an unsuccessful mother. Some skepticism is expressed that she alone can free her children from her. To do this, the children's father must exercise his main child-bearing responsibility; he must help his children establish distance and independence from their mother (Halpern, 1979). After her children become adults, a woman may live some 30 more years with her spouse. A mother should, therefore, not expend all her energy on her children.

In spite of the cultural theme that the ideal woman is a mother, there is little overt support for her in this role. It earns no money in a culture that measures status by salaries. Little formal socialization for parenting is provided in contrast with, for example, subsidized driver's or occupational education. Nor, at times, are a mother's activities given much credence. According to one politician, a mother of three children is apt to be " . . . watching TV all day" (Helms, 1978). If a mother's "finished product," the grown independent person, turns out creditably, he or she is complimented for personal achievements. If the individual turns out badly, the mother is blamed for poor parenting. The maternal hormone has many supporters.

What, then, might be gained from taking on a role for which one may be ill-trained and for which she will receive little credit? Child-bearing can be a physically rewarding experience, perhaps comparable to the peak experience of the mountain climber. A woman needs to prepare her body as it is pushed to a command performance that recognizes and uses its physical capabilities. Children may provide the health benefits of closeness. However, the data about the risk of isolation for adults were gathered from male and from senior citizen populations. Mortality and morbidity rates do not compare mothers of young children with women of similar ages who do not have children.

Child-rearing can be a maturing experience. A mother often treats her children as she was treated by her parents. Her child may, thus, behave as she did in her childhood. She then has an opportunity to review some of her past by seeing herself simultaneously as both a child and an adult. Becoming more aware of her past may help a woman gain some control over the influences from her past. A mother who does not have another occupation can devote more time to the demands of child-rearing and not have as many conflicting time demands.

The role of being a mother does not necessarily end when the children are adults. In spite of the American cultural belief that grown children are totally independent and separate from their parents, ties between adults and their parents can be strong and rewarding. The years labeled "postparental" by growth and development textbooks could more accurately be called the "interdependent" years when both generations exchange advice, goods and services, and affection with each other. Older women may not readily admit to participating in such exchanges, for "Mom" is a stock image of a clutching, castrating, mentally crippling woman who will not let her grown children become independent (Halpern, 1977). However, maintaining close ties with adult children may benefit an older woman, who can anticipate an average of 8 to 10 years as a widow. There seems some connection between isolation and illness in older females (Lynch, 1978).

There is, of course, no guarantee that close ties will be maintained. The results of being a mother cannot be predicted in advance. A woman in the United States has few opportunities to practice before assuming the obligations of being a mother. She learns these skills by doing them, and her learning may come too late to benefit her children. Not all children are healthy—some are handicapped, a few die—and the costs of being their mother are even higher. The chances that a woman will maintain beneficial ties with her grown children have not been measured. Impressionistically, however, the odds seem higher than cultural themes imply. It speaks well for the strengths of family relationships that close interdependent contacts persist in a culture that tends to discredit them.

THE NONMOTHERHOOD CHOICE. If a woman chooses not to be a mother, she will please some and displease others. She may be accused of being selfish. She is not doing her "natural" duty; therefore, she is an "unnatural" female. On the other hand, she may be applauded for demonstrating that a woman can "do her own thing," even if this "thing" is not being a mother. She avoids the costs of childbearing and rearing—time, energy, and money. She has more freedom to devote to her career, which can be uninterrupted. Working mothers often have discontinuous careers, interposed between pregnancy and child-rearing. A woman who is not a mother can gain cultural rewards for being independent and distant, for being available to changing opportunities.

There are costs. She will lose the benefits already described—a physical experience, a learning opportunity, family ties with children. However, other peak experiences are available. One can also learn about the past from encounter groups or open discussions with close friends. Family members are not the only possible cure for isolation in old age. Significant long-term relationships can be formed with kith as well as kin.

THE WORKING MOTHER'S CHOICE. If a woman chooses to be a mother and to have another occupation, she adds to her costs rather than changing them. Most often, she assumes the major responsibilities of child care as well as those of her job. If these obligations intersect, her conflict is major. For example, preschool children have, on the average, seven upper respiratory infections a year. If her child is minimally sick, she must balance his or her short-term needs for her attention with long-term work needs. If her child is very sick, she has little recourse but to defer to that priority. Child care for sick children is virtually nonexistent.

Working mothers face, in addition, the animosity or the indifference of professionals such as health care and social welfare providers. Many offices and clinics are open only during weekdays; a mother whose child needs care is assumed to be free during those hours. Professionals are still debating: *should* a mother work (as though all mothers who work have this option); is day care a hazard to the mental health of children? The debaters have, apparently, not yet realized that mothers *do* work and have worked for decades. Such mothers need help with their tasks, not a deferred diagnosis.

Working mothers compound their load by continuing to perform most household chores; fatigue and overwork are real hazards. Implications that she can and should do it all compound her guilt. A recent advertising campaign blithely described a woman, aided by a perfume, who could feed the kids and the pets in the morning, work all day, bring home the bacon, cook it, and still make her spouse "feel like a man." Since she can do so much, one wonders how *he* spends his time—perhaps in buying more perfume for her.

The rewards for a working mother may also be additive. She can derive benefits from both work and children. If time is limited, one may make better use of it. Working mothers receive at least one cultural commendation. In terms of dominant themes, these mothers contribute to the development of their own independence and to that of their children (Greenleaf, 1978).

THE SINGLE PARENT CHOICE. If she is a single parent, a woman often has a costly and lonely role, one not necessarily chosen, but often incurred. This chapter makes little reference to a father's contributions to child-rearing, for that is not its focus. But those contributions can be sizable. Two parents can assist each other and share the costs as well as the benefits. A single parent does not have this support, but must manage home, children, and work alone. If she works (66 percent of single parents do), she may be independent (a cultural plus), but she, more than working mothers with a spouse, is vulnerable to her children's needs. If she does not work, she and her children may exist on minimal welfare subsistence. The single welfare mother is another disvalued cultural figure who is often portrayed as a social parasite breeding for the benefits of the dole.

What rewards accrue to her? One can sur-mise that her compensations are those of other mothers and workers, relationships with children and returns from work. Studies have surveyed the satisfactions of mothers and of working mothers (Wright, 1978). The conclusions vary. By and large, however, single parents are an unstudied population. How they deal with the maternal hormone is unknown.

increasing the benefits, decreasing the costs

The main suggestions for women in this section are: know yourself and "enemies"—those who engender guilt; place yourself where you wish to be and avoid, as much as possible, those individuals who are somewhere else. To do so, one needs to recognize two characteristics of American cultural patterns. The first is a proclivity to organize and interpret data in an either/or fashion. The second is a tendency to champion the "either" or the "or."

In the 1940s and '50s, the current middle-aged adults (who now control much of the financial and political resources in the United States) were making their decisions about parenting. In those decades popular songs such as "Ballerina," "Accentuate the Positive," and "It's Gotta Be This or That" underscored dichotomized thinking by posing choices such as: something was either good or bad; love was either completely present or it was totally absent; a woman was either an old maid or a wife, a career woman or a wife. There were no mixed states or roles. Song styles have changed, but this mentality persists. If an individual is not independent, she is dependent; and it takes very little contact with parents, for example, for an adult to be considered dependent. Either a woman works, or she stays home; there is *no* in-between.

This either/or mentality also leads to an at-tempt to identify one single cause of a complex problem. The suggested single cure for the problem is based upon this identified cause, and other facets are ignored. This cure is advocated until a reaction occurs. Then, the pendulum of recommended action swings toward the opposite direction. Throughout these swings, advocates of one point or another remain vociferously at various positions along the arc.

Medical treatment of childbirth in the United States illustrates these characteristics. As medical technology increased, maternal and infant mortality rates decreased significantly. Based on this success, the solution to the remaining mortality rates seemed to be more technology—a point of view that ignores other factors contributing to lowered mortality. Childbirth became more and more a mechanical process of sedation and manipulation, reaching a peak of instrumentation in the 1950s and 1960s. Then, a reaction occurred. Some consumers, nurses, and doctors began stressing other aspects of obstetrical care, ways in which the childbirth experience could be enhanced rather than manipulated. Such methods included natural childbirth (usually defined as childbirth without medication) and providing increased early contact between mother and newborn infant. What began as an enhancement has, at times, become a bandwagon. Some mothers (who may be tired or who may be experienced mothers) find that they must "bond" (maintain the expected contact with their infants after delivery) or risk being considered poor mothers. For some women, experiencing natural childbirth may be the required proof that they are adequate and "natural" mothers.

Some physicians, concerned with the 5 percent of women who are at risk for childbirth complications, apply more technology—fetal monitoring and quick intervention—to all births, including those of the 95 percent who may not need it. Debates rage about the best location for birth. Those concerned about the risks of hospital care discount the real benefits of a hospital. Those troubled about the risks of home delivery discount the real benefits of such deliveries.

Similarly, child-rearing advice tends to concentrate on one major argument and to ignore how much this advice may be influenced by environmental factors, such as economic conditions. It is enlightening to note the parallels between professional theories and changing economic and demographic factors. During World War II, women were needed in the work force. The economy was expanding, production was increasing, and men were leaving civilian work to enter military service. Women were urged to work. The federal government subsidized day care centers so that women *could* work. Day care was described as beneficial, even " . . . marvellous" for children (*Day Care*, 1943). David Levy's (1943) book warned against "maternal overprotection," intense mothering that caused problems for children. These problems could be helped by some separation of mother and child.

After the war, returning soldiers filled the labor market. Federal subsidizing of day care stopped. Young women were warned that those who worked risked becoming that dreaded figure, the old maid (Jarman, 1952). Professionals in the early 1950s were influenced by the concept of maternal deprivation vividly described by John Bowlby. He defined this as an unhealthy syndrome caused in a child by any separation from the mother, including separation incurred by a mother's work (Bowlby, 1953). In that decade some women chose careers, some mothers worked, but their existence was overshadowed by the numbers of women who stayed home and produced the baby boom.

In the 1960s, the numbers of the baby boom became evident, and concerns about overpopulation were voiced. In a very popular book, Betty Friedan (1963) asked, "Is being a mother and a housewife sufficient?" Her answer of "no" was echoed more strongly a decade later by Betty Rollin (1970), who queried, "Motherhood, who needs it?" Most professionals did not follow this challenge to the domestic and maternal. Rather, professional literature continued to express concern about maternal deprivation. However, more mothers and other women were working. The economy was expanding, in part because of the needs of the increasing numbers of young children in the population. The obstacles that these women encountered, because of cultural themes that a good mother stays home with her children and that a good woman has children, created part of the format for the women's liberation movement.

During the 1970s, the bulge of the baby boom reached young adulthood. In that decade the economy declined. The labor market at present does not have enough jobs for all who can work. Discussions about the roles of women today contain both pronatal (she should be a mother) and antinatal (she should not) commentary. The admonitions against motherhood are somewhat muted by the scarcity of jobs. When these are more difficult to find, women in the past (and the future looks similar) have been the more expendable workers. The arguments for motherhood are also fostered by the decline in birth rates. Professionals have added a new concept to their literature about women, that of maternal bonding, a process of early and close contact between mother and child—a process with which a mother's work could interfere (Klaus, 1972).

This commentary is not meant to negate the validity of these cited theories. Rather, it is to point out that situational factors influence what, in a complex and varied environment, is being observed. In the past or in the present there has not been one monolithic stance. Arguments were and still are made for and against day care for children, for and against close linkage of mother and child. How, then, should a woman plot her own course in the midst of these various themes and trends?

First, she needs some relatively objective information, relatively because each source has its bias. There are, nevertheless, references that are less polemic. Some of these include:

1. Descriptions of historical trends in professional advice given to women and of the environmental trends influencing this advice (Ehrenreich & English, 1978).
2. Discussion of both the positive and negative aspects of parenting and of cultural patterns influencing the decision to become a parent (Veevers, 1973).
3. Statistical analysis rather than opinion about working women (Women's Bureau, 1975).

Second, a woman must read between the lines and look for the assumptions and biases of the author. A member of the American College of Obstetricians and Gynecologists concludes that the results of home deliveries are " . . . worrisome to disastrous" and he dismisses such deliveries as " . . . a fad" (Pearse, 1979). He is thinking primarily of physical health and past successes of medicine, and he is ignoring some of the arguments for home deliveries. Similarly, an article that might indict physicians for their cruel treatment of women during hospital deliveries may be overlooking the valid concerns these doctors have about physical safety.

Brazelton (1979), an influential authority on early infant care, answers the question "Must you have more than one child?" with a "no." But he adds, of course, an only child may achieve less and have more trouble with independence than will a child with siblings. He is both a pronatalist and influenced by the cultural values of independence. A newspaper editor concludes that discipline problems in public schools in 1977 began when mothers went to work during World War II (Angelos, 1977). A speaker addressing 200 child welfare specialists juxtaposes comments about working mothers, incest, and child abuse (Bryant, 1977). A working mother *should* shudder; she is being scapegoated and other factors affecting discipline and family welfare are being ignored. Growth and development textbooks may tuck a commentary about working mothers in a section about maternal deprivation or follow a paragraph about working mothers with a lengthy treatment of sudden deaths in infants. The bias of the authors should be taken into account before the reader makes similar parallels.

Third, a woman who has decided on her posture toward being a mother should look toward what supports her choice. If that choice is not to be a mother, Rollin's (1970) article and Ellen Peck's (1971) conclusion that pronatalism is a "baby trap" are helpful readings. Those who are or who wish to be mothers can find much support, including that of Peck (1978), who suggests ways of being a "happy parent." This particular author illustrates the point that a choice once made is not necessarily permanent. A working mother should definitely avoid Fraiberg (1978); she goes beyond Bowlby in equating working mothers and day care for children with deprivation. More appropriate reading would be surveys of the effects of maternal employment on children and families, which conclude that no damaging results can be documented (Howell, 1973).

Meeting with other women who have made the same choices can also be supportive. Groups such as the National Organization for Nonparents and Parents Without Partners can help a woman to find validation of her interests. Working mothers have, as yet, no national organization, but these women can be found. They are the majority of mothers.

Finally, women need to recognize one current source of the maternal hormone. They are requiring a rethinking of dominant cultural values, and they are making it apparent that other modes of resolving unresolvable dilemmas are needed for *both* men and women. Women will be faulted (and, therefore, encouraged to feel guilty) for making it obvious that the dilemmas can no longer be settled by simply allocating one complex of patterns (closeness, dependence, stability) to women and the other (independence, distance, and change) to men. As women increasingly move into the work force, as they debate publicly their roles as women, they are eroding the segregation of work from home. They are seen to be damaging the stability of the home by leaving it to work (an example of the "either/or" mentality, either a woman is at home or she isn't). Women are threatening the independence to be gained from work by bringing dependent relations with them to work; for a working mother is not as separated in work from her home environment as is a working father—if he has a woman at home to tend to home concerns. Thus, women are requiring more than simplistic dichotomous thinking. This is a difficult demand in a culture that is characterized by a desire to find one solution to any question. It is, then, not surprising that one simple solution to the issues raised by women is to encourage more secretion of the maternal hormone.

Women have both worked and been homemakers longer than have men. Women now risk moving solely toward the male model of distance and independence. This model is tempting; it is culturally valued and a source of power and prestige. But it incurs the risks of isolation. Dealing simultaneously with both poles of the unresolvable dilemmas makes resolution more difficult. Women have been considering for themselves both sides of these dilemmas longer than men have. Men are, perhaps, a generation behind in their liberation from cultural stereotypes. They tend to interpret women's reconsiderations of roles as a threat rather than as an opportunity for men to examine themselves also. Until men have more freedom to debate and to choose their roles, women will still have to cope with the maternal hormone. That they can cope with it has been demonstrated. Perhaps men will also discover a "paternal hormone" of guilt and will begin successfully to deal with that.

Angelos, C. Florida school chose discipline basics. *Seattle Times*, B-1, June 22, 1977.

Binstock, R. H., & Shanas, E. (Eds.). *Aging and the social sciences*. Van Norstrom, 1976.

Bowlby, J. *Child care and the growth of love*. New York: Van Nostrand, 1953.

Brazelton, T. B. Must you have more than one child? *Redbook Magazine*, March 1979.

Bryant, H. The undermined U.S. family. *Seattle Post-Intelligencer*, A-1, July 22, 1977.

Day care—Marvelous for Terry. *Time*, March 22, 1943, p. 40.

Ehrenreich, B., & English, D. *For her own good: 150 years of the experts' advice to women.* Anchor, 1978.

Fraiberg, S. *Every child's birthright: In defense of mothering.* New York: Basic Books, 1978.

Friedan, B. *The feminine mystique.* New York: Norton, 1963.

Greenleaf, B. Help: *A handbook for working mothers.* New York: Crowell, 1978.

Gregor, T. Social relationships in a small society: A study of the Mehinacu Indians of central Brazil. PhD dissertation, Columbia University, 1969.

Halpern, H. *Cutting loose: A guide to adult relationships with your parents.* New York: Simon & Schuster, 1977.

Helms, J. The proposed hardship index is a statistical gimmick. *Dun's Review*, April, 1978, *111(4)*, 125–128.

Howell, M. Employed mothers and their families, I. *Pediatrics*, August 1973, *52(2)*, 252–263. Effects of maternal employment on the child, II. *Pediatrics*, September 1973, *52(3)*, 327–343.

Jarman, R. It's tougher than ever to get a husband.

Saturday Evening Post, February 23, 1952, *244. 34. 30*, 152–154.

Klaus, E. et al. Maternal attachment. *New England Journal of Medicine*, March 2, 1972, *286(9)*, 460–463.

Levy, D. *Maternal overprotection.* New York: Columbia University, 1943.

Lynch, J. *The broken heart: The medical consequences of loneliness.* New York: Basic Books, 1978.

Pearse, W. Home birth. *Journal of the American Medical Association*, March 9, 1979, *241(10)*, 1039–1040.

Peck, E. *The baby trap.* New York: Pinnacle, 1971.

Peck, E. Results of an important new survey: How to be a parent. *Family Circle*, September 27, 1978.

Rollin, B. Motherhood: Who needs it? *Look*, September 22, 1970.

Veevers, J. E. The social meanings of parenthood. *Psychiatry*, August, 1973 *(36)*, 291–310.

Women's Bureau. Bulletin 297: *1975 handbook on women workers.*

Wright, J. Are working women really more satisfied? Evidence from several national surveys. *Journal of Marriage and the Family*, May, 1978, *40(1)*, 301–313.

MARCIA GRUIS KILLIEN, R.N., Ph.C.

16

women and childbirth

The experience of pregnancy is a significant process in the life cycle of a woman. It involves major changes in the body's functioning, intensified feelings and moods, and often alters relationships with friends and family. Each woman experiences pregnancy and childbirth in her own unique way. For some, the pregnancy may be unexpected and perhaps unwelcomed; for others it is an event long anticipated and planned. The impact of the pregnancy may differ according to one's life situation: if it occurs in the teens or in the twenties or thirties; when single or married; if it is a first or subsequent pregnancy; if other relationships and circumstances are stable or undergoing upheaval, and so on.

Despite these differences, most women share some common experiences during the childbearing year. Some of these experiences are a source of joy and wonder, while other events are unfamiliar and may cause concern. All women share the desire to have an enjoyable pregnancy, to stay healthy, and to produce a healthy child. Every woman has the right to find pleasure and a sense of accomplishment through the experience of pregnancy. For some women, lack of accurate information, good health care, and adequate support interfere with attaining these goals. This chapter gives information that will assist women in having a healthier, happier pregnancy. Getting ready for pregnancy, common experiences of pregnancy, labor, and postpartum, and ways to take an active role in the pregnancy are discussed.

getting ready for pregnancy

A woman can increase her chances for a positive pregnancy by trying to achieve the best physical condition before becoming pregnant.

nutrition

As a woman begins to plan for a pregnancy, she needs to take a good look at her nutritional status. Women who are underweight (10 percent or more below the ideal weight for their age and height) when a pregnancy begins are more likely to deliver low birth weight infants, who have a more difficult beginning in life. Women who are overweight (20 percent higher than the ideal weight for their age and height) have more health problems during pregnancy, such as high blood pressure and infections. Losing weight during pregnancy is not recommended because dietary restrictions can interfere with the baby's growth and development.

Learning to have and maintain a well-balanced diet will also make it easier to meet the body's nutritional needs during pregnancy. Beginning pregnancy with a healthy, well-nourished body can reduce some of the discomforts experienced during early pregnancy and prevent the demands of pregnancy from causing undue strain on the body. The Department of Agriculture suggests that a well-balanced diet includes:

1. Milk and cheese: 1 quart of milk, 2 ounces of cheese per day.
2. Meat, eggs, or dried beans, peas or nuts: 2 or more servings each day.
3. Vegetables and fruits: 4 or more servings a day, including deep yellow vegetables and dark green leafy vegetables at least every other day.
4. Breads and cereals: 4 or more servings each day.

The first three months of pregnancy is the period when the baby's basic organs are being formed. It is very important that the baby receive adequate nutrients during its development. Since a woman often is not aware that she is pregnant even until several months after conception, maintaining a healthy diet at all times is a good practice.

exercise

Pregnancy puts many demands on a woman's body as it stretches and changes to accommodate the growing baby. Labor and delivery can be as strenuous as any athletic event. Muscles that are in good tone tend to work with better efficiency. Therefore, women who are in good physical condition tend to have fewer discomforts during pregnancy, quicker labors, easier deliveries, and faster postpartum recoveries.

Prior to becoming pregnant is a good time to find an enjoyable type of physical activity. Walking, jogging, biking, and swimming are all excellent forms of exercise that can be continued throughout pregnancy.

A word of caution—a fever (temperature

above 38.9°C, or 102°F) can cause birth defects in the baby and increases the chances of spontaneous abortion, stillbirth, and premature labor. Investigations suggest that hyperthermia (increased body temperature) can occur in situations other than illness. Sohar et al. (1976) found that after 20 minutes in a sauna bath, 22 percent of women studied had a body temperature of 39°C (102.2°F) or above. During strenuous exercise, the body temperature may also increase. Women who are considering pregnancy should be alert to these potential hazards and avoid becoming overheated.

medical and dental care

The physical demands placed on the woman's body cause no problems if she is healthy. However, pregnancy can cause pre-existing diseases or health problems to become worse. These conditions can also interfere with a normal pregnancy. Some health problems such as infections like rubella (German measles), herpes virus type II, and syphilis, can be particularly devastating to the developing baby. Before pregnancy a woman should have a thorough medical and dental examination to identify any conditions that might interfere with a healthy pregnancy or be endangered by the pregnancy. If possible, these conditions should be treated before the pregnancy begins.

use of toxic substances

The baby undergoes critical development during the first three months of pregnancy. During this period, exposure to some substances can have deleterious effects on the fetus, ranging from mild to severe.

MEDICATIONS: Almost any drug that affects the woman will be transmitted across the placenta to the baby. It is very important not to take any unprescribed medication when there is a possibility of pregnancy. There is some evidence that even over-the-counter drugs such as aspirin, sleeping preparations, antacids, and excessive amounts of vitamins may be harmful. The effect of oral contraceptives is still under investigation. Becoming pregnant soon after discontinuing oral contraceptives has been associated with increased incidence of twins, chromosomal abnormalities, and folic acid (a vitamin) deficiency during pregnancy. A woman may want to use an alternate method of contraception for several months after discontinuing birth control pills before attempting to become pregnant.

ALCOHOL. Alcohol is now recognized as a powerful teratogenic agent (causes malformations in the fetus). Women who consume more than six alcoholic drinks a day are considered to be at major risk and should not become pregnant until they can reduce their alcohol intake. Current research also indicates that women who are moderate social drinkers (two or three cocktails a day) are also at risk. Alcohol use *prior to* as well as during pregnancy has been associated with low birth weight infants and behavioral differences in infants. Alcohol should be considered dangerous to the developing baby prior to, during, and after conception.

TOBACCO. Smoking during pregnancy has been associated with low birth weight infants, increased spontaneous abortions, stillbirths, and pregnancy complications. Women should stop or at least cut down on smoking prior to becoming pregnant. Reducing smoking at any time during pregnancy can have a positive effect on the health of the baby.

CAFFEINE. The effects of caffeine on the fetus

are under study. There is some evidence that high consumption of caffeine (eight cups of coffee per day) is linked with spontaneous abortion, stillbirth, and premature labor. When planning a pregnancy, it is wise to limit consumption of caffeine drinks such as coffee, tea, and colas.

ADDICTIVE AND RECREATIONAL DRUGS. Using addictive drugs such as heroin and methadone during pregnancy most often results in the baby being addicted. Almost all psychogenic drugs have been found to cause malformations in animals, but the effects in humans are not clear.

environmental hazards

Exposure to certain chemicals such as zinc, lead, and pesticides in the environment and to radiation increases the risk of chromosomal abnormalities in present and future pregnancies. Our environment is becoming increasingly contaminated with these substances. Although it is impossible to know what chemicals are in one's environment in order to avoid possible unhealthy contact, a woman planning a pregnancy should be alert to possible hazards in her work and home surroundings and should not expose herself to known risks.

the childbearing year

Pregnancy is a normal process. The growth of the baby and the accompanying changes in the expectant mother that occur during the 40 weeks of gestation are largely predictable. The feelings and behaviors that go along with these changes are more diverse and are dependent upon the situation and characteristics of the individual woman. Reading about pregnancy and talking with other women can be helpful and reassuring. At the same time, each woman discovers that her experience is uniquely hers. Indeed, each pregnancy for the same woman is different. Learning about and being sensitive to changes in pregnancy can give the woman a sense of control and can help make the experience one of growth.

finding out
if you're pregnant

Some women have many symptoms that lead them to suspect they are pregnant; for others, it is difficult to be sure. Common physical changes that may signal a pregnancy include:

1. MISSING A MENSTRUAL PERIOD (AMENORRHEA). If a woman has regular menstrual periods, this is usually a reliable indication she is pregnant. However, some women do have some bleeding for the first months of pregnancy. These "periods" are usually shorter and bleeding is lighter than a regular menstrual period. If menstruation fails to occur within 10 to 14 days of the day expected, the woman should suspect pregnancy and arrange for a pregnancy test and physical examination.

2. BREAST CHANGES. Often the breasts seem to swell and may tingle, throb, or feel tender, due to increased levels of hormones early in pregnancy.

3. NAUSEA. Some women experience severe nausea and vomiting in early pregnancy, while others have none at all. The nausea occurs most often in the morning (thus, the name "morning sickness"), but some women experience it at other times of the day or throughout the day. This symptom often begins about the time of the first missed menstrual period and disappears by the end of the third month of pregnancy, after the body adjusts to different hormone levels. Eating small amounts of food rather than large meals may help, as will eating crackers or dry toast before rising in the morning.

4. FREQUENT URINATION. Hormones and the growing uterus pressing on the bladder sometimes make

the pregnant woman urinate more often early in pregnancy. Since this can also be a sign of a bladder infection (especially if accompanied by pain or burning), it should be investigated promptly.

5. FATIGUE. As the body adjusts to changing hormones and physical changes, the pregnant woman usually feels *very* tired, often constantly. This symptom usually disappears after the first months, but until then she needs plenty of rest.

Since all these changes can be caused by conditions other than pregnancy, the woman should have a pregnancy test and physical examination to determine if she really is pregnant. The most common pregnancy tests depend on the presence of a hormone, human chorionic gonadotropin (HCG), found in the blood and urine of pregnant women. Most tests are sensitive to HCG after three or four weeks of gestation, or 42 days following the first day of the last menstrual period.

Pregnancy testing equipment is now available in drugstores so that the woman can perform the test herself at home. If the procedure for the test is followed *completely* as directed, the tests are quite accurate. However, it is easy to make an error when performing the test and have a false negative (test incorrectly indicates nonpregnancy when you really are) or false positive (test incorrectly indicates pregnancy) result. Tests can also be done by your doctor or at a local clinic such as Planned Parenthood. The first urination of the morning should be tested. If the test is negative, it should be repeated in a week if pregnancy symptoms persist.

The woman should also have a physical (pelvic) examination to confirm the pregnancy. Thus, certain physical signs of pregnancy can be detected: (1) softening of the cervix, (2) softening of the uterus, and (3) changes in uterine size and shape. The examination will help determine how far the pregnancy has advanced and when the baby is likely to be due.

Detecting pregnancy as soon as possible is important. If the pregnancy is unwanted and the woman elects to have an abortion, this should be performed as early in pregnancy as possible to insure the healthiest outcome for the woman. If the woman chooses to continue the pregnancy, knowing she is pregnant will help her arrange for health care and assist her in planning her pregnancy experience.

so you're pregnant—
what now?

INITIAL REACTIONS. Most women respond to the confirmation of pregnancy with mixed emotions. Its discovery can bring special feelings of excitement and anticipation. At the same time, doubts and fears may also be present. What will it be like to be a mother? Am I really ready for parenthood? What will this mean for myself? For my partner? How will pregnancy and parenthood change my life and my plans?

At first, it may be hard to believe that the pregnancy is real. Although some women have the physical symptoms already mentioned, others feel much the same as when they are not pregnant. If nausea and fatigue make the woman uncomfortable, or if she has anxiety about being a mother, the woman may not always feel very happy about being pregnant, even if the pregnancy was planned. Women often feel that now is not the "right time" to be pregnant. It is important to recognize that these feelings are all normal and are part of the process of adjusting to the changes that pregnancy brings. It helps to share feelings of conflict as well as feelings of excitement and joy with those around you.

PHYSICAL CHANGES. As pregnancy progresses, the physical changes in the woman's body become more evident. Some of the discomforts that accompany early pregnancy have already been mentioned—breast tenderness, nausea, tiredness. Some women also have more irregular bowel movements and become constipated because of the pressure of the growing uterus and increased amounts of progesterone (a hormone). Taking iron supplements can also increase problems with constipation. Increasing exercise and drinking more fluids (5 to 7 glasses of fluid per day) can help remedy this problem. Adjusting the diet to include bran cereals, vegetables, and fruits can also help. Vaginal secretions also increase. If secretions become itchy, irritating, or odorous, an infection may be present and should be treated.

At about the fourth month of pregnancy, the baby starts to increase significantly in weight, and the uterus enlarges. The woman will start to gain weight and as the waist thickens, clothes no longer fit. The uterus continues to grow throughout pregnancy, but figure changes become evident at different times for different women. As the uterus grows, the skin on the abdomen stretches and pink lines ("stretch marks") may appear. These are a normal occurrence and cannot be prevented. However, if they become dry or itchy, adding oil to the bath or applying oil to the skin may relieve the discomfort.

In the middle of pregnancy, many of the discomforts experienced in the early months disappear and the woman feels especially healthy. Between the eighteenth and twentieth week, she may feel the baby move ("quickening"). The breasts may begin to secrete a thin yellow substance called colostrum (milk does not appear until several days after the baby's birth).

The final months of pregnancy can again bring some discomforts. The pressure of the growing baby and uterus may cause heartburn, constipation, and difficulty in breathing. Eating small portions of food, regular exercise, and frequent rest periods can help

the woman feel more comfortable. Some women have difficulty sleeping. Resting on one side, with a pillow to prop up the uterus and head, may make sleeping easier. During the last weeks of pregnancy, the woman may notice that her uterus becomes hard at periodic intervals. The uterus actually contracts irregularly from the early weeks of pregnancy on, but the woman usually does not become aware of this until the end of pregnancy. These contractions may cause concern; the woman may worry that she is beginning labor and sometimes contractions cause discomfort or prevent relaxation and rest. Although the contractions differ from labor contractions in that they are irregular and do not cause the cervix to thin and dilate, they do help prepare the cervix and uterus for labor. If the contractions persist, walking or relaxing in a warm bath often stops them.

EMOTIONS. It is not surprising that emotions fluctuate during pregnancy—it is a time of great change. The mixed feelings that accompany the discovery of pregnancy return throughout the months ahead as the woman adjusts to the changes in her body and in her life. Even in the happiest of pregnancies there are moments of depression, confusion, and fear. Women worry abut their babies; will they be healthy? They worry about their relationship with their partners; will parenthood change the relationship? Conflict between partners is common as the man and woman each undergo emotional changes during pregnancy. Women find that they feel more intensely during pregnancy. They experience rapid mood swings—happy one moment, sad the next. Dreams become more vivid and are sometimes frightening. As labor approaches, concerns center around delivery. The final weeks of waiting can be especially difficult. The woman often feels tired and awkward and no longer wants to be pregnant. During this time, it helps to remain active, but it is also important to avoid becoming fatigued, since labor can begin at any moment.

It helps to discuss feelings with others. Some feelings that may seem strange or silly are usually experienced by other women also. It can be reassuring to know that her experiences are common. Fears are often alleviated by discussing concerns with her nurse or doctor, a special relative or friend, or by getting information from reading or attending classes.

taking care of yourself during pregnancy

PRENATAL CARE. Health supervision during this period is an essential part of staying healthy and having a successful pregnancy. The type of health supervision should fit the woman's individual needs and desires.

During the early part of her pregnancy care, factors that will determine the type of care she needs should be assessed. Some women, because of pre-existing health conditions or situations that arise during pregnancy, are at higher risk for complications with pregnancy than are others. These women need special attention during this time.

In most situations, the pregnant woman visits her doctor or nurse monthly during the first half of pregnancy. The frequency of visits increases to biweekly and then to weekly as the time of delivery approaches. During each of these visits, several factors should be assessed:

1. WEIGHT GAIN. Weight gain during pregnancy is an indicator of fetal growth and maternal health. Both the amount and pattern of weight gain are important. The pattern should be regular, with the major increase occurring during the second half of pregnancy. Weight gain should not be more than 2 pounds in one week. A total of between 22 to 28 pounds should be gained during pregnancy. Weight gain comes from the following sources:

Baby	7.5 pounds
Placenta	1.0 pound
Amniotic fluid	2.0 pounds
Uterus	2.5 pounds
Breast tissue	3.0 pounds
Blood volume	4.0 pounds
Maternal stores	4.0–8.0 pounds

The body needs additional calories (about 300 more per day) and nutrients during pregnancy. Part of prenatal care should be advice about what kinds of foods to eat. Sometimes iron and vitamin supplements are recommended.

2. BLOOD PRESSURE. One of the most frequent complications of pregnancy is a condition called toxemia (or pre-eclampsia). One of the early signs of this problem is an increase in blood pressure. Detecting signs early can help prevent severe problems.

3. URINE. The urine should be checked at each prenatal visit to determine if it contains an unusual amount of sugar or protein, which signals potential problems with the pregnancy.

4. UTERINE GROWTH. Measuring the size of the uterus (usually with a tape measure) at each prenatal visit is one way of determining if the baby is growing adequately.

5. FETAL HEARTBEAT. The baby's heartbeat can usually be heard with a special stethoscope, called a fetoscope, at 18 to 20 weeks. The heartbeat can be heard earlier with an ultrasound device called a dopler. Listening for the heartbeat is one way of determining an accurate "due date" for the delivery. The baby's heartbeat is usually about twice as fast as the mother's (about 120 to 160 beats per minute).

6. PELVIC EXAMINATION. A pelvic examination is usually done at the first prenatal visit and then toward the end of pregnancy. The purpose at the end of pregnancy is to determine if the cervix has started to thin out (efface) and open up (dilate) in preparation for delivery.

7. CONCERNS OR PROBLEMS. At each visit the woman should be given the opportunity to discuss any concerns or questions she has at the time. It may be a good idea to write these down during the time between visits to help her remember to discuss them with the physician or nurse.

SEXUAL ACTIVITY. Sexual feelings may vary during pregnancy. Some women feel especially sexual at this time. Sometimes, if the woman is anxious or not feeling well, she may lose interest in making love. Men's feelings during pregnancy vary, too. The woman should be aware of her feelings and discuss them with her partner. Many people have received conflicting or inaccurate information about the safety of making love during pregnancy. There is no evidence that sexual intercourse should be restricted during a normal pregnancy. Sometimes intercourse, especially orgasm, will bring on uterine contractions. These are normal and nearly always stop when the woman is lying down and relaxing. Labor will start only if the time is right.

There are some circumstances under which intercourse is not recommended: (1) if there is vaginal or abdominal pain, (2) if there is vaginal bleeding, (3) if the amniotic sac (membranes) has broken, or (4) if the woman has been warned against intercourse because of danger of miscarriage or premature labor.

During pregnancy some coital positions are more comfortable than others. Late in pregnancy the traditional "man on top" position may be uncomfortable. Experimenting with ways of making love that are satisfying to both the woman and her partner is suggested. The baby is well protected and cannot be harmed by pressure. Oral-genital contact is also safe, as long as air is not blown into the vagina, as it may cause an air embolism.

CLOTHING helps the woman to feel comfortable and attractive during pregnancy. Clothing should be functional and not constricting. Use of stockings with bands that restrict circulation in the lower leg should be avoided. Low-heeled shoes tend to be more comfortable and are safer. As the breasts enlarge, a bra that provides adequate support will be needed for comfort and to prevent stretching. If the woman plans to breastfeed, a nursing bra can be purchased for use during pregnancy as well

as later. Excellent practical suggestions on clothing for pregnancy are found in *Birth* (Harmony Books, 1974), by Catherine Milnaire.

labor

PREPARATION FOR LABOR. Being prepared for labor includes learning about your body and what to expect during labor. It can also involve learning techniques of breathing and relaxation that will make the woman more comfortable during labor. Information can be acquired in several ways: reading, talking with other women, and attending prenatal classes.

A wide choice of classes is available; some provide only information, while others teach specific techniques for breathing and relaxation (often called natural childbirth). To select a class that fits specific needs, the doctor, nurse, or other women may have useful information about classes that are available. Getting several opinions may be useful. Classes vary in cost and length of time offered. Some classes are available that meet throughout pregnancy; others prepare the woman only for labor and delivery. A partner or a selected support person can usually attend classes with her. (They need to know what is happening, too!) If an unmedicated labor and delivery are planned, classes that teach breathing and relaxation techniques are highly recommended.

ONSET OF LABOR. No one really knows why labor begins when it does. Sometimes the onset is sudden and definite. At other times, it is difficult to determine if labor has begun or if the symptoms are "false labor." True labor contractions tend to be regular, evenly spaced, and occur at increasingly frequent intervals. As labor progresses, the contractions increase in duration and strength. Labor contractions will not stop if the woman relaxes or lies down. They usually become stronger with walking. Some women have labors that do not follow the usual pattern. If there is any reason to suspect that labor has started, notify the doctor or midwife. They can determine if labor has started by examining the cervix to see if it is progressively thinning and dilating.

EXPERIENCE OF LABOR. Every woman experiences labor in her own way. Some women have long labors, other labors are rapid. The amount of pain also varies.

The beginning of labor is usually the longest part. The woman is usually quite comfortable and can be up and about, keeping distracted from her contractions. As labor progresses, contractions become stronger and closer together. The woman now may need to work with the contractions, using relaxation and breathing techniques to maintain control. She may be more comfortable in bed or walking. Once the amniotic sac has broken, the woman should be lying down to prevent prolapse (falling) of the umbilical cord.

The amniotic sac contains about a quart of fluid. It may break with a painless large gush of fluid from the vagina, or a small trickle. Since the membranes protect the baby from infection, once they have broken, it usually is important that the baby be delivered within about 24 hours. If labor does not begin, an induction of labor may be indicated.

As delivery approaches, the contractions become very strong and close together. This is the most difficult time of labor (called "transition"). The woman may become irritable and may develop hiccoughs or nausea. Pressure from the baby in the vagina creates an urge to push, and in time the baby is delivered. Soon thereafter, the placenta is delivered.

It helps to have a person whom the woman trusts with her in labor. That person (the partner or another special person) can assist her in remaining relaxed and working with her contractions.

postpartum

The childbearing experience is not complete after the delivery of the baby. The weeks that follow are a time of adjustment.

physical restoration

The uterus continues to contract following delivery, reducing its size and preventing bleeding. About 10 days after delivery, the uterus is so small it can no longer be felt in the abdomen. When this occurs, the woman no longer looks "still pregnant." The uterus continues to become smaller until about six weeks after delivery when it has returned to approximately its prepregnant size.

The lining of the uterus is discharged after delivery. The woman will notice a vaginal discharge (called lochia), which changes in color and amount over the first postpartum weeks. Initially, the discharge is red and is similar to a menstrual period. Over the weeks the discharge becomes pinkish, then yellow-white. The discharge should not continue to be bright red, nor should it have a bad odor. Lochia continues for 4 to 6 weeks after delivery.

Milk comes into the breasts during the second or third day after delivery. This may be accompanied by engorgement; the breasts are hard, hot, and swollen. This usually only persists for about a day. If the woman is breastfeeding her infant, the engorgement is eased by nursing. Sore nipples can be another source of discomfort for the breastfeeding mother until the nipples toughen and no longer are irritated by the infant's vigorous sucking. Prenatal preparation of the nipples and gradual initiation of breastfeeding after delivery can help prevent this problem. Prenatally, the nipples can be toughened by rubbing them briskly with a towel for one or two minutes several times daily. The woman's partner can also suck on the nipples during lovemaking.

After delivery, the woman should nurse her infant for only short intervals, initially, gradually increasing the nursing time. Since the infant sucks most vigorously at the beginning of the feeding session, the breast that is offered first should be alternated. Leaking of milk from the breasts between feedings (especially during lovemaking) can be a common annoyance and can also contribute to nipple soreness. This problem is usually remedied when the milk supply becomes stable, adjusting to the infant's demands between 4 and 8 weeks postpartum. Until then, an effort should be made to keep the nipples as dry as possible to prevent soreness and infection. Exposing the nipples to the air after feeding is one way to aid in drying.

Fatigue is a common postpartum experience. This comes from the physical adjustment that is taking place and from the loss of sleep that often accompanies the arrival of a new baby. It is important to get as much rest as possible, both to help the body heal and to reduce the feelings of depression that are accentuated by fatigue.

learning to care for the baby

Fatigue and tension in the weeks following delivery are caused in part by the incessant care demanded by an infant. Our mobile society, with friends and family frequently far away, often forces the mother to begin to care for her baby unassisted at a time when her own physical and emotional needs are great. Few opportunities are provided for people to learn about infant care through their own experiences before they become parents. Thus, infant behavior and care giving is a new and sometimes confusing and awkward experience. Prenatal classes and baby classes are ways to learn more about the baby. Advice from friends can also be beneficial, although possibly conflicting. In time, the new mother will learn to trust her own judgment and understand the signals that the baby is sending.

Feeding the baby is a major part of early infant care. The comfort and satisfaction of the mother and the baby during feeding sessions have significance for the development of a healthy mother-infant relationship. Breast and bottle feeding each have advantages and disadvantages, but either method can be equally satisfying to the infant. Each method has been "fashionable" at different times among different groups of women. When making a choice, the woman should consider her life-style and activities, plans for sharing infant care, and attitudes of people significant to her.

Human milk is ideally suited to an infant's needs. Colostrum, the substance that the baby feeds on before the milk comes into the breast, is high in antibodies that protect the newborn from many infections. Breastfeeding provides the infant with a natural immunity to common diseases for the first months of life. There are few medical contraindications to breastfeeding, and this method is recommended when the family has a history of severe allergies. Breastfeeding can be very demanding of the new mother's time, however, especially during the early weeks. Until the milk supply is stable, the mother should miss as few feedings as possible. Some women find this too limiting of their other activities or responsibilities to work or to other children. Sharing child care is easier when bottle feeding.

The attitude and desires of the woman's spouse or partner are particularly important to consider. Some men are very supportive of breastfeeding, while others are jealous of the special closeness that breastfeeding brings the mother and child. Some men view the breast as part of the couple's sexual relationship and have difficulty being comfortable with breastfeeding. The woman who breastfeeds needs the support and encouragement of those around her. When selecting an obstetrician and pediatrician (or other health professional), the woman should be sure that person will be supportive of her desired method of feeding and that he or she can offer needed information. Additional encouragement and practical suggestions can be obtained from other women who have nursed their infants or from organizations like the LaLeche League. Books can be another source of information.

It sometimes takes time for the mother to become comfortable with her infant during feedings. She needs to learn her baby's unique rhythms and cues of hunger and satiation. As she learns about her baby, feeding becomes easier and more enjoyable.

forming a relationship with the baby

A mother's relationship with her infant begins long before birth as she plans the pregnancy and experiences the movements of the baby prenatally. Mothers have fantasies about their infants and dream about what they will be like. After birth, the mother adjusts her image of her infant based on the real characteristics she notices. Each infant is unique, just as every mother is unique. Developing knowledge and understanding of a baby's patterns of crying, sleeping, feeding, and other behavior takes time, just as getting to know any other person does.

accommodation to a new family member

The needs of the baby must be regulated with the mother's needs as an individual and the demands of other family members. Many women are not prepared for the changes in life-style that result from having a baby. The woman must learn to alter her activities and to incorporate new activities related to the baby, while at the same time not neglecting her own needs. New mothers frequently feel tied down and isolated from friends. They have difficulty finding time for personal needs and interests. Changing relationships in the family can also cause concern. The attention required by a new baby often makes older brothers and sisters jealous of the newcomer; their needs for reassurance and affection increase. The woman's relationship with her partner may also suffer from neglect. It is important that she plan time for meeting her own needs and developing relationships with others important to her. As a result, she will feel better about herself and enjoy being with her baby more.

other considerations

Each woman adjusts to having had a baby at her own pace and in her own way. She should be sensitive to her own needs and seek advice and support from those around her. In her community, she will likely find formal or informal groups to support her with breastfeeding concerns, career adjustments, and child care. She will make decisions about when to resume sexual intercourse, how long to continue breastfeeding, and if or when to return to work outside the home. Each of these decisions largely depends on what is comfortable for the individual.

It takes time for the body to return to a nonpregnant state. Contraception is one thing to consider after the baby is born. A woman can become pregnant at any time she resumes sexual relations; most women do not have the resources, either physical or emotional, to experience another pregnancy immediately. The method of contraception chosen may be different from the one previously used. Oral contraceptives are not recommended for women who are breastfeeding. If a diaphragm was used previously, it should be refitted after delivery. Foam and condoms are a good choice while waiting to visit the doctor or to use another method.

choices

Women are finding increased satisfaction in their childbearing experiences as they take an active role in their own care. Considering options and making choices based on individual needs and desires help to maintain a sense of control over experiences.

One of the major decisions to be made is the selection of a provider of prenatal care. Some types of professionals who can care for women during pregnancy are:

OBSTETRICIAN. A medical physician who specializes in the care of women during pregnancy and childbirth. An obstetrician should have the knowledge and skills to care for women during normal or complicated pregnancies.

FAMILY PRACTICE PHYSICIAN. A medical doctor who cares for family members of all ages. He or she can care for a woman during a normal pregnancy, but will probably consult with or refer her to an obstetrician if complications arise. The family practice physician can also provide care for the baby after delivery if desired.

NURSE-MIDWIFE. A registered nurse who has specialized education in the care of women during pregnancy and childbirth. The nurse may care for women during normal pregnancy and childbirth. Some nurse-midwives work with a physician in providing a team approach to care of women during pregnancy.

When selecting a health care provider, a major consideration is what is desired for the childbirth experience. Several different physicians or nurses should be interviewed until one is found with whom the woman feels comfortable and trusts. It is important to know their qualifications, experience, and philosophy about childbirth. Some areas to be explored might be their attitudes toward medication in labor, natural childbirth, breastfeeding, home births, father and sibling participation in labor and delivery (including during cesarean deliveries), and rooming-in. If the professional is in practice with a group of other health care providers, it should be noted whether the other individuals will be involved in the care. If so, what are their attitudes concerning the childbirth experience?

Prenatal care may be available in a private doctor's office, clinic, or hospital. Sometimes the situation includes other resources such as prenatal classes, nutritional counseling, social workers, and body conditioning classes. These resources can be helpful, and their availability should be explored.

Another decision may be about the setting in which the baby will be delivered. Several alternatives may be available.

TRADITIONAL HOSPITAL SETTING. This is the most common option available to women in the United States. About 95 percent of all births in this country occur in hospitals. The hospital experience is highly dependent on the philosophy of that hospital and of the physician or nurse who will be providing care there. Usually, labor rooms and a separate delivery room are provided. Following delivery, 2 to 5 days are spent in the hospital for recovery. Hospitals differ in their policies about who can be present during labor, types of anesthesia available, use of fetal monitors, and how much the family can be together after delivery. When a doctor or nurse is selected, delivery care facilities should be discussed, including the policies of that institution.

ALTERNATIVE BIRTH CENTERS. In response to women's demands for a childbirth experience that seems less "sickness-oriented," many physicians or nurse-midwives practice in a setting that is more homelike. An alternative birth center may be in a clinic or a separate part of a hospital. The available facilities vary. Some alternative birth centers have facilities and equipment to handle emergencies and complications that may arise with the mother or baby during labor and delivery. In other situations, the mother or baby must be transferred to a hospital if complications arise. In most alternative birth centers, the woman's partner and other significant people can be with her during labor and delivery. Labor and delivery usually occur in the same room, and the baby remains with the mother after delivery. The mother may stay at the center for some time after delivery or may go home as soon as her condition has stabilized after delivery.

HOME BIRTH. Home birth allows the woman to labor and deliver in familiar surroundings, free from routines and strangers. Home birth is an appealing alternative that many women consider. When thinking about a home birth, there are several things to consider related to the safety of the experience.

1. What type of screening is available prenatally to determine if the woman is a good candidate for a home birth? Home birth is not a safe alternative for anyone who runs a risk of anything other than a normal labor and delivery.

2. Who will be present during labor and delivery? The doctor or midwife must be aware that a home birth is planned and must agree to this. Will they be present throughout labor or do they plan to arrive just before the delivery? Since the course of labor can be quite unpredictable and complications can arise suddenly, it is much safer if a knowledgeable, skilled person is in attendance throughout labor. The professional must have the medical and legal qualifications to handle emergencies should they arise. He or she should be able to resuscitate a newborn, use oxygen, recognize and temporarily treat complications like hemorrhage, cord prolapse, or abnormal labor. Especially, she or he must have easy and quick access to hospital facilities should they become necessary.

3. What type of provisions for emergencies have been made? This includes availability of emergency equipment such as oxygen and medications and consideration of how near hospital facilities are. It is desirable for the woman to visit the hospital to which she would be taken in case of complications so that it will be somewhat familiar to her.

The majority of women experience a normal labor and delivery. However, complications cannot always be predicted prenatally and serious problems can arise suddenly. When choosing a home birth, the safety of the option should be seriously considered. For many women, the risks are greater than the benefits. For these women, there are increasingly better options available in alternative birth centers and in hospitals.

Childbirth should be a positive experience. Many of the recent advances in technology have made childbirth a safer experience for mothers and babies, but may also interfere with the naturalness of the experience. Use of fetal monitors, intravenous fluids, anesthesia, and induction of labor are reassuring to some women, but disturbing to others. When making choices about the type of experience desired, the woman's knowledge about these practices should be developed by reading and discussing their advantages and disadvantages with others. When specific desires are decided, a birth plan (in writing) for the doctor or nurse should be made. Having this on hand for birth plan prenatal visits and labor and delivery serves as an important means of communicating wishes to others.

Above all, the woman should work with her health care provider in planning the childbirth experience and utilize his or her knowledge and skill to assist in planning. Many events of pregnancy, labor, and postpartum cannot be planned. It helps to be flexible and open to things as they occur. Each childbirth is a unique experience that should be a source of satisfaction and growth. There is much a woman can do to have a healthy, happy childbirth.

Boston Women's Health Book Collective. *Our bodies, ourselves* (2nd ed.). New York: Simon & Schuster, 1976.

Caplan, G. Psychological aspects of maternity care. *American Journal of Public Health*, 1957, *47*, 25.

Eastman, N., & Jackson, E. Weight relationships in pregnancy: The bearing of maternal weight gain and prepregnancy weight on birth weight in full term pregnancy. *Obstetrical and Gynecological Survey*, November 1968, *23*, 1003.

Fraser, A. C. Drug addiction in pregnancy. *Lancet*, October 23, 1976, *7991*, 896.

Kaminski, M. et al. Alcohol consumption in pregnant women and the outcome of pregnancy. *Alcoholism: Clinical and Experimental Research*. April 1978, *2*, 155.

Killien, M., & Poole, C. Prenatal care. In K. Kowalski & B. Jennings (Eds.), *Primary Health Care of Women*. Forthcoming.

Poole, C. Health maintenance. In K. Kowalski & B. Jennings (Eds.), *Primary Health Care of Women*. Forthcoming.

Rossi, A. Transition to parenthood. *Journal of Marriage and the Family*, February 1968, *30*, 26.

Rothman, K. Fetal loss, twinning and birth weight after oral contraceptive use. *New England Journal of Medicine*, 1977, *29*, 486.

Rush, D., & Kass, E. Maternal smoking: a reassessment of the association with perinatal mortality. *American Journal of Epidemiology*, 1972, *96*, 183.

Sohar, E. et al. Effects of exposure to Finnish sauna. *Israel Journal of Medical Science*, November 1976, *12*, 1275.

Turner, G., & Collins, E. Maternal effects of regular salicylate ingestion in pregnancy. *Lancet*, August 23, 1975, 335.

Wethersbee, P. et al. Caffeine and pregnancy: a retrospective survey. *Postgraduate medicine*, September 1977, *62*, 64.

Worthington, B. et al. *Nutrition in Pregnancy and Lactation*. St. Louis: C. V. Mosby, 1977.

CAROLE BROWNER

induced abortion:
the risks and the myths

Since the 1973 Supreme Court decision that guaranteed American women the right to legal abortion, the number of pregnancies purposely ended each year has increased. In 1973, nearly 750,000 abortions were performed; by 1978, the figure grew to 1.4 million; and by 1979, estimates are that 1.5 million legal abortions were performed. In 1978, 29 percent of pregnant women in the United States ended pregnancies; between 1967 and 1978, 1 out of every 8 women of reproductive age, a total of 6 million women, obtained at least one legal abortion.

Many view the rising number of induced abortions with alarm. They fear an "abortion mentality" taking hold among Americans with an increasing reliance on abortion as the preferred means of birth control rather than as the method of last resort. Why, they ask, with highly effective contraceptives widely available, do so many women seek abortion? A related concern they often express is that ready access to an easy means to end unwanted pregnancies encourages promiscuity since the "price" of sex outside of marriage is no longer great. They point to the rapidly rising rates of pregnancy and abortion among teen-agers as evidence to support their position.

The fear at the core of many of these issues stems from more than the ethical aspects of the problem. Ready access to induced abortion frees women from mandatory motherhood. It undermines some of the social supports for the nuclear family by minimizing the need for a division of labor based on the requirements of child care. With women tied to pregnancy and childbearing throughout most of their adult lives, half the population is removed from the sectors of society where rewards, power, and influence are allocated.

Proponents of the position to restrict access to abortion generally remove the event from its context. Their perspective typically overlooks both the historical role abortion has played in limiting population growth and the personal meaning abortion has for the individuals involved. This kind of information is needed if we are to understand the significance of the seemingly "high" rates of induced abortion in the United States.

Until the early 1970s, induced abortion was the most widely practiced method of fertility control in use throughout the world. It is now ranked third after voluntary sterilization and oral contraceptives. The actual number of pregnancies ended each year by abortion is not known. Many women practice it in countries where its use is restricted by law or outlawed completely, such as throughout Latin America and in parts of Asia where other means of fertility control are not widely available. Population experts estimate that between 30 and 55 million abortions are performed annually. This means that 1 out of every 4 pregnancies ends in abortion.

The widespread practice of induced abortion is not a new phenomenon. Anthropologists have documented its existence in virtually every society, despite differences in the reasons for its use, extent of its practice, and degree of social disapproval. During the 2 million years of human history before the invention of agriculture, abortion and infanticide were commonly practiced. It was impossible for a woman to carry more than one small child the long distances that the nomadic lifestyle required. In the absence of other effective means of birth control, abortion and infanticide were often essential.

The frequency with which abortion was used declined with the development of agriculture and the possibility of feeding more people per unit of land. In every society, however, some pregnancies were aborted. Abortion was often used in tribal societies to maintain purity of the kin group, such as when a pregnancy occurred and the father was not known or an alien, or when pregnancy was due to incest. Other reasons for abortion included not wanting to become a parent yet or wishing to protect one's beauty. In peasant societies, abortion was probably most often used by women pregnant but not yet married or because of illness or old age. Bringing us to present times, Potts, Diggory, & Peel (1977) have shown that no society has modernized economically without a significant number of its members relying on abortion as one of the means to regulate fertility.

It is not possible to discuss in depth the interplay of all factors responsible for present abortion rates in the United States. Instead, we will concentrate on three critical issues that surround the present controversy: (1) the social circumstances that lead to unwanted pregnancies and how decisions to end pregnancies are made, (2) the procedures used to end unwanted pregnancies, and (3) the factors that influence postabortion adjustment.

preabortion considerations

It is not very meaningful to classify pregnancies into two non-overlapping categories of "wanted" and "unwanted" since this greatly oversimplifies the reality for most people. Continuing any pregnancy will have both advantages and disadvantages. Women sometimes undergo late abortions because of the difficulty deciding whether a pregnancy is more wanted than not. Although it makes more sense to discuss degrees of unwantedness, it is conceptually difficult to do so. For the purposes of this discussion, we will assume that pregnancies can be classified in this simple, one-dimensional way.

An unintended but wanted conception occurs when the conscious desire to become pregnant is absent, but the reality of pregnancy is easily accepted. Examples of this are when pregnancy occurs to an engaged couple prior to the wedding or when efforts at child spacing are unsuccessful and pregnancies closer than the ideal for the couple result. Although objective life conditions would dictate a different timing, only minor accommodations are required for the pregnancy to be integrated into the couple's life situation.

Under other conditions, unintended conceptions are simply unwanted because continuation would necessitate radical changes in the life plan. A pregnancy that occurs when a woman is in school or at a stage of her career that cannot easily be resumed if interrupted, or one that takes place after a couple has all the children they wish are examples of unwanted pregnancies. Some women in these and similar situations will continue the pregnancy in any event, but many will seek abortion. Although a conception may have been unintended, not all unplanned pregnancies are unwanted. Nor will every unwanted pregnancy end in abortion. Women, therefore, do not experience equal risk of abortion throughout their entire reproductive careers. A mixture of social and psychological factors make them more likely to experience unwanted pregnancy during particular periods in their life cycle.

social characteristics of women seeking abortion

Each year social characteristics of women who obtain abortions throughout the United States are compiled for further study. They reveal important information about the circumstances under which women are likely to end pregnancies.

Abortion *rates* are the number of abortions performed per 1,000 women in a particular social category, such as the number of abortions per 1,000 white women in the United States or the number of abortions per 1,000 women between the ages of 15 and 44. Abortion *ratios* are the number of abortions per 1,000 pregnancies (excluding miscarriages and stillbirths) in a particular social category. In recent years, the highest abortion ratios have been found among poor, nonwhite, unmarried women under the age of 20.

Women at the extreme ends of the reproductive years are more likely to seek abortion than those in the middle. In 1978, 58 percent of pregnant women under 15 and 45 percent of those between 15 and 17 obtained abortions, as did 47 percent of women aged 40 and over. This contrasts sharply with the proportion of pregnant women in their twenties who underwent abortions: 30 percent of those between 20 and 24, and 21 percent of those between 25 and 29. Age, then, was one factor that women considered when deciding a pregnancy's course.

The lesser frequency of abortions among women in their twenties, however, is a function of age and marital status combined. A much greater proportion of women in their twenties than below are married when they become pregnant or use the pregnancy as an impetus for marriage. In 1978, only 22 percent of married pregnant women chose abortion, as compared with 66 percent of unmarried pregnant women. This pattern differs from such eastern European countries as Czechoslovakia and Hungary, where abortion rates are higher among married women, but is more similar to England and Wales, which show higher abortion rates among the unmarried. These data indicate that, in the United States, abortion is often used to delay the onset of childbearing or when couples want no more children. Its use to influence the number of years between pregnancies is not very common. Nearly half the abortions in 1977 were performed on women who had no living children.

Race and socioeconomic status seem closely linked in their influence on pregnancy outcome. While 26 percent of white pregnant women sought abortion, 40 percent of nonwhite pregnant women did so. These data on socioeconomic status are inferred rather than direct, but during 1976 when federally funded Medicaid abortions were available, the rate of Medicaid abortions per 1,000 women aged 15 to 44 was three times higher than the non-Medicaid rate. This indicates that poor women often choose to end rather than to continue their pregnancies, probably because of economic reasons.

However, the ability of poorer women to obtain abortions in the United States has been a matter of recent intense controversy. In 1977, Congress passed the Hyde Amendment, legislation that prohibited the use of federal funds to finance abortions unless the pregnancy was due to "promptly reported" rape or incest or its continuation would endanger the pregnant woman's life or result in serious physical injury. Although the constitutionality of the law was promptly challenged, the Supreme Court upheld the right of states to refuse to use Medicaid monies for abortion sought for reasons other than those outlined above. The effects of this legislation were promptly and dramatically felt: during 1979, the number of Medicaid financed abortions fell to about 2,400; nearly 295,000 had been performed the previous year.

As this chapter is written, proposals to further restrict poor women's access to abortion are pending in the executive and legislative branches of the government. The intent is to eliminate federal financing of abortions needed in cases of incest and rape and fund only those that would save the mother's life. These political battles clearly show how poor women are especially vulnerable to a changing political climate, which may force motherhood on those who lack the economic resources to make a personal choice. (See Hayler, 1979, for an excellent discussion of the sociopolitical context in which decisions about the availability of abortion for all women are made.)

psychological characteristics of women seeking abortion

The role of psychopathological factors in seeking an abortion is only a minor one. It is no longer accepted that women who undergo abortion are different from other women with regard to personality characteristics or manner of psychological functioning. Until about 1965, psychiatrists, physicians, and abortion researchers generally believed that women who sought abortion were immature, neurotic, or acting out unresolved psychic conflicts.

No data have been collected to support this point of view. Studies that attempted to determine women's preabortion mental states have been challenged because they examined psychological measures in a superficial way without also considering the objective reasons for the abortion. These earlier studies have also been discounted because, during the 1960s, mental health grounds were the surest way for women to be authorized for an abortion. This led them to exaggerate the extent of psychological distress so they could "qualify" for the procedure.

To determine what factors influence how women themselves perceive an impending abortion, 22 women were interviewed, mainly unmarried, white, and middle-class, who came to a California family planning clinic in 1972 for abortion referral. Less than half the women (41 percent) felt that the event was a major emotional crisis for them. This woman's feelings were typical of those in this group: "I guess you can call it a crisis. I never had such a problem before. I never considered this the last time I was pregnant. . . . I've been very confused; I want to cry all the time. I hate to have to do it, but there doesn't seem to be any other way."

Only nine of the women were ambivalent about abortion. They could easily imagine circumstances under which they would continue the pregnancy, such as if they were earning more or if their partners were encouraging. A second characteristic the women shared was an inability to find an effective social support system to help them resolve their situation. They lacked what they considered satisfactory emotional relationships with their sexual partners, and most disagreed with the partner on whether the pregnancy should be continued. In addition, they received conflicting advice on how to proceed from the other relatives and friends who were consulted. This, too, contributed to their own uncertainty. A combination of a weak social support system and personal ambivalence led to a preabortion period characterized by confusion and distress. Although all continued to function on some level (none quit their jobs, for example, or sought psychiatric help), they found the experience a very difficult one.

The majority of the women (59 percent) did not consider the pregnancy to be a crisis. Although they did not differ from the others in terms of such social characteristics as age, number of living children, educational experience, or marital status, there were important factors in these women's life situations that enabled them to deal effectively with the pregnancy. The women in this group expressed no ambivalence about having the abortion; they could not imagine any circumstances under which they would continue the pregnancy at this time in their lives. They strongly felt that the trauma would have been greater were abortion not readily available. One woman put it directly: "Being pregnant is not such a serious thing because I can get an abortion. If I couldn't, then it would be a real crisis. I believe it involves a certain responsibility to make a decision one way or the other, but I believe that it's my decision to make."

In addition to a lack of ambivalence, these women had strong social supports to help them through the abortion period. Most had emotional relationships with a sexual partner that they described as happy and satisfying. In the overwhelming majority of the cases, both agreed on the decision to end the pregnancy. Those few who chose not to consult with the partner found friends or relatives who offered emotional support. Lack of personal ambivalence and the absence of interpersonal conflict together created an atmosphere in which the decision to end the pregnancy could be quickly made and easily carried out. Evidence for this was the fact that more than half the women in the "noncrisis" group came for abortion referral in the first seven weeks of pregnancy, while only one-third of those in the "crisis" group did so. The noncrisis women saw the

pregnancy as a significant life event, but they did not find their lives completely disrupted.

abortion techniques

Pregnancy occurs when a fertilized egg attaches itself to the lining of the uterus (the endometrium) and begins to grow. Six weeks after the woman's last menstrual period, the embryo is a month old and about the size of a pea. It rests in the amniotic sac, which contains clear fluid to protect the embryo from injury and maintain it at an even temperature. By the end of the second month, the fetus is about an inch long, and the placenta, the tissue that nourishes the fetus, is well developed. Fourteen weeks after the last menstrual period, or the end of the third month of gestation, the fetus is 2 to 3 inches long and weighs less than an ounce.

Abortion involves removing the fetus, placenta, and built-up endometrium from the uterus. The size of the fetus determines the method used. Abortion is easier, less physically and emotionally stressful, and safer the earlier it is done. At the present time, techniques that do not require a hospital stay are performed mainly during the first 12 weeks after the last menstrual period. The abortion methods most commonly used in the United States are discussed in the next section.

early abortion

Suction dilation, also known as vacuum aspiration (dilation and evacuation, D & E) is now the most widely used abortion method in the United States. Its use is mainly limited to the first three months of pregnancy. The cervix is slowly stretched or dilated by inserting nonflexible rods (dilators) of increasingly

larger size until the opening is wide enough for the tip of the aspirator to enter the uterus. Women sometimes feel cramping during the dilation, but otherwise do not experience pain during the procedure. Those who have been pregnant in the past or are in the very early stages of pregnancy may not require dilation. A thin tube of either flexible or hard plastic or metal, called a cannula, is passed through the cervix into the uterus. The tube is then attached to a suction source, usually an electric or mechanical pump. During the 2 to 5 minutes of suctioning, the contents of the uterus are removed and deposited into a container within the aspirator.

The entire abortion takes about 10 minutes, and women generally return home within a few hours of the procedure. The abortion may be done in a doctor's office, clinic, or hospital under local anesthesia or with none at all. For both these reasons, the cost is generally low. The advantages of suction abortions include a very low rate of complications, especially if a flexible cannula is used, limited blood loss, and rapid recovery. Complications, although rare, include perforating the uterus with one of the instruments used in the abortion, infection, incomplete abortion, where the entire contents of the uterus are not removed, and hemorrhaging.

Until the mid-1960s, most abortions were performed by *surgical curettage* (dilation and curettage, D & C). It continues to be used in cases of incomplete abortions and to treat infertility, menstrual irregularity, and very heavy menstrual bleeding. The cervix is dilated as in suction curettage. A long-handled, spoon-shaped metal loop is then inserted into the uterus and used to scrape loose the uterine lining. The contractions caused by the stroking action of the curette causes the uterus to empty. Although the abortion may be done under local anesthesia, general anesthesia is more commonly used in America. Surgical curettage has no advantage over suction curettage, and complication rates, especially due to uterine perforation and anesthesia effects, are higher.

later abortion

Abortion was rarely performed between the thirteenth and fifteenth week of pregnancy because the likelihood of complications such as uterine perforation and excessive bleeding was thought to increase. During this time, the uterus is expanding and its walls are becoming thinner and more spongy to accommodate the growing fetus. Women who requested abortions at the end of the first trimester of pregnancy had to wait several weeks until an intra-amniotic injection abortion (see below) could be performed. This was unfortunate since injection abortions are much more painful, physically dangerous, emotionally traumatic, and expensive than first trimester abortions. Recently, suction curettage has been found to be an acceptable option for early second trimester abortions. Most performed between 12 and 15 weeks of pregnancy now make use of this technique.

Intra-amniotic infusion (saline abortion, salting out, prostaglandin abortion) is the next most commonly used second trimester (16 to 24 weeks) abortion method. A solution is injected through the abdominal wall into the amniotic cavity, causing an abortion to begin 10 to 36 hours later. Contractions last another 8 to 15 hours. The injection may be done un-

der local anesthesia with the woman remaining home until the contractions begin or the entire process may take place over a 2-to-4-day hospital stay. Intra-amniotic infusion is more painful than earlier abortion methods since the contractions may be of similar intensity and duration to full-term delivery. Although complication rates are about the same as for delivery, they are higher than for first trimester abortions. Risks include hemorrhage, retained placenta, which must later be removed by curettage, and infection. The emotional impact may also be greater than in earlier abortion since the fetus is more developed and is "delivered" as in full-term pregnancy.

Until recently, hypertonic saline (salt) solution was injected to cause the abortion. Prostaglandins, hormonelike substances that naturally appear during labor and delivery, are now also used in some parts of the United States, although their expense inhibits widespread adoption. Saline abortions have fewer side effects than prostaglandins, although the abortion process is longer and there is the very slight possibility of shock or death due to changes in the salt concentration of the blood or cerebral hemorrhage in the base of the brain. Prostaglandins work more quickly than saline, but may be accompanied by such side effects as nausea, vomiting, and diarrhea. There is a slightly higher incidence of incomplete abortion with prostaglandins and an increased risk of cervical tearing due to too rapid dilation. With prostaglandins, too, there is the possibility that the fetus will be expelled with signs of life and for this reason they are not usually used after 20 weeks of pregnancy.

In abortion by *hysterotomy*, the fetus is removed through an incision in the lower abdomen. The procedure is similar to a caesarean delivery and is used in the second trimester of pregnancy when abortion by intra-amniotic injection is not possible. Although hysterotomy alone does not directly affect the reproductive system, it is commonly used when sterilization by hysterectomy (see below) is planned following the abortion. Six to 10 days of hospitalization are required. Hysterotomy has one of the highest complication rates of all abortion techniques, particularly the risks of hemorrhaging and incomplete abortion. Use of general anesthesia for the procedure also increases the chances of complication. In some

cases, subsequent pregnancies must be delivered surgically by caesarean section.

Abortion by *hysterectomy*, or surgical removal of the uterus (but not the ovaries), is done in cases when pregnancy accompanies a known uterine disease, such as fibroid tumors or a uterine prolapse, or when sterilization following abortion is desired. The procedure is performed under general anesthesia and requires 6 to 10 days of hospitalization. Because hysterectomy is major surgery, the rate of complications is relatively high.

physical effects of induced abortion

In every country where abortion has been legalized and is widely available, the number of deaths due to abortion and childbirth and the amount of illness caused by infection and other abortion complications have declined. The possibility of death after legal abortion is now very slight, as is the risk of serious complications. It is universally true, however, that the *earlier* in pregnancy an abortion is performed, the less the chance of injury and death.

illness and injury

Nonserious abortion complications such as mild fever or nausea following the application of anesthesia are not unusual. Complications of this type tend to last only a short time and have no lasting physical repercussions. Women are advised to refrain from strenuous activity for a day or two after an abortion to minimize the possibility of minor complications.

Two types of major complications are recognized: those that occur at the time of the abortion or within the following month and those that occur more than a month later. Injuries that may occur at the time of the abor-

tion include perforating the uterus with one of the instruments used in the procedure, hemorrhaging, laceration of the cervix, problems with blood coagulation, and anesthesia side effects such as fever and convulsions. The most common major complications occurring more than a month after the procedure include retention of placental tissue, mild to severe infection, pulmonary embolism, and sensitization of Rh-negative women by blood from an Rh-positive fetus.

In the 1970s, about 10 percent of the women who had abortions had one or more complications, although most were minor. One percent had major complications. Rates for both total and major complications were lowest for abortions done by suction curettage, followed, in order of increasing frequency of complications, by surgical curettage, intra-amniotic infusion, hysterotomy, and hysterectomy. Less than 1 woman in 100 had any complications from abortions by either suction or surgical curettage. Between 2 and 3 per 100 experienced complications from intra-amniotic infusion abortions; nearly 7 in 100 from hysterotomy; and more than 15 per 100 from hysterectomy. Because these last two are major surgery, the risk of complications is greater.

There is a definite relationship between status and abortion complications. Complication rates are higher for women receiving public funds to finance abortions than for private patients. These differences are seen especially clearly in the women who had second trimester abortions. Investigators suggest a number of reasons for the differences, including the possibility that the women who use public funds are in poorer health prior to the abortion and that there are fewer opportunities for rest and aftercare upon return home than there are for women who finance their abortions by other means.

Findings are contradictory concerning the long-term physical effects of induced abortion. Early studies suggested a relationship between abortion and a variety of physical hazards to both the fetus in later pregnancies and the woman herself, including premature delivery, low birth weight babies, increased incidence of infant mortality, and the greater possibility of spontaneous abortions of subsequent pregnancies. More recent research has shown no evidence of any of these effects. Nor is there evidence that induced abortion increases the risk of sterility.

mortality

With regard to mortality rates, abortion is safer than most other types of surgery. It is also much safer than childbirth unless it is performed after the sixteenth week of pregnancy. The death rates for abortion complications are: 1 death/100,000 abortions for suction curettage, 17/100,000 for intra-amniotic infusion, and 45/100,000 for hysterectomies. This compares with a death rate of 5/100,000 tonsillectomies, 74/100,000 simple mastectomies, 352/100,000 appendectomies, and 14/

100,000 childbirths. The most important factor affecting abortion mortality is the duration of the pregnancy. Abortions performed on women who have been pregnant for eight weeks or less had a mortality rate of .5 death/100,000 abortions. This rate rose to 3/100,000 for abortions performed during the eleventh and twelfth week of pregnancy. The rate increased even more drastically for second trimester abortions to 19/100,000 during the sixteenth through twentieth week of pregnancy and 40/100,000 for abortions performed on pregnancies of more than 20 weeks gestation.

The legalization of abortion resulted in a remarkable drop in the total number of deaths from abortion complications, with the sharpest decline related to illegal abortion. In 1970, 158 women died from abortion complications; at least 106 died after illegal procedures. Fifty-five women died following abortions just three years later in 1973, the year the Supreme Court removed restrictions on first and second trimester abortions. This same year, 19 women died from illegal procedures. Another sharp drop in abortion-related deaths occurred by 1978. A total of 27 women died, seven from illegal abortions.

Like the higher rates of injuries poor and nonwhite women suffer as a result of abortion, they also suffer much higher death rates from illegal procedures. Between 1972 and 1974, 70 percent of the women who died following illegal abortions were nonwhite. Half the women who died after legal abortion were also nonwhite, although less than one-third of abortion patients at the time were in these racial categories. Reasons for the higher death rates include their poorer health prior to the abortion and their lack of access to safe legal abortion services. The maldistribution of abortion services throughout the United States means that poor, nonwhite, rural women are more likely than others to have to travel long distances outside their home communities to obtain a legal abortion. They are often forced to resort to an unsafe illegal procedure instead.

psychological effects of induced abortion

Three areas must be considered when examining the psychological effects of abortion: effects on women who have had abortions, effects on women who have been denied abortions, and effects on children of women who have been denied abortions. This discussion is restricted primarily to the first of these areas since very little is known about the other two.

The distinction between severe psychological illness and mild, passing emotional reactions must clearly be made when looking at psychological effects of induced abortion. This is especially important because abortion can represent psychological stress on at least two levels—not only is it an end to pregnancy, but, like any surgical procedure, it can spark complex feelings related to invasion of body boundaries. Sadness, depression, anxiety, shame, and regret are among the normal responses. A society's attitude toward abortion will help intensify feelings each woman experiences.

severe
psychological reactions

Concern about the possibility of extreme psychological reactions to abortion grew out of the psychoanalytic orientation that dominated the field of abortion research prior to the 1960s. The woman who sought abortion was seen as mentally inadequate because she did not wish to continue the pregnancy. But this refusal could take a further psychological toll in the form of a "postabortion psychosis." As influential as this position was throughout our society, it was based on polemics rather than fact. After examining the postabortion mental states of thousands of American and British women, researchers concluded that psychotic episodes following abortion are very rare, much rarer, in fact, than postpartum psychosis. Women at greatest risk have severe psychiatric conditions that predate the abortion; those in good mental health run little risk from the procedure. It should not be surprising that childbirth is more psychologically stressful than abortion. When a woman returns to the nonpregnant state after an abortion, she can proceed with her life as before. But childbirth dramatically changes her entire existence. If the pregnancy is unwanted, this change may be especially difficult to endure.

milder
psychological reactions

The nature of the less severe psychological effects of abortion is more difficult to determine. Much of the existing research has serious shortcomings in design and execution, making it hard to evaluate and compare their findings. Seldom have studies compared the reactions of women who had abortions with control groups of "ordinary" women or ones who carried pregnancies to term. Examinations of women's mental status prior to the unwanted pregnancy and again after the abortion have not been done. Instead, investigators have evaluated women just before the abortion, when their emotional reactions may be exaggerated by the stress of the abortion decision. And with the abortion controversy continuing at an intense pitch, research findings are especially likely to be interpreted in accordance with the investigator's own bias on the subject.

Another problem with assessing the psychological effects of abortion is the difficulty in separating what women feel from what they believe they *should* feel. Women whose predominant feelings following an abortion are happiness or relief may wonder if they are "normal" or why they are not having a more extreme reaction.

It is rare for a woman to have an extreme negative emotional response as a result of an abortion. The occasional woman who has a mental reaction serious enough to require hospitalization invariably had severe psychological problems before her pregnancy. Immediately after an abortion, many women simultaneously feel both negatively and positively about their decisions. They feel tremendously relieved that the situation has been remedied and that they were able to respond in a positive way. Most report being happy and satisfied with the decision. At the same time, some women feel a certain amount of regret—to have been pregnant and forced to end it is a difficult choice to have made. A sense of loss, accompanied by depression, anger, or sadness, is common, although these feelings become less acute with the passage of time.

There are some circumstances under which women experience a greater than normal risk of negative emotional reaction to an abortion. In part, this is a function of how the abortion decision is made. Women who are confused or ambivalent about the best course for them and lack an opportunity to express their feelings are more apt than others to experience negative psychological aftereffects. Most find it

helpful to discuss the alternatives with a friend, relative, or professional, such as an abortion counselor, social worker, or clergy person, so they can come to terms with their emotions. Women who feel they have been pressured into ending the pregnancy by parents or others close to them may also have difficulty accepting their feelings of anger or regret during the postabortion period. A social situation that allows the woman to make her own decision in an environment of warmth and support increases the ease with which she will recover emotionally from an abortion.

Women who have second trimester saline or prostaglandin injection abortions are also more likely than others to have negative postabortion reactions. This is true for a number of reasons. These women are usually younger and more apt to be single than women who seek abortion in the first trimester. They are likely to be less experienced with the signs of pregnancy and not know how to go about arranging for an abortion. Because the pregnancy is in a more advanced state, they may also have a greater attachment to the fetus and may, therefore, experience a stronger sense of loss or grief after the abortion. Injection abortions are also more prolonged and more painful than early ones and they require hospitalization. Delivering a recognizable fetus, as is the case in injection abortions, is very traumatic for some women, especially if they are very young themselves or on the maternity floor of a hospital where injection abortions are sometimes performed. All of these factors may contribute to the intensity of the postabortion reaction for women who have them later in pregnancy. The earlier a woman can end her pregnancy, the more likely she will do so with a minimum of emotional distress.

It is generally the case, however, that women who feel very anxious when they learn they are pregnant start to feel better once the abortion is over and they can begin to return to their life as it was before. It often takes months for the complex array of feelings that women experience during pregnancy, abortion, and recovery to be fully integrated and accepted. In most cases, however, the abortion becomes an important maturing experience. Women see themselves as having resolved a stressful situation in a decisive way.

Many use the abortion as an opportunity to re-evaluate aspects of their present life circumstances. This may involve a second look at available contraceptive alternatives or a reassessment of the romantic relationship in which the pregnancy occurred. Most women find an abortion is a learning experience that, with time, they assimilate into their total perspective.

effects of abortion denied

What about the effects of the inability to obtain an abortion when one is desired? Although the short- and long-term effects on women from pregnancies they were forced to continue have not been studied in the same detail as have the effects of induced abortion, a few comments may be made. These considerations are especially important since greater legislative control over the conditions under which abortions are available for *all* women is becoming more common throughout the country. Social observers believe that the decade of the eighties will see even greater restrictions on the availability of legal abortion. Many of the women denied legal abortion will undergo the danger, anxiety, and expense of illegal abortion because they are determined to end their pregnancies. For them, the inevitable result will be a greater likelihood of infection, injury, and death from abortion complications. The situation will also be difficult for women unable to obtain any kind of abortion as their career, marriage, education, and life plans undergo radical change. In some cases, the outcome will be particularly unhappy. Studies show that about half the women forced to bear children they do not want several years later continue to have preferred an abortion; many never accept the situation or

grow to love the child. And when a group of women with unwanted pregnancies who sought abortion was compared with a group who gave their children up for adoption, more of the adoption group had long-term difficulty adjusting emotionally to their decision.

It is also necessary to consider the effects on children born when their mothers are not able to obtain abortions. One study indicates that these children, especially the boys, seem to have more difficulties with all-around adjustment. They have a greater number of illnesses, are more likely to need hospitalization, do more poorly in school, need more psychiatric treatment, experience more difficulty relating to their peers, and engage in more delinquent behavior than children of wanted pregnancies. The authors conclude that maternal love does not automatically grow in every woman who becomes a mother. Children born to women who do not want them are born into a situation that is potentially handicapping to both.

Forrest, J. D., Sullivan, E., & Tietze, C. Abortion in the United States, 1977–78. *Family Planning Perspectives,* 1979. (11), 32–341.

Haylor, B. Review essay: Abortion. *Signs: Journal of Women in Culture and Society,* 1979. (5), 307–323.

Henshaw, S., Forrest, J. D., Sullivan, E., & Tietze, C. Abortion in the United States, 1978–79. *Family Planning Perspectives.* Jan.–Feb. 1981. (13), 6–18.

Institute of Medicine. *Legalized abortion and the public health.* Washington, D. C.: National Academy of Sciences, 1975.

Moore-Cavar, E. C. *International inventory of information on induced abortion.* New York: International Institute for the Study of Human Reproduction, 1974.

Potts, M., Diggory, P., & Peel, J. *Abortion.* Cambridge, Eng.: Cambridge Univ. Press, 1977.

JEANNE QUINT BENOLIEL, R.N., D.N.Sc.

women and loss:
the many faces of grief

Loss is so much a part of human existence that its contribution to personal development is often unrecognized. Yet, how any woman responds to the major losses she encounters as an adult has origins in experiences of infancy and childhood. These early encounters with loss directly influence her sense of personal identity, trust in other people, and capacity to cope with serious losses encountered later in life—including those produced by death and dying.

human development and relational ties

By definition, loss is a state of being deprived of something that once was available and important and now is gone. For human beings, loss is associated with the disappearence of emotional attachments to people and things that give meaning to life. A loss can be major or minor depending on the importance of the relationship to the person involved. In a profound sense, birth can be viewed as a major loss that makes great demands on the human organism for responsive adaptation. The newborn infant moves from a protective, warm intrauterine world into a new and sometimes precarious environment in which needs for

221

warmth, food, and comfort are not automatically provided through physiologic processes, but instead depend on the whims and wishes of other people. Birth introduces the infant to separation, and the infant learns to experience withdrawal by others as a threat to personal gratification and survival.

attachments and separations

The extreme helplessness of the newborn infant makes her utterly dependent on the choices and actions of the key adults around her. In great measure they influence her chances for physical survival. More than that, they become the recipients of the infant's primary emotional attachments, and they provide the social milieu through which she learns to interact with other people. Out of interactions with these important figures, she begins the process of developing an autonomous self and learns to associate her responses with counterresponses from other people. Ironically, experiences with separation and loss are essential for learning the meaning of personal autonomy and a sense of mastery over the world. Yet, without active counterresponses, from the mother in particular, a newborn can suffer serious physical and psychosocial deprivations that interfere with the establishment of feelings of security and self-worth. The extreme effects of maternal deprivation on infants in the first year of life were shown by Spitz (1946) to result in extreme depression, withdrawal from interactions, and failure to thrive.

The importance of a responding environment to the development of personhood and the capacity to cope with adversity and change has been espoused by all of the major theories in this area. Theories vary, however, in the emphasis given to intrapersonal, inter-

personal, and social components of the adaptive process. Those who favor the psychoanalytic view are likely to emphasize reactions to loss and separation as the result of psychic conflict including the reactivation of feelings that remain from the first year of life (Brenner, 1976). Not uncommonly, writers in this school refer to grief (the reaction to loss) as a poor adaptive response and the grieving process itself as a form of illness (Peretz, 1970). Those who back the attachment theory emphasize grief as an adaptive response that takes account of present as well as past meanings of the lost relationship and sees the environment as a critical factor affecting the process of coping with loss (Bowlby, 1973; Parkes, 1972). Although both sets of theories note the importance of early childhood experiences for the development of effective coping capacities, attachment theorists led by Bowlby (1969) place considerable emphasis on the human capacity to modify behavior at later ages in response to discrepancies between performance and already established goals.

The influence of early childhood experiences on personal development is twofold. It is through these early experiences with adults that a baby learns to trust other people and to anticipate adult availability in times of crisis and strain. It is through a process of identification with the feelings, thoughts, and behaviors of the significant adults around her that a girl (or boy) learns to think and feel about herself as a person capable of coping with change. Seligman (1975) believes that a child's sense of mastery about self requires her to synchronize her voluntary responses to the world and the outcomes she experiences and sees as positive in nature. In his concept, the absence of mother, loss of stimulation, and nonresponsive mothering in infancy all contribute to learning a sense of helplessness and inability to influence the environment.

types of significant loss

A girl's capacity to cope with loss begins during the same period that she is learning to attach value to herself as a separate being. Thus, her capacity to cope with change is closely intertwined with her feelings of personal worth. Both are affected by her experiences with loss during these formative years.

The normal process of growth and development in and of itself brings both gains and losses. The process of learning to walk creates a new capacity for mobility and active exploration, but it may also cause the significant adults to impose constraints on the use of that mobility. Some changes in living can be trivial; others can involve the severing of important relationships. A child who has been breastfed from birth will at some point learn that this form of feeding and comfort is no longer available. The birth of a second child will cause the firstborn in any family to lose a position of central importance to a newcomer who is likely to require a large amount of parental attention. These changes are losses of valued relationships for children, but their importance for individual children can vary depending on the child's attachment to that relationship and the attitudes and actions of other people toward the change. Through experiences with these kinds of changes in relationships, a girl learns ways of adapting that eventually become part of her basic personality and coping style.

Throughout life, each individual experiences losses. Some require a minimal amount of adaptation. Others are major changes, making heavy demands on the personal and social resources of the individual. The extent to which any given loss is major in its effects depends on the type of loss, its special meaning to the individual, and the circumstances under which the loss takes place.

Probably the majority of those writing about grief believe that the most important type of loss for human beings is the departure of a human relationship to which the individual had strong emotional bonds and from which came personal gratification and significant meaning. Loss of a key relationship through death is viewed by many experts as the most critical of loss experiences because the change is permanent in effect. The significance of such losses in the lives of women provides the core of this chapter. It is important to be aware, however, that human beings form attachments to other forms of relationships, including external objects and material possessions, physical and social aspects of the self, and social roles that are central to an individual's sense of esteem and personal value.

Changes in physical appearance may be particularly important losses for women, especially those who base personal and social worth on the external physical attributes of womanhood. Personal investigation of women's adjustment after mastectomy gave evidence that women's perceptions of self are strongly affected by removal of a breast, but discussion about the topic is not easy, perhaps because breast loss is experienced as a lessening of sexual identity (Benoliel, 1971).

The point is that women's ties to their bodies, their homes, and their social competencies predispose them to loss experiences, some of which may be serious and severe. These losses precipitate the need for grief and mourning just as much as do losses produced by the death of a significant person. Yet, as Werner-Beland (1980) has sensitively shown, loss of a part of the self—whether physical or psychosocial—is different from losses produced by death because the source of grief remains as a constant reminder of the change that has taken place.

Physical losses producing changes in appearance or interference with social competency are particularly potent life experiences because they contribute to shifts in the attitudes and behaviors of other people toward the disabled person. A woman faced with serious physical changes in herself also must respond to and cope with the effects of the reactions of others to the change and the impact of their grieving on her social interaction with them. Werner-Beland (1980) believes that coping with the loss imposed by physical disability or disease requires adaptive behaviors that are different in quality from those associated with the loss of a significant person. Even so, there is ample evidence in the literature that loss of a significant person creates intense grief reactions and makes heavy demands on a woman's established coping capacities. Significant loss by death means change that affects all levels of human adaptation—physical, emotional, cognitive, existential, and social.

loss, grief, and bereavement

Because loss plays such a central part in human development, the capacity to cope with loss exists at different levels. In fact, a woman's pattern of coping with personal and social changes throughout life is made up of integrated coping mechanisms that could be described as separate entities, but that, in response to real crises, function together as a total response.

mechanisms for coping with loss

Perhaps the earliest coping behavior learned by infants in response to loss is aggressive activity and loud protest, which, if successful, get the attention of concerned adults and bring relief. Important parts of these early learnings are sensations such as pain and first-order emotions such as tension, appetite, fear, rage, and satisfaction, which involve the baby as a total being and are associated in negative or positive ways with a sense of safety and comfort (Arieti & Bemporad, 1978). These protoemotions are closely tied to physiological changes that help the baby to survive in response to various types of stimuli. They stimulate the infant's perception of her world and function as motivating forces for early learning about the meanings of danger, threat, and pleasure.

Threatening situations in which loss exists appear to play an important part in the learning of trust in self and in others. Infants who are only partially successful in getting satisfactory responses to their protests about a lost relationship may develop a general pattern of angry and aggressive behaviors, according to Bowlby (1973). Those who experience little success may retreat into patterns of helplessness and withdrawal (Seligman, 1975). Whatever the pattern learned in these early years, it becomes part of an adaptive response that continues through the remainder of a woman's life.

Psychologic coping mechanisms become more complex as the human mind develops, and learning about the world is influenced by symbols as well as stimuli and signals. Images about people and things become representations that allow the person to anticipate the future and review the past. Symbolic thinking paves the way for new emotional reactions—anxiety in response to the expectation of danger, anger in response to images that earlier would have caused rage, and wishing in response to an image that is attractive. Language is central to recognizing these changes and it facilitates the development of what Arieti and Bemporad (1978) call the complicated third-order emotions of sadness, hate, love, and joy. The importance of these emotions is how they depend on the thinking processes. They appear in response to a complicated interplay among thoughts, feelings, images, and experiences. They connect the past with present and future, and they do not disappear in response to simple measures. They are complex results of human-to-human interdependence. Sadness, in particular, is a frequent result of significant loss.

The psychological defense mechanisms that evolve in the unconscious mind to protect the human psyche from information that it is not ready to face are highly important. Developed during the formative years as another protection against real and perceived threats, these mechanisms function to guard against excess anxiety and to secure gratification. They take a variety of forms and include repression of thoughts and feelings, displacement of feelings onto other people or things, projection of ideas, rationalization of behavior motives, substitution of attachment, denial of feelings or reality, and regression to earlier patterns of behavior.

The set of psychologic mechanisms learned by a particular girl is probably both a unique pattern in response to the socializing influences of her parents and other people and a common or typical pattern reflecting cultural and social values as these are learned through the family (Palgi, 1976). Both conscious and unconscious responses to experiences with loss are heavily influenced by what the child learns about social norms and rules governing proper behavior in public and private places. Thus, a girl learns that crying behavior may be appropriate in one situation and not in an-

other. She learns how children are expected to behave with adults, and she learns from watching adults what is expected of them under various circumstances—including the death of another person. In other words, the child is socialized to respond to death losses in terms of the values and beliefs of the family and the society. One of the problems for children in the twentieth century in Western societies is that social norms governing proper behavior for coping with death have emphasized denial of its reality and have provided ambiguous and unclear guidelines for social conduct in the presence of death and dying (Benoliel, 1978). As a result, many young women have developed few social skills for coping effectively with the impact of these situations.

At the broadest level are institutionalized cultural patterns of response to death, which reflect the basic values and beliefs of a society or segment of society. The importance of cultural values, beliefs, and practices is that they determine in great measure the bereavement behaviors that members of a society or a subgroup learn are expected before and at the time of death. They influence the how, whether, and when of emotional expression that is acceptable, including variations permitted by age, sex, and position (Rosenblatt, Walsh, & Jackson, 1976).

Commonly, religion is a significant influence on attitudes toward death as well as bereavement behaviors, but religious beliefs and customs must be understood in the context of the larger culture of which they are part. Bereavement behaviors tend to be a complex intermingling of culture and religion, as Palgi (1976) has shown in her analysis of bereavement practices in Israel. The Jewish religion has clearly defined rules of behavior for all stages of the mourning process. Yet, the actual behaviors of the Israelis in response to the deaths of sons, husbands, and fathers in the war in 1973 varied by country of origin and represented cultural modifications of the basic Jewish practices. More than that, some behaviors—for example, wailing and lamentations—practiced by some ethnic groups from the Middle East were seen as shocking and inappropriate by Ashkenazi families, who are prone to maintaining control over the overt expression of emotion. The point is that people are ill at ease and easily embarrassed by behavior that is different from their own. They can also misinterpret the extent to which grief is experienced by lack of understanding of the meaning of various culturally expressed modes of mourning.

The relationship between the inner experience of grief and the outward expression of mourning is a complicated mixture—an intertwining of coping levels from the biologic to the cultural. There is strong evidence that grief is a universal human response to the loss of a significant person. The actual process of adaptation to the loss can vary greatly in its behaviors and in its outcomes.

factors affecting the impact of death

The impact of loss through death depends on a combination of circumstances and not simply on loss per se. The impact is determined by an interaction among several important elements: the special meaning of the person who is gone; the degree to which the relationship is replaceable; the amount of personal and social disruption produced by the death; the time in the life cycle when the death occurs; and the availability of adaptive capacities and coping resources to respond to a changed life situation.

The very young and the very old are particularly vulnerable to the impact of losing a significant person: the young because their coping capacities are undeveloped and limited; the old because their personal and social resources for coping are diminished or diminishing, and they are likely candidates for the heavy burden of multiple losses (Benoliel, 1971). The impact of loss can also be affected by the type of death, the circumstances surrounding it, and the opportunities available to the survivor for bringing the experience to a close.

grieving as adaptation to change

Significant loss through death brings a state of sorrow and deprivation. Grief refers to the total response a woman makes to this important loss. Grieving is the psychobiologic process whereby this change in relationship is assimilated in her mind and a new definition of reality emerges. Grieving is a process that takes time to complete, but successful resolution of grief requires more than time. It requires emotional and cognitive work that eventually leads to "giving up" the relationship that is gone and moving on to new relationships and life activities (Lindemann, 1944; Parkes, 1972).

Because grief encompasses the woman as a totality, it affects her well-being physically as well as mentally. In his now classic study of grief reactions following an acute loss due to violent death, Lindemann (1944) observed five characteristics that he viewed as part of grief. These are: (1) physical distress and body tensions; (2) feelings of guilt; (3) a preoccupation with an image of the lost person; (4) hostility and anger; and (5) changes in usual behaviors and established patterns of social conduct. In other words, the process of grief affects the body and the mind, and it demands energy and attention.

From systematic studies of adult bereavement, Parkes (1972) clarified the changes in response that take place as part of the grieving process. The first phase is a period of numbness that lasts for a few hours to several days. Commonly, widows at this time describe themselves as shocked, blunted, dazed, or numb. Often the death itself does not seem real, and the woman reports a sense of disbelief. Glick, Weiss, and Parkes (1974), in a study of widows under 45 years of age, found that the initial reactions of shock and disbelief were generally extremely intense when sudden death threw women without warning into the state of widowhood.

The second phase of grieving is characterized by a separation anxiety and a preoccupation with thoughts of the person now gone. Women at this time pine for the lost relationship and engage in what Parkes called searching behavior—a tendency to focus attention and activity on objects and places associated with the deceased. Emotions at this time are a mixture of sadness, anger, and sometimes guilt and fear. Not uncommonly, women in this period feel a sense of helplessness and a wish to be helped.

Parkes (1972) identified the "pang of grief"—an episode of severe anxiety and psychological pain associated with missing the person—as the most characteristic feature of grieving. He saw pining as the emotional and subjective component of the urge to search for the lost object. The adaptive behaviors of human beings in response to the pangs of grief are crying and searching. Both behaviors can be viewed as efforts to recover or find the person who is lost. They are at their strongest during the early weeks following the death.

The actual manifestations of grief during the early phases are often surprising and disconcerting. Physiologically, women are likely to experience loss of appetite, insomnia, extreme fatigue, headaches, and various muscular pains and tensions. In the psychological realm, feelings of panic are frequent, along with difficulties in concentrating on anything but the loss. Feelings of restlessness and anger are commonplace, and many women are struck by the emotional instability and behavioral unpredictability that they experience. Suddenly bursting into tears in front of strangers, for instance, can be an unsettling experience for a woman who has always viewed herself as in control of her feelings.

Although searching behavior probably serves an important adaptive function toward the resolution of grief, it is not initiated by conscious processes and may not be recognized by the woman in grief. Searching behavior can take many forms. It is shown in a preoccupation with thoughts about the lost relationship and in memories about the past. It can result in dreams about the person who is gone. It can show itself in the development of strong attachments to personal belongings of the dead individual. It can produce a need to return to places once shared with the lost person. Searching probably plays a part in altering the perceptions of the grieving woman toward the deceased individual and in moving the process of grief into another phase (Parkes, 1972).

After the early phases of acute grief, the experience of yearning for the lost person gives way to feelings of apathy and despair, accompanied by a general aimlessness in behavior and a disorganization of usual patterns of activity. The most characteristic feeling associated with this period is depression and a sense that life is now empty of meaning. Despite the sense of aimlessness, most women are able to organize their lives into reasonable routines and to mobilize their personal resources toward resolution of the loss. The process of moving through and out of this feeling of depression takes place with cognitive and emotional effort, whereby perceptions and feelings of the past are brought into a new perspective and the pain associated with the lost relationship gives way to a new orientation to self and relationship with others.

resolution of grief

The process of "grief work" is not an easy matter. It requires a willingness to experience fully the complex emotional reactions that significant loss brings into being. It requires active mental activity to come to terms with the impact and meaning of the lost relationship. Often the process requires a woman to relive the death itself in a kind of obsessional review until such time as she can integrate what happened into her ongoing life. For many, the process includes coping with feelings of guilt and shame about past actions and thoughts in relation to the deceased. It may mean shifting back and forth between a tendency to idealize the lost person and feelings of anger for being left. Ultimately, the resolution of grief means internal acceptance of the reality that the relationship is gone and a lessening of intense emotional ties to the image of the deceased.

The process of finding resolution for the loss of a significant relationship may take a year or more of active work at grieving. It is a gradual process through which ties to the past are slowly let go and reconstruction of a future without that person emerges. According to Schmale (1973), the process of "giving up" the lost relationship necessitates the experience of depression, which includes a low point of helplessness and hopelessness; it is at this point, he believes, that the grieving person has increased psychic and physical vulnerability to disease and other disabling predispositions.

During this period of adaptive change, the behaviors of grieving women reflect their basic methods of coping. Some will have strong needs to be with other people. Others will make efforts to reorganize their lives to accommodate the change. Still others will accommodate their personal efforts and wishes to the realities of the needs of other people, a situation most commonly observed in women left with children in the home.

The extent to which the personal burden of sorrow is shared with others during this period depends on a woman's basic inclinations to do so in combination with the availability of people who are willing to listen. A great deal of grief work takes place within the mind of the grieving woman. Yet, because a significant death is a stress-producing situation, many coping mechanisms are at work at the unconscious level. Not surprisingly, physical symptoms of various kinds may continue for weeks or months, including headaches, menstrual irregularities, problems in sleeping, and many others. Some women continue to have frequent spells of weeping. Others are troubled by irritability and feelings of intense anger. The behavioral patterns of women as they move through the process of grief resolution vary considerably and reflect basic coping capacities and changes in conduct associated with new perceptions on the meaning of life.

Although much is not understood about the processes whereby resolution of grief is achieved, there is considerable evidence that the availability of emotional and social supports from other people plays an important part in helping the grieving person to move toward successful resolution. Support systems serve two important functions for the grieving woman. They provide outlets for sharing the experience of grief with others. They provide help with the readjustments in ongoing living that the death of a significant person necessitates. Lack of social supports may well contribute to inadequate resolution of loss and the development of prolonged grieving and other atypical patterns of reaction.

bereavement and mourning styles

The process of grieving is also affected by the bereavement behaviors that a woman is permitted to use. A problem in Western societies comes from an emphasis that fosters a social role of a bereaved person preoccupied with needs for grief expression but fails to provide socially sanctioned outlets for the external expression of the many strong feelings that grief incurs. Yet, within this broad cultural context, there are many differences in bereavement behaviors practiced by people from various ethnic backgrounds. Some groups give both women and men permission to grieve, whereas others proclaim the importance of maintaining control over emotions, regardless of internal feelings.

The need to say farewell to the deceased individual is expressed in funeral rituals and other types of leave-taking activities, most commonly derived from a combination of religious and ethnic beliefs. The aid in adapting to grief provided by participation in rituals was noted by Glick, Weiss, and Parkes (1974) in their study of widows' reactions during the postbereavement year. One of the major problems in the twentieth century may well be the disappearance of many rituals of transition and the removal of prescribed activities that assisted grieving individuals to share publicly in these important changes in social status. There is much to suggest that the lessening of bereavement practices in the United States and other Western societies has created a discrepancy between the personal needs of people for help in learning to mourn and the availability of social mechanisms to assist them in coping with this major transition.

significant losses in women's lives

Death causes a significant loss when its effects are intense and long lasting. Such deaths would generally include the loss of a parent, the loss of a spouse, and the loss of a child.

death of a parent

A woman's age at the time of parental death is a factor of some importance, for her age has important relationships to her past experiences with loss and her present capacity to cope with the stresses of change. Children are particularly vulnerable to the loss of a parent for two reasons. Their ideas about themselves are closely intertwined with identification with the parent, so that loss of the parent is felt as a loss of part of the self. In addition, children are dependent on their parents for direct care and services, and the removal of a parent produces a deficit in these services. The problem faced by children when a parent dies is not solely a matter of grieving for the lost relationship, although this activity is very important. Removal of a parent with whom the child identifies closely can interfere with the maturation of personality and the development of important coping capabilities.

Furman's (1974) work with children has shown how the loss of a parent in childhood or adolescence can have long-lasting effects unless the adults in the situation behave in ways to counteract the shock of the loss experience. Children need to know what has happened, to be allowed to express their feelings, and to participate in family activities related to the death. At the same time, children need to be in contact with a concerned adult who sees to it that their basic needs for food, attention, and care are met. Children in times of stress need the comfort of daily routines, and they need permission to acknowledge their pain and the stresses they experience. The extent to which the surviving spouse or other adult can be sensitive and responsive to these needs of grieving children depends on the maturity of that parent or person and the assistance she or he receives in coping with personal responses to the death. The multiple problems faced by the widow with children living at home has been tellingly detailed in Caine's (1974) description of her personal experiences in coping with life as a surviving spouse.

A more common problem today is loss of an aged parent by a woman in her middle years. Such deaths can occur suddenly, but more frequently follow a prolonged period of living and dying. Losses associated with prolonged dying produce more than the need for grief and mourning. Women in these circumstances are faced with many difficult decisions—about care-giving at home, about the use of a nursing home, about the impact of a sick parent on other family relationships. In other words, these women are faced with the conflicts and distress associated with reversal in roles as their aged parents become increasingly dependent on them for help with many things.

Loss of a parent following prolonged illness can bring relief as well as grief. Such experiences take a tremendous toll in energy and emotional investment, and grieving is only one part of a larger set of reactions and concerns. Coming to terms with parental loss under these circumstances means coming to terms with the impact and meaning of the total situation. Women who find resolution after these difficult and often painful transitions with their parents must somehow come to terms with any unfinished business that they carry about past relationships with parents and the present situation. These processes of resolution may be difficult to achieve without a socially supporting network of concerned people.

death of a spouse

Loss of a spouse is viewed by many experts on grief as the most significant loss in a woman's life. The complexities of the grieving process for that lost relationship have been detailed earlier. The importance of this loss for women, however, may well rest with the fact that loss of a husband often results in other social changes that radically affect a woman's life. Lopata's (1973) study of widows in Chicago showed their identified problems as loneliness, financial difficulties, child-rearing, decision-making, shortage of time, and self-pity. This study also showed that loss of a husband brought some compensations—such as freedom and independence from the care of another.

Lopata's study showed that widows' adaptations to the experience of bereavement were greatly affected by the personal and social resources at their disposal. Particulary disadvantaged were widows who tended to be lower class and dependent on ascribed social relationships. These women had developed few skills for coping with new situations in living, and many were psychologically handicapped by their suspicions of strangers and even acquaintances. For a variety of reasons, many such women found themselves relatively isolated from other people. In contrast, women who were able to modify their lives in response to the reality of widowhood were capable of dealing with the changes in their living situation, had supportive friends and relatives, or a combination of both.

The particular problems faced by a woman after the loss of her husband are determined in great measure by the time in life at which death occurs. Young women with small children face the general problem of taking care of themselves and their children; young women without work experience are often handicapped in seeking financial improvements. In contrast, an older woman may find herself "on her own" for the first time in her life, and she may have few social skills for moving out into new kinds of relationships. The point is that loss of a spouse brings multiple changes into a woman's life, and some women are better prepared than others to respond to the demands of those changes.

death of a child

Although some experts believe that loss of a spouse is the most important loss faced by a woman, others think that loss of a child is the most distressing and long lasting of griefs because it is untimely in its coming (Palgi, 1976). Loss of a grown child is particularly likely to be distressing because the parent anticipates being dead before the child. More importantly perhaps, the depth of distress may well be related to the importance attached by the parent to her role as parent (Benoliel, 1971). In other words, any woman whose self-concept is heavily invested with her image as mother may well encounter difficult problems in resolving the grief associated with loss of a child.

Much has been written about the importance of the relationship between mother and child, and women's thinking about themselves as mothers cannot help but be influenced by these many writings. In addition, however, a woman's feelings about a child are undoubtedly influenced by the experience of carrying the infant within her body. Given this closeness of mother and child, it is easy to understand that the death of a child can be difficult to resolve. Yet, many women do have the capacity to allow themselves to experience the full gamut of the grieving process and to find resolution to this most important loss.

Death of a child can also be brought about through a woman's decision to have an abortion. Research by Pasnau and Farash (1977) showed that virtually all of the women in their sample responded to the experience of abortion with some sense of loss. The findings also showed that the older women with living children showed a greater degree of loss than did the younger group who did not have children. The findings suggest that attachments to unborn children are directly related to personal maturation and social experiences. Gilligan (1977) studied the process of decision-making in women contemplating abortion and identified a sequence of moral judgments whereby decisions were reached to have the procedure performed. Both studies showed that decisions about abortion do not come easily to many women and often involve them in the pain of loss and grief.

risk factors and unresolved grief

The normal process of grieving is an effective and necessary means for resolving the impact and outcomes of lost relationships. Yet, there are times and circumstances under which grief is inhibited or does not take place within a reasonable length of time. Parkes (1972) saw atypical grief as manifest by an intense separation anxiety coupled with an effort by the person (usually only partially successful) to avoid the grieving process. Other factors thought to contribute to atypical grief are an ambivalent relationship with the deceased, the shock of unexpected death, death that occurs under catastrophic circumstances, and inflexible behaviors for coping with stress and change.

Failure to resolve the loss means that the woman carries the loss inside in a form that interferes with her capacity to function in a maximally effective way. Poor adaptive grief reactions take a variety of forms, including prolonged depression, alcoholism or other drug dependence, psychosomatic illness, hypochondriasis, and neurotic and psychotic states. The extent to which maladaptive grief can be prevented by programs of early intervention has yet to be established, but research into bereavement has helped to direct and guide these efforts. Vachon (1976) reviewed research bearing on grief and bereavement following the death of a spouse and identified five factors predictive of greatest risk: (1) poor social support, (2) person under age 45 whose spouse died suddenly or over 65 whose spouse had illness of six months or longer, (3) ambivalent marriage relationship, (4) minimal funeral ceremony associated with denial of the impact of death, (5) and previous psychiatric history.

Relationships with other people are increasingly recognized as important contributors to the process and outcomes of bereavement. Silverman and Cooperband (1975) have shown that the widow-to-widow program of mutual help can be beneficial to the widowed elderly by encouraging grief and providing peer supports. Women have long been contributors to various systems of helping relationships such as these, but much remains to be learned about the kinds of social supports that are needed to facilitate normal grieving and the successful resolution of loss under different sets of circumstances.

Arieti, S., & Bemporad, J. *Severe and mild depression.* New York: Basic Books, 1978.

Benoliel, J. Q. Assessments of loss and grief. *Journal of Thanatology,* 1971, *1,* 182–194.

Benoliel, J. Q. The changing social context for life and death decisions. *Essence,* 1978, *2(2),* 5–14.

Bowlby, J. *Attachment and loss, vol. 1: Attachment.* New York: Basic Books, 1969.

Bowlby, J. *Attachment and loss, vol. 2: Separation, anxiety and anger.* New York: Basic Books, 1973.

Brenner, C. *Psychoanalytic techniques and psychic conflict.* New York: International Univ. Press, 1976.

Caine, L. *Widow.* New York: Morrow, 1974.

Furman, E. *A child's parent dies.* New Haven: Yale Univ. Press, 1974.

Gilligan, C. In a different voice: Women's conceptions of self and of morality. *Harvard Educational Review,* 1977, *47,* 481–517.

Glick, I. O., Weiss, R. S., & Parkes, C. M. *The first year of bereavement.* New York: Wiley, 1974.

Lindemann, E. The symptomatology and management of acute grief. *American Journal of Psychiatry,* 1944, *104,* 141–148.

Lopata, H. Z. *Widowhood in an American city.* Cambridge, Mass.: Schenkman, 1973.

Palgi, P. Death, mourning and bereavement in Israel arising out of the war situation. In S. Feinstein & P. Giovacchini (Eds.), *Adolescent psychiatry, developmental and clinical studies,* Vol. IV. New York: Avonson, 1976.

Parkes, C. M. *Bereavement.* New York: International Univ. Press, 1972.

Pasnau, R. & Farash, J. Loss and mourning after abortion. In C. E. Hollingsworth & R. O. Pasnau (Eds.),

The family in mourning. New York: Grune & Stratton, 1977.

Peretz, D. Reaction to loss. In B. Schoenberg et al. (Eds.), *Loss and grief: Psychological management in medical practice.* New York: Columbia Univ. Press, 1970.

Rosenblatt, P. C., Walsh, R. P., & Jackson, D. A. *Grief and mourning in cross-cultural perspective.* New Haven, Conn.: HRAF Press, 1976.

Schmale, A. H. Adaptive role of depression in health and disease. In J. P. Scott & E. C. Senay (Eds.), *Separation and depression: Clinical and research aspects.* Washington, D.C.: American Assoc. for the Advancement of Science, 1973.

Seligman, M E. P. *Helplessness: On depression, development and death.* San Francisco: Freeman, 1975.

Silverman, P. R., & Cooperband, A. On widowhood, mutual help and the elderly widow. *Journal of Geriatric Psychiatry,* 1975, *8,* 9–27.

Spitz, R. Anaclitic depression, *The psychoanalytic study of the child,* 1946, *2,* 313–342.

Vachon, M. L. S. Grief and bereavement following the death of a spouse. *Canadian Psychiatric Association Journal,* 1976, *21,* 35–43.

Werner-Beland, J. A. *Grief responses to long-term illness and disability.* Reston, Virginia: Reston Publishing Company, Inc., 1980.

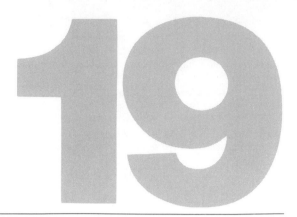

ANN WOLBERT BURGESS, R.N., D.N.Sc.

women and abuse:
rape and battering

The subject of rape (and battering) . . . has thrived on prudery, misunderstanding, and above all on silence. Nothing which so profoundly affects the lives of at least half of our population ought to be locked out of public consideration because of ancient concerns with "nice sensibilities."

The opening quote is taken from one of the first—if not *the* first—city council reports on the problem of rape in Washington, D.C., in 1973. Although the problem of battering was not addressed, it is likely that both forms of violence against women have been cloaked in secrecy and that the most helpful result for victims has been that the issue is now quite visible. The subsequent years have seen prog-

ress in terms of other cities looking at the problems of victimization of women and developing plans of action, usually in providing services for victims and their children.

Abuse, defined as improper treatment or use, may be experienced by a woman through a variety of mechanisms, including biological abuse (drugs, alcohol) and psychological abuse (verbal harrassment, sexual). The term *abuse*, when used in connection with behavioral abuse, is frequently used in combination with the concept of the "victim." Victimology—the study of the victim—has dramatically expanded since the early 1970s to become increasingly important in the health and social science literature. The term *victim* is often

234

used to refer to a person who has suffered either as a result of ruthless design or by accident (Viano, 1976).

Two types of physically abusive situations encountered by women in our society include forced sexual relations (rape) and battering. It is generally well accepted that the reported abusive acts against women are significantly less than the number of acts actually being committed. Thus, we are dealing with two social problems that generally go unreported, undetected, and undisclosed.

This chapter will discuss rape and battering in terms of traditional and contemporary views, characteristics, and motivational intent of the abuser, as well as sources of help for the victim of rape or battering.

rape

traditional views

Forced sexual assault—rape—is a sexual offense, illegal behavior, and proscribed in the criminal codes of every state. Being convicted of rape constitutes a felony, which is a capital offense punishable by varying degrees of penalties.

One of the ways to understand traditional views is to describe briefly the myths or images that exist regarding the rape victim. One of the most popular images, and one of the most difficult to disabuse people of, is that rape is primarily motivated by a need for sexual gratification. This myth is often reflected in jokes made about rape. For example, a man says: "I wouldn't complain about being raped by a group of girls." Or the frequent question, can a woman rape? To be discussed further under the motivational intent of the offender, rape is more often an expression of nonsexual needs, such as power and aggression in which the weapon used to express the aim is sex. Just as the overweight person is not eating because he or she is hungry or the alcoholic drinking because he or she is thirsty, neither is the rapist raping because he needs sexual activity. Very often the rapist is married or has access to a sexual partner. And, as illustrated in the following example, the child was sexually assaulted by the man who was in a sexual relationship with the mother:

> Amy, age 3½, was brought to Children's Clinic because of a foul-smelling discharge. When questioned about the situation, Amy said, "After my mother goes to bed, Bobby (mother's boy friend) comes in and touches me down there."

A second myth is that rape victims are hysterical. This myth is important because if the victim does not show this expected demeanor, people such as police and hospital staff may not believe she has been raped. However, in studying the reactions of rape victims admitted to one emergency floor, victims, in fact, demonstrated two emotional styles. About half of the victims were verbal and talkative, and half were quiet and guarded. Feelings of fear, anger, or anxiety were expressed verbally or shown by such behavior as crying, shaking, smiling anxiously, being restless, and being tense. In the controlled style, feelings were masked or hidden, and a calm, composed, or subdued bland affect was seen (Burgess & Holmstrom, 1979). The following case of a public health nurse who was raped illustrates the controlled style of emotion.

Emily: I have been visiting this mother and her five children for two years now. On my last visit, while I was there, she started having a spontaneous miscarriage. I made arrangements for her to be admitted to the hospital and for the children to stay with neighbors in the project. The next day, the mother's boy friend called and said there were some papers that needed to be filled out and asked for me to stop by and pick them up. I had another client to see in the project and said I would. After I was in the apartment, he locked the door and took out a knife. He threatened to kill me and said I wasn't to visit there any more and that a group was going to get me if I didn't stop the nursing visits . . . he ripped off my clothes and raped me twice . . . I was petrified he was going to kill me or the gang was going to get me. I promised I wouldn't tell the police. I made the other home visit in the project; went to lunch and back to the office and sat through a class. On the way home I cried. I had company for the weekend and managed to get through that . . . Went home for the holidays and my parents realized something was wrong but didn't ask any questions. I went back to work . . . While I was away I found out another nurse had been called to the woman's home by the boy friend to pick up papers. He tried to assault her. She was able to fight him off and got away to the police. Then I told what had happened to me.

Contrary to the hysterical myth, this victim showed an extremely controlled style that allowed her to function until the second nurse was assaulted. At that point she was able to talk about her experience and to express her feelings. Both nurses pressed charges and testified in court against the assailant, who was convicted.

Another myth is the notion that if the woman really wanted to, she could prevent the rape. People misunderstand cooperation with the rapist in order to survive as consent. Victims overwhelmingly report that they felt their lives were in danger, and they submitted in order to live. Clinicians who deal with the rapist will be the first to warn that in some situations—perhaps in many—the rape assault cannot be avoided. A study of the coping behavior of rape victims indicated that although victims use a variety of strategies to survive, "going along with the assailant" was an adaptive mechanism to remain alive when there was threat to her life (Burgess & Holmstrom, 1977). As one victim said, "I realized it was going to happen when he smashed me across the face. I realized what was going to happen so I gave in." In another case, one can see the number of strategies the victim tried prior to submitting to the rapist.

Irene: I must have fallen asleep . . . the next thing I knew I saw a leg and an arm coming in my bedroom. I screamed and screamed and screamed. I was kicking at my covers to get out of my apartment. I grabbed at his hair and he said, "I'm escaping from the police and I'm hiding out in your apartment." I said, "OK—I will let you out the door." Then he said, "How do you think I got in babe. I climbed the tree." I still had his hair and he slugged me in the head and told me to be quiet. He had black leather gloves over my mouth and I thought I would suffocate. He kept telling me not to look at him. I tried to look at his hair, listen to his voice . . . trying to think of everything I had read and heard. Then he said, "I'm here to screw you." I kept fighting. My feet were at the head of the bed. He took his gloves off and was feeling my body. He told me to stand up. No one was coming to help me and I was panicking. Mentally I decided I had tried everything I could think of. He ripped my nightgown off and grabbed me from the back and said, "I want you from behind." I said, "OK, if you will leave." He said OK and I kept trying to stall. He said he wouldn't hurt me. Then he changed his mind and pushed me onto the bed. He started to pull his pants zipper and there was a knock at the door . . . it was the police.

In this case, the victim had resigned herself to comply with the assailant's demands after she had tried all the strategies she could think of. But her screams did alert her neighbors, who called the police. However, after the man was arrested and a date was set for court, he defaulted—that is, never appeared at court.

Another myth is that prostitutes cannot be raped. To the contrary, we know that prostitutes are sometimes victims of rape since they may represent everything the rapist finds threatening and which he resents in a woman. For a man who wants to rape a woman, the prostitute is an easy mark. The hours that the prostitute works and the knowledge that she will have an extremely poor chance of bringing charges successfully against him in court also contribute to her vulnerability to be raped. In the study of the 109 adult women admitted to the emergency department of Boston City Hospital with the complaint, "I've been raped," 18 were prostitutes and three of them were raped while the remaining women were victims of such situations as nonpayment, perversion, robbery, and violence (Burgess & Holmstrom, 1977).

In one case involving a prostitute who was raped, the following testimony was recorded during the trial.

> *Laura:* We had a talk. He called me a bad name. He wanted to give me money to use my body. The waitress came over and told him to get away . . . my girl friends and I left and I was walking down the street. The next thing I knew I was grabbed by the neck into an alley. I screamed and someone put his hand over my mouth. I was pushed into a room. He ripped my clothes off and I was screaming. I got up and ran to the window but he threatened all the other guys would come in if I kept screaming. I heard the guys outside telling him to hurry up.

In this case, someone heard the woman's screams and the police arrived on the scene and arrested the offender. He stated he paid her 20 dollars. The police, with permission of the victim, checked her wallet and found 7 dollars. Unfortunately, this case, at trial level, resulted in a hung jury. The defense lawyer was successful in arguing that, although it was true that the men intended a cruel joke on the woman, it was not an act deserving to be called rape. The hung jury required an entirely new trial. By that time, the defense lawyer had learned of the victim's prostitution history and, with that knowledge, the victim decided to drop charges.

contemporary view

In the late 1960s and the 1970s, the medical literature began to take the woman's claim of rape more seriously than before. Especially notable in this regard is the work of physician Charles Hayman and his colleagues. Hayman, associated with the District of Columbia Department of Public Health, describes the intent of a follow-up program initiated by nurses in the department to assist victims of sexual assault by providing emotional support in conjunction with medical assistance. They anticipated that the measures would be particularly helpful for the prevention and management of pregnancy, venereal disease, and injury following an assault (Hayman, Lewis, Steward, & Grant, 1967).

This beginning change in medical care was further supported by the strength of the women's movement in bringing the problem of rape to the attention of the public. The first move to help rape victims came from outside the standard institutional structure. Victims and potential victims created rape crisis centers on their own because established institutions such as hospitals and police were unwilling to do so (Csida & Csida, 1974). The centers typically operated on a very limited budget and with nonprofessional volunteer staffs. Perhaps one of the reasons the District of Columbia was as effective as it was in providing aid to victims is the fact that it developed one of the very first rape crisis centers in the United States and that Hayman's work was being conducted in that same geographic area.

battering

Battering—forcible physical assault—up until the late nineteenth century was considered a "necessary aspect of a husband's marital obligation to control and chastise his wife" (Dobash & Dobash, 1978). This behavior, in the twentieth century, is now proscribed by law. However, cultural attitudes continue to endorse such practice and legal efforts to enforce the laws have failed to lend much aid.

Two psychological views are currently proposed regarding battering. In the first, Walker (1977–78) conceptualizes the relationship between the battering experience and learned helplessness. This view presents a psychological rationale for the reason the battered woman becomes a victim, and how the process of victimization further traps her and renders her psychologically paralyzed, unable to leave the relationship. It is precisely this psychological rationale that is the construct of learned helplessness. This theory builds on Seligman's (1975) empirical studies with animals and humans in which he observed that helplessness is learned and once it is learned, it taxes the coping capacity to initiate a response to relieve any current distress. Encouragingly, Seligman also observes that helplessness can be unlearned.

Walker (1977–78) believes that the social pressures placed on women to behave in certain ways may be a salient component for the learned helplessness behavior observed in adult women, especially battered women. Drawing from past as well as current research with her colleagues, Walker suggests the following hypotheses regarding learned helplessness.

1. It is difficult for battered women to change their way of thinking and to believe assertive actions will make a difference in what happens to them.
2. Helplessness is learned on a continuum; that is, a woman learns from an interaction of traditional female role standards and individual personality development.
3. Battered women will be ambivalent about the women's movement.
4. Battered women believe it is their role to make their marriage successful; they cover up the violence for the sake of the "happy family" cultural stereotype.
5. Battered women value men's approval more than that of other women.

In summary, Walker states:

> Battered women tend to isolate themselves so that friends and family do not find out how bad their life really is. They lie to others so much that they begin to confuse reality themselves. They make excuses for their men and assume self-blame for many battering incidents. They begin to believe all the negative comments made by the batterers to them. This pattern seems to occur even with successful career women and may be explained partially by the cognitive dissonance between their home life and professional life. Their need for others to view them as successful is stronger than their need to escape from violence [p. 530].

The second psychological theory proposed for battered women is female suffering.

Waites (1977–78) argues that this concept is inadequate as an explanation of actual behavior since many situations involve women having little choice in whether they can leave the abuser. Waites points out that when the options available to battered women are examined, it is not clear that the alternative that would provide a retreat from the distressful situation is available. For example, the negative consequences of staying, which imply the possibility of repeated abusive behavior, must be weighed against the negative consequences of leaving. Waites describes four incentives as important to the woman's decision.

1. Identity vs. identity loss. The role of wife is most often viewed as a cornerstone of identity; to leave may threaten the wife with identity loss.
2. Social approval vs. stigmatization. Marriage is socially approved in our culture, while singleness is more often viewed as a stigma. This stigma attached to the "broken home" may be shared by the woman.
3. Economic support vs. economic deprivation and downward social mobility. The woman with children is especially vulnerable to economic loss; downward social mobility is often viewed as a consequence of marital separation; and stigma is attached to being on welfare.
4. Love vs. loss of attachment. Battered wives may love their husbands and the prospect of losing these ties may threaten the wife with isolation from any close relationship.

characteristics and motivation of the abuser

Since the 1970s, clinicians and researchers have begun to redefine violence against women. They have questioned the literature and as a result new perspectives have begun to emerge. Rather than continue the "blame the victim" view, they are beginning to look at (1) the behavior, characteristics, and motivation of the abuser, and (2) the impact of the violent behavior on the victim.

motivational intent

The accounts of victims of both rape and battering suggest that issues of power, anger, and sexuality are important in understanding the abuser's behavior. A study of rapists' motivation, in fact, revealed that rape serves primarily nonsexual needs (Groth, Burgess, & Holmstrom, 1977). Rape was found to be motivated more by retaliatory and compensatory motives than by sexual impulses; it was a pseudosexual act, complex and multidetermined, but addressing issues of hostility (anger) and control (power) more than desire (sexuality). The defining issue in rape and battering is the lack of consent on the part of the woman. Sexual relations are achieved through physical force, threat, or intimidation.

Rape and battering are acts of aggression. In some offenses, the assault appears to constitute a discharge of anger. In other cases, the aggressor seems to react to resistance on the part of the victim. When the victim resists the advances of her abuser, he retaliates by striking, hitting, or hurting her. Hostility is quickly triggered and released sometimes in a clear, consciously experienced state of anger or, in other cases, what offenders will describe as a state of fear or panic. In still other offenses, the aggression is expressed less as an anger motive and more as a means of dominating, being in control and in charge of the situation, an expression of mastery and conquest. In a fourth variation, the aggression itself is intrinsically gratifying. It becomes eroticized as the abuser finds excitement and pleasure both in control over his victim and in hurting her, whether or not actual sexual contact is achieved. In such cases, the outcome may be the murder of the victim.

typology of rape

POWER RAPE. In this type of rape assault, the offender seeks power and control over his victim through intimidation by means of a weapon, physical force, or threat of bodily harm. Physical aggression is used to overpower and subdue the victim, and its use is directed toward achieving submission. The aim of the assault usually is to effect sexual intercourse as evidence of conquest. To accomplish this, very often the victim is kidnapped, tied up, or rendered helpless in some fashion.

This type of offender often shows little skill in negotiating interpersonal relationships and feels inadequate in both sexual and nonsexual areas of his life. Having few other avenues of personal expression, sexuality becomes the core of his self-image and self-esteem. Rape becomes the means by which he reassures himself of his sexual adequacy and identity, of his strength and potency.

Since it becomes a test of his competency, the rape experience for this offender is one of anxiety, excitement, and anticipated pleasure. The assault is premeditated and preceded by an obsessional fantasy in which, although his victim may initially resist him, once overpowered, she will submit gratefully to his sexual embrace. She then will be so impressed with his sexual abilities that she will respond with wild abandon. In reality, this offender is often handicapped by impotency or premature ejaculation. If not, he still tends to find little sexual satisfaction in the rape. The assault is disappointing for it never lives up to his fantasy.

Often he must convince himself that his victim became "turned on" to him, really wanted sex but could not admit it, clearly consented nonverbally, and enjoyed the sexual contact. Yet, at some level he realizes that he has not found what he is looking for in the offense: something he cannot clearly define he senses is lacking. He does not feel reassured either by his own performance or by his victim's response to the assault and, therefore, he must go out and find another victim—this time the "right one."

The offenses become repetitive and compulsive. The amount of force used in the assault may vary and there may be an increase in aggression over time as the offender becomes more desperate to achieve that indefinable experience that continues to elude him. Usually there is no conscious intent on the part of this offender to hurt or degrade his victim. The aim is to have complete control over her so that she will have no say in the matter. She will be submissive and gratify his sexual demands.

> Steve is a 24-year old married man, He pleaded guilty to six charges of rape. In every case he approached the victim in a shopping mall with a gun. His fantasy was that the woman would say, "You don't need a gun. You're just what I've been waiting for" and then "rape" him. He would kidnap them, tie them up, force them to submit to intercourse, and then question them as to whether he was as good as other sex partners they had. Except for the sex offenses, Steve had no criminal history.

The victim of this assault is often within the same age group as the offender or younger. Hospital examination generally will show minimum or inconclusive evidence of physical or sexual injury. Concurrently, clinical evidence of intercourse—presence of active sperm—may be absent. The victim will often report being questioned by the offender regarding her sexual life and her reaction to his sexual performance. He may ask her name as well as if he can see her again. She is fearful that the offender will attempt to return and is upset about the forced conversation and sexual assault. Her coping behavior is often for the purpose of trying to talk her way out of the rape or resisting intimidation initially by being assertive and confrontive to the offender.

> Nancy is a 45-year old divorced woman. While at home on a Friday evening, a former boy friend came by with a bottle of gin and asked her to share some drinks with him. Nancy agreed to. Later in the evening she refused to have sex with him and her account of what happened follows: "He messed me over the street way. I'm not supposed to tell. He said he'd beat me if I tell and he gave me a sample tonight to show me. They work you over to control you so they can have you sexually anytime they want. He hit me on the ear, pulled my hair, hit me in the back of my kidneys—very strategic. But it's not the physical part that's the thing. It's mental—to control you."

ANGER RAPE.   In this type of sexual assault, the offender expresses anger, rage, and contempt and hatred for his victim by physically beating her, sexually assaulting her, and forcing her to perform or submit to additional degrading acts. More force is used in the assault than would be necessary simply to subdue his victim. The assault is one of physical violence to all parts of the body. He often approaches his victim by striking and beating her; he tears her clothing and uses profane and abusive language.

The aim of this type of offender is to vent his rage on his victim and to retaliate for perceived wrongs of rejections he has suffered at the hands of women. Sex becomes a weapon, and rage is the means by which he can use this weapon to hurt and degrade his victim.

This offender displays a great deal of anger

and contempt toward women. He sees them negatively as unloving, ungiving "whores and bitches." Sex itself is regarded at some level of experience as base and degrading, and this offender typically finds little or no sexual satisfaction in the rape. His subjective reaction to the sexual act is frequently one of repulsion and disgust, and often he experiences difficulty in achieving an erection or an ejaculation during the assault.

His relationships to important women in his life are fraught with conflict, irritation, and irrational jealousy. He is often physically assaultive toward them. His sexual offenses tend to be episodic and sporadic, triggered by conflicts in his relationships to the women in his life (mother, girl friend, wife), but frequently displaced onto other individuals.

The rape experience for this type of offender is one of conscious anger or sadistic excitement. His intent is to hurt his victim, and his assault is brutal and violent. The motive is revenge and punishment and in extreme cases this may result in homicide.

He finds it difficult to explain his assault when he cannot deny it except to rationalize that he was drunk or on drugs. Often the details are lost to his memory in that he becomes "blind with rage" during the assault. Satisfaction and relief result from the discharge of anger rather than from sexual gratification. Pleasure is derived from degrading and humiliating his victim.

> Derek is a 25-year old married man and the father of four. He had an outstanding military service and after discharge was married. His marriage was not approved by his father, who told his sons that "women were no good." Following a dispute with his history teacher and feeling humiliated by her in front of the class, Derek stormed out of the class, very angry, thinking "women are dirty, rotten bastards" and went to a bar for a few drinks. On his way to his car he spotted a 40-year old woman

(whom he described as looking older) in the parking lot. He grabbed her by the throat and hit her in the mouth; ripped off her clothes and raped her. Prior to this offense, Derek's only criminal record consisted of arrests for gambling, loitering, and being drunk.

Victims may be older or elderly as target victims for this type of rapist, although they may be of any age. Medical examination will generally reveal considerable trauma to all areas of the victim's body, often requiring X-rays and consultation with other medical specialists. Victims report experiencing the rape as a life-threatening situation, and the symptoms following the rape will be disruptive to their physical, behavioral, social, and sexual life-styles.

Victims will describe a blitz style of attack or a sudden and dramatic switch in the offender's behavior. Having used a confidence ploy to entrap his victim, the offender then exhibits a behavior change in which he assaults her in a fury of anger. Victims may be physically immobilized and unable to use any coping strategies during the rape. Abusive and humiliating language by the offender may be used and often "perverted" acts become a major aspect of the assault.

The sadistic rapist is the most dangerous type of offender. He finds pleasure, thrills, and excitation in the suffering of his victim. His aim is to punish, hurt, torture, and destroy his victim. Aggression becomes eroticized.

> Mary, a 33-year-old single woman, was returning to her apartment around 9:00 p.m. one evening. Suddenly she was jumped from behind, knocked to the ground, and remembered nothing until she awoke in the assailant's apartment. She was held captive there for two days during which time reported being continually beaten, raped, and forced to perform fellatio. She said, "He bit me and burned me. He had pictures of rattlesnakes on his wall." The medical exam re-

vealed multiple injuries to her face and eye; multiple bruises and lacerations to her body, and human bite marks and cigarette burns to her chest. Mary was hospitalized for several days.

characteristics of the offense

GAINING ACCESS. The rapist's first goal is a practical one. He must find a victim and get her sufficiently under his control in order to rape her. Victims generally report two styles of attack: the blitz and the confidence. The blitz rape is a sudden attack in which the rapist confronts the victim without any prior warning—out of the blue. The emphasis is on physically based strategies. For example, the rapist may grab a woman walking on the street and shove her into a car. His physical action may be reinforced by verbal means. In the confidence rape, the emphasis is more on linguistically based strategies (Holmstrom & Burgess, 1979). The rapist gains access by winning the confidence of the victim and then betraying it. His "line" may be supplemented by physical action or maneuvering the victim into a position or place from which it is difficult to escape.

Two main styles of linguistic strategies occur at the point when the rapist is trying to obtain a victim. One is that of threats and orders (I'll kill you if you don't do it), the other the confidence line. The confidence line strategy is most frequently used with victims known to the rapist, but it also occurs with strangers. If the rapist already knows the victim, his conversation builds on this existing relationship. If the victim is a stranger, he uses a conversation to gain trust. His talk creates an image of normalcy and everyday experience that belies what is to follow. Some of the confidence lines include offering assistance (Do you want a ride home?); requesting assistance (I need a ride); promising social activities (Let's go and talk); promising material items (We can go to the house and get it); promising information (Joe told me to tell you something); requesting her company (I need someone to help me do that); referring to someone she might know (Joe will be there, too); trading on social niceties (I just wanted to come and say goodbye).

The linguistic strategies are most closely related to the power component of an assault. All the statements by the assailant are used to control the victim verbally before, during, and after the assault. The analysis of rapists' talk suggest that many rapists simultaneously exploit and attempt to "normalize" or "conventionalize" their exploitation.

GAINING SEXUAL CONTROL OF THE VICTIM. The sec-ond goal of the rapist, after gaining physical access to a victim, is to gain sexual control. As previously discussed, rapists' goals on the psychosocial level are to demonstrate their power over the victim and to vent their anger at the same time. Sexuality is a component, but not the dominant factor. The rapist's power and anger may be directed at the individual victim, at the male perceived to own her, or at the group she is perceived to represent. Rapists' goals in pair and group rape may also include impressing their fellow rapists. Linguistic strategies are one means used to achieve these goals. For example, threats and orders may continue throughout the rape. Most frequently, the victim is ordered to be quiet and is told what to do sexually.

sources of help for the victim of rape or battering

A woman who is raped or battered is placed in the position of having to make a decision of whether to tell or not to tell. The issue of disclosure becomes especially important. If the woman choses not to disclose, she alone must silently bear the symptoms of trauma. The woman who chooses to be silent about her victimization cannot be helped unless someone detects her suffering and is able to get her to disclose her secret. However, for the woman who decides to disclose, there are sources of help. This section discusses a case illustration of a rape victim's experience and the framework of victim counseling that was provided. The steps followed for victim health care are outlined as well as the legal process.

It started out an ordinary day. I had been shopping in Cambridge and was going home to make an apple pie. It was about 3:00 p.m. I had the keys to my apartment out . . . I heard footsteps behind me; they came up the steps and this man grabbed me. I thought he was just trying to pick me up. I said, "I'm busy and can't talk to you now." I continued into my apartment and he followed . . . backed me against the apartment buttons and asked me for money. I told him I didn't have any, that I spent it all. He hit me across the face. I pulled out my purse and gave him $37 and he said I must have more . . . He asked me if I had keys. I said I was living with someone. He said he would kill them.

He held one arm over my mouth and one arm behind my back. I opened the door and he looked around the apartment. I said, "There's the TV—take it and go." He said that wasn't what he wanted. He grabbed a knife from my kitchen and told me he was a gangster and that he had raped three other women and killed them and that was what was going to happen to me. He waved the knife around and told me to undress and said, "If you don't hurry, I'll kill you. If you're not quiet I'll kill you."

For the next three hours, this 23-year-old woman was forced to have oral, anal, and vaginal penetration, received physical beating to her head and body and knife lacerations to her face, eye, and arm. The assailant then took her to a strange neighborhood, showing her off as "my woman." After several attempts, she was finally able to free herself from him and sought protection in a fire house.

This case is discussed in the context of counseling the victim and presents the conceptual framework for such counseling that developed out of a clinical nursing-sociological study with 146 adult, adolescent, and child victims of sexual assault who were admitted to the Boston City Hospital emergency services over a one-year period (Burgess & Holmstrom, 1979). These concepts have been useful in teaching hospital staff as well as interdisciplinary groups who work with victims in the hospital and in the community.

conceptual framework underlying victim counseling

short-term model

Victim counseling is a short-term crisis treatment model. The focus of the initial interview and follow-up is on the rape incident, and the goal is to aid victims to return to their previous life-style as quickly as possible. Previous problems that are not associated with the rape are not considered priority issues for discussion in counseling. This would include individual or family problems, academic problems, drinking, and drug abuse problems. Victim counseling is not considered psychotherapy. When other issues of concern are identified by the victim, which indicates another treatment, referrals are suggested to the victim if so requested.

crisis request of the victim

The victim is considered "normal"; that is, an individual who was managing adequately in a life-style prior to the crisis. In this context, the victim is viewed as a customer of emergency services who has an immediate crisis request, seeking a particular service from the professional. A study of the crisis requests of the 146 sexual-assault victims admitted to Boston Hospital revealed five categories (Burgess & Holmstrom, 1973):

1. Police intervention: I need police help.
2. Medical intervention: I need medical help.
3. Psychological intervention: I need to talk to someone.
4. Control: I need to get back into control.
5. Uncertain: I'm not sure I need anything.

In the example, the victim had serious physical injuries when she was admitted to the emergency floor. Her eye was severely swollen, bruised, and there was a question of injury to the cornea. Her clothes were disheveled, and she was physically exhausted. It was very clear that her immediate crisis request was for medical intervention. The police had been called by the firemen, provided aid in the immediate scene, and brought her to the hospital. Her comment following the medical examination expresses her relief to be free of the assailant and the circumstances:

> I feel so safe here. I wish I could stay forever. He can't get me here—too many layers of concrete; too many people who care.

The crisis request is the common ground of

communication between the victim and counselor. For the counselor, identifying and understanding the request at the initial interview reduce and contain the sense of helplessness and powerlessness one may feel in dealing therapeutically with the victim. Something *can* be done for the victim provided that one first, jointly with the victim, determines what needs to be done and in what order.

assessing coping behavior

Assessment of coping behavior and strategies used before, during, and after the rape is an essential step in crisis intervention. This assessment can be used as a supportive measure. Counselors, in listening to the victim recount the rape, can identify the coping behavior and help the victim to recognize it. This support tells victims they have coped as a positive adaptive mechanism in a life-threatening situation.

The case example illustrated early awareness of danger ("I heard footsteps behind me"). The victim tried to cope verbally with the assailant. He used physical force and she complied by giving him the money when she realized the seriousness of the situation (phase two, or prerape). Still not aware that the man also intended to rape as well as rob, she tried verbal bargaining ("Take the TV and go"). The assailant then bragged about his previous violent behavior. The victim thought of ways to escape and attempted action (almost got to her apartment door) following the first rape. The victim was unsuccessful in the coping task of escaping and complied with his order to go with him out of the apartment. She tried to calm him verbally, tried to elicit help from people she passed (a bus driver, friend of the assailant, store woman). She complied with his demand for oral penetration to survive ("If you don't get it up, I'll kill you"). She verbally

convinced him to leave an especially frightening isolated area to which he had taken her and finally physically escaped, fleeing to a fire station, telling the firemen of the rape and her fears, and then hiding until the assailant was gone.

crisis intervention

In the Boston City Hospital Victim Counseling Program, telephone counseling was used as a primary intervention tool after seeing the victim for the initial interview at the hospital. There are several reasons why telephone counseling was effective. It provides relatively quick access to the victim; it places the burden on the counselor to seek out the victim, rather than on the victim to seek help at a time when she is in crisis and having difficulty making decisions; it allows the victim considerable power in the situation; it encourages the victim to resume a normal life-style as quickly as possible; it is not costly; and it provides an alternative way to discuss difficult issues rather than face-to-face.

In this case, telephone counseling was quite effective because the victim moved several times in the first few months and found it useful to be able to talk with the counselor about the changes that were occurring. There were landlord problems regarding breaking a lease, decisions to make about where and with whom to live, as well as her thoughts and feelings about identifying the assailant, then continuing through the court process.

negotiating
the counseling request

Negotiating the follow-up counseling request is a key factor in the clinical work as the counselor states what services are available. In studying the counseling requests of the 146 victims on telephone followup— that is, what services they were asking from the crisis counselor—five categories were identified:

1. Confirmation of concern: It's nice to know you are available.
2. Ventilation: It helps to get this off my chest.
3. Advice: What should I do?
4. Clarification: I want to think this through.
5. Wants nothing: I don't need the counseling services.

By learning what the victim wants in terms of follow-up, an important alliance is made because the victim has been listened to carefully and with respect. The term *respect* is used in the same sense of paying attention to, carefully observing, and appreciating the worth and dignity of the person. The counselor communicates this to the victim by taking her seriously, by being honest, by listening well, and by regarding the victim as a person instead of an object.

In the case example, the victim requested both ventilation and advice. She was concerned and anxious about the court process, such as whether she needed a lawyer and her ability to identify the assailant. She asked many questions about which she herself had to made decisions. The counselor's role was to listen and point out any alternatives that were possible for her to consider.

rape trauma syndrome

Assessing, understanding, and evaluating the reactions and feelings of the victim following a rape are the essential skills of the counselor. A rape experience triggers a two-phase reaction: an acute, highly confusing and disorganized state followed by a long-term period where the victim attempts to put her life back into the order it had prior to the rape. The acute phase includes many physical symptoms and a wide range of emotional reactions, which result from being faced with a life-threatening or highly stressful situation. The long-term phase includes changing residence, seeking social network support, dealing with nightmares and daymares, and the development of phobic reactions.

In this case, the young woman experienced moderate symptoms of rape trauma syndrome. She had difficulty eating and said, "I'm getting a hole in my stomach because I can't eat." The lacerations to her face were painful, and additional medical consultations were necessary, especially for her eyes. Fearing seeing the assailant again, she said, "I just expect him to be everywhere." Minor mood swings, such as outbursts of crying when a man came around a corner fast at work and frightened her, were experienced. Because the neighborhood reminded her of the places she was forced to go with the assailant, she feared returning to work. She said she could hardly walk the two blocks from the trolley to work: "I never thought I could make it . . . panting when I got to work . . . had to talk to myself to calm down and cool it . . . just sheer panic walking that far in broad daylight."

She had to change residence, stating she would never be able to return to her apartment alone. She experienced further trauma from the landlord who said she would have to sublet. "He seemed to think it was my personal problem . . . said it happens every day."

The court experience reactivated the original crisis. She had difficulty identifying the assailant. Confident in selecting his picture from police photos, when confronting him in court, she was confused "because he seemed so cowed . . . not bragging and boasting as he was before." After court she was concerned that all his friends now knew where she worked and was "always looking around to see if they were around." The mother of the defendant was observed to be walking around the hallway before court to find out who was the "one out to get my son." The counselor intervened and took the victim into a private interviewing room. However, after court when everyone was walking out, the mother came right up to the victim and, pointing her finger in her face, said, "You bitch, you're going to suffer." This was said in a very intimidating manner. The victim's reaction was "another face to memorize."

hospital procedure

The hospital can be a vital force in either aiding victims or contributing to their further distress. It is generally advised that all victims receive immediate medical attention because of the physical and emotional trauma to which they have been exposed. Treatment and follow-up include the following:

1. Make a careful medical examination, including documenting all signs and symptoms of trauma to the body as well as to the genital area.
2. Take a menstrual history and test for pregnancy. Information regarding last date of consenting sexual intercourse may be asked if tests for sperm are to be done.
3. Explain the pregnancy prevention alternatives. The alternatives include: waiting to determine whether her next period begins or until such time as the results of a pregnancy test are known; menstrual extraction if the next period is late; diethylstilbestrol—a synthetic estrogen—provided it is within 72 hours after the assault; postcoital IUD inserted within five days after the assault and retained for at least seven days.
4. After testing for venereal disease, explain the dangers and modes of transmission of venereal disease. Schedule follow-up appointments to test for gonorrhea (one week) and syphilis (4 to 6 weeks). Be sure to question what body orifices were penetrated, because oral gonorrhea is found increasingly among child sexual-assault victims. Discuss prophylactic antibiotic therapy in terms of keeping follow-up appointments for detecting penicillin-resistant forms of gonorrhea.
5. Follow-up appointments should include antivenereal disease testing as well as pregnancy prevention. If diethylstilbestrol is prescribed and taken, careful instructions and follow-up should be provided so that she is well advised of potential consequences.*

psychological treatment

Sexual assault creates a crisis for the woman and she should be offered psychological care. The emotional trauma should be acknowledged, support for the feelings and reactions provided, explanations of all procedures to be performed should be made, and the informed consent of the woman in all decisions affecting her care should be obtained.

Many hospitals in the United States now have psychological services for rape victims and battered women. If services are not available at the hospital, referrals to advocacy or rape crisis groups should be offered.

The treatment of choice in acute crisis situations such as sexual assault is crisis counseling. A favorable prognosis for treatment of the acute crisis state is enhanced if the woman is seen immediately following the assault. In

---

*High doses of diethylstilbestrol seem to change the inner lining of the uterus so that a fertilized egg passes out of the uterus and pregnancy cannot continue. Side effects of the drug include nausea and vomiting, headache, menstrual irregularities, and breast tenderness. There is also concern over studies that suggest that when pregnant women took high doses of DES for a long time, daughters from those pregnancies had a far greater than average number of tumors of the vagina. This has caused so much concern that it is now strongly recommended that if a woman taking DES is later found to have been pregnant or becomes pregnant despite DES treatment, abortion should be considered. If the menstrual period is two weeks late after taking DES, a pregnancy test should be done. There is no evidence that a short course of DES causes any long-term harm to the woman herself. Women who should not receive DES even after being raped include: women who know they are pregnant, women who have tumors of the breast or reproductive organs or who have strong family histories of these cancers, and women who have had vein clots.

designing treatment, therefore, consideration should be given to the speed of intervention. Crisis counseling may not be effective when a counselor is not right on the scene, whether it be in the emergency room or the police station.

Intermittent crisis states are more frequently seen in battered women where the burden of keeping the activity secret for weeks, months, and years was placed with the woman. Such situations imply an unresolved trauma, whereby the individual has not told anyone of the assault, has not settled her feelings and reactions on the issue, and is carrying a tremendous psychological burden. Very often, a second trauma will reactivate the woman's reaction to the prior experience.

When a diagnosis of intermittent crisis is made, the woman has three therapeutic tasks: (1) to discuss the previous assault in considerable detail and with a full range of feelings, (2) to identify the reasons for not disclosing the assault, and (3) to talk of the current traumatic situation and look at the similarities and differences. The task for both client and counselor is then to work out a therapeutic plan of action that is present- and future-oriented.

the legal process

The legal process can be very confusing to someone who has never been involved in any type of legal action. For example, victims often think that they will have to go to court just once and that will be the end of it. They do not realize that there are many steps involved. The crime must be reported to the police, after which the victim will be interrogated. Then the woman must decide whether to press charges and go to court. A series of court steps and appearances are necessary. Initially, a public hearing is held before a judge to determine if the case should be "bound over to the Grand Jury." If the process continues, the next step is the trial at superior court, which usually lasts several days.

Throughout this process, women and their families develop a multitude of intense reactions. Many stressful situations can be dealt with more easily if the person thinks them through ahead of time, has accurate information about what to expect, and has done some anticipatory coping. This also seems to be the case with testifying in court. Thus, many of the techniques for preparing a rape victim for court have in common the idea of providing her with more information about what to expect and of having her think through some of the issues ahead of time.

The woman needs support at the courthouse. The counselor needs to help her deal with the reactions to the court and prepare her for dealing with the verdict. The most distressing problem arises when the defendant is found not guilty. Victims of rape frequently are not believed and, in general, it is very hard to get a conviction for rape. The victim needs to be told it was still important for her to try (Burgess and Holmstrom, 1980).

summary

The women's liberation movement must be fully credited: (1) for bringing these two neglected target populations—rape victims and battered women—to the attention of professionals as well as to the public, and (2) for providing the model—the structural or institutional analysis of behavior—within which to discuss the public issues and why they lead to violence against women (Bart, 1978). Herman and Hirschman (1977) comment on the need for grassroots organizations or feminist model interventions.

> The Women's Liberation Movement has demonstrated repeatedly to the mental health profession that consciousness raising has often been more beneficial and empowering to women than psychotherapy. In particular, the public revelation of the many and ancient sexual secrets of women (orgasm, rape, abortion) may have contributed far more toward the liberation of women than the attempt to heal individual wounds through a restorative therapeutic relationship . . . The same should be true for incest. The victims who feel like bitches, whores, and witches might feel greatly relieved if they felt less lonely, if their identities as the special guardians of a dreadful secret could be shed [p. 755].

The interventions for physical and sexual abuse of women should begin at the level of primary prevention. Such interventions to be considered would be: delegitimizing rape in our society, providing refuge facilities for women and children in crises, providing equitable child care facilities, equalizing the power balance of finances, encouraging women to participate actively in their own health care, and isolation of abusers and rapists until they can pay back the damage done in trauma to the victim.

Bart, P. B. Victimization and its discontents or psychiatric ideologies of violence against women. Paper presented at the annual meeting of the American Psychiatric Association, Atlanta, 1978, p. 9.

Burgess, A. W., & Holmstrom, L. L. Crisis and counseling requests of rape victims. *Nursing Research* May–June 1973, *73(3)*, 196–202.

Burgess, A. W., & Holmstrom, L. L. Coping behavior of the rape victim. *American Journal of Psychiatry*, 1977, *133(4)*, 389–404, 413–147.

Burgess, A. W., & Holmstrom, L. L. *Rape: Crisis and recovery*. Bowie, Md.: Brady, 1979.

Burgess, A. W., & Holmstrom, L. L. Rape victim counseling. *Journal of the National Association for Women Deans, Administrators, and Counselors*, 1980, 38(1), 24–30.

Csida, J. B., & Csida, J. *Rape: How to avoid it and what to do about it if you can't*. Chatsworth, Calif.: Books for Better Living, 1974.

Dobash, R. E., & Dobash, R. P. Wives: The "appropriate" victims of marital violence. *Victimology: An International Journal*, 1978, 2, 426.

Groth, A. N., Burgess, A. W., & Holmstrom, L. L. Rape: Power, anger, and sexuality. *American Journal of Psychiatry*, November 1977, *134*, 11.

Hayman, C. R. Lewis, R. R., Steward, W. F., & Grant, M. A public health program for sexually assaulted females, *Public Health Reports*, June 1967, *82*, 497–504.

Herman, J., & Hirschman, L. Father—daughter incest, signs: *Journal of Culture & Society*, 1977, 2, 755.

Holmstrom, L. L., & Burgess, A. W. Rapists' talk: Linguistic strategies to control the victim. *Deviant Behavior*, 1979, *1(1)*, 101–125.

Seligman, E. *Helplessness: On depression, development, and death*. San Francisco: Freeman, 1975, p. 28.

Viano, E. Victimology: The study of the victim, *Victimology*, 1976, *1(1)*, 1–7.

Waites, E. A. Female masochism and the enforced restriction of choice. *Victimology*, 1977–78, *2(3/4)*.

Walker, L. E. Battered women and learned helplessness. *Victimology*, 1977–78, *2, 3/4*, 530, 525–534.

TY HONGLADAROM, M.D.

women
and musculoskeletal pain

The body has eight major systems: cardiovascular (heart and blood vessels), endocrine (glands), gastrointestinal (digestion), genitourinary (sex organs/elimination), hematopoietic (blood), respiratory (lungs), and musculoskeletal (muscles and bones). The musculoskeletal system is the largest of our body systems. The entire skeleton consists of 200 or more distinct bones that articulate (join) with other bones and provide the rigid structure for our body. A *joint* occurs where bones meet (see Figure 20.1). It is covered by a *capsule*, which is formed from dense fibrous tissue in continuity with the lining of the bone, called the *periosteum*. Inside the joint and covering the articulating surface of the bone is *cartilage*. The rubber resiliency of

cartilage reduces pressure on the joint, and its smooth surface minimizes friction. Articulation (or joining) allows motion and stability. *Ligaments* are tough fibrous tissues that connect the bones. A healthy ligament is pliant and flexible to allow freedom of movement, yet is strong and inextensible to provide static (passive) support.

Muscles are specialized contractile tissues that connect to bones through *tendons* or *aponeuroses*. They provide the power that moves bones, and, at the same time, they stabilize the joints (active support). When muscles contract, tendons glide. Wherever there are surfaces that move upon each other, a delicate membrane of connective tissue, called a *synovial membrane*, is formed. The function of the cells of this membrane is to secrete a lubricating fluid to reduce friction between these moving structures. This membrane is found surrounding tendons as well as on the inner surface of joint capsules. Synovial membranes also line cavities called *bursae*. The muscles are covered with *fasciae*, which separates them from one another or other structures. Fig. 20-1 shows the main parts of the musculoskeletal system and how they work together.

Even from this short review, it can be easily seen that this complex system, composed of thousands of moving parts, is easily and frequently subject to disease and injury.

figure 20.1
cross section of the knee showing components of the musculoskeletal system

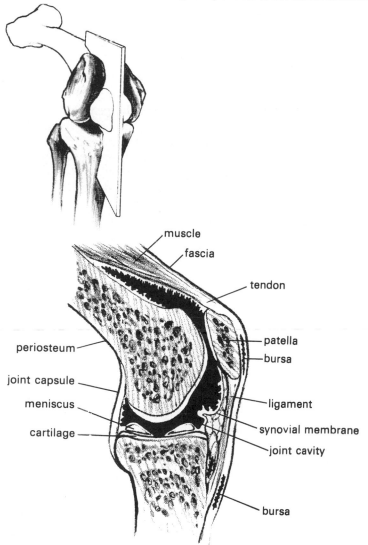

causes of musculoskeletal pain

The causes of musculoskeletal pain are numerous. Many readers will remember the cartoon strip "Bringing Up Father," which frequently showed Jiggs with his feet propped up, suffering from gout, a condition that causes painful joints, especially the big toe. Women have a higher incidence of collagen disorders, such as systemic lupus erythematosis and scleroderma, whose cause is not yet definitely agreed on, but appears to be related to the body's immune or defense system. *Infection* can certainly cause musculoskeletal pain, and with the rise in sexually transmitted diseases, gonococcal arthritis is becoming more common. Fortuantely, *tumors* of the musculoskeletal system are rare, but they can cause pain.

The most common cause of musculoskeletal pain is *trauma. Strain* is a damage to some part of the muscle-tendon unit. It is usually due to overuse (chronic strain) and infrequently due to overstress (acute strain). It ranges from minor (first degree), to severe (second degree), to complete tear (third degree). *Sprain* is a damage to the ligament. It can also be due to overuse or overstress and can also be classified as first, second, or third degree. *Subluxation* implies that the joint or tendon has moved out of its usual location. If it is complete, it becomes a *dislocation.*

When bone is traumatized, its covering (periosteum) can be bruised and inflamed (periostitis) or the bone itself can be broken (fracture). Fractures can be classified as simple (one break) or comminuted (more than one) and closed or opened, if the bone penetrates the skin.

The treatment of fractures and dislocations is quite straightforward. They are returned to their usual place and maintained there by either internal fixation (screws, pins, plates, nails), or external fixation (casts, braces, traction). If the fracture is properly set and remains undisturbed, it should heal. The rate of healing depends on the age and health of the individual as well as the bone involved.

Acute strains and sprains also should heal without difficulty. Third-degree strains or sprains may need to be repaired surgically, whereas first- and second-degree injuries are treated with cold, a pressure dressing, and elevation for 24 to 48 hours to decrease bleeding and swelling. The body part is immobilized and protected to prevent further injury. This can be done by rest, strapping, or casting. As the pain and swelling decrease, the part should be gently and actively moved within the limits of the woman's pain. This is very important since trauma will cause inflammation and edema, which is a fluid that acts like glue and will bind down the moving part. Furthermore, rest will allow the soft tissues (joint capsule, ligament, tendon, muscle, fascia, skin) to shorten and become weak. Active movement will prevent adhesion (binding down) and maintain the length of the soft tissues, as well as their strength and endurance. Neglecting this phase of treatment commonly results in a prolonged recovery period.

Syndromes of musculoskeletal pain are extremely varied. They can be classified by etiological causes—trauma, infection, metabolic or immunological disorders. They can also be classified by the structures involved—arthritis, tendinitis, bursitis, and myositis. The suffix, *itis*, means inflammation. Arthritis, thus, means inflammation of the joint and usually indicates red, hot, swollen, and painful joints. Most women who believe they have arthritis do not have it. Rather, they have arthralgia, that is, pain in the joint but without inflammation (*algia* means pain).

Although most women have experienced pain, it is not easily defined or conceptualized. Pain is an unpleasant experience that is entirely subjective. It can only be defined by the individual in terms of past experience and the meaning it holds for that individual. Pain is the most common reason for seeking help from physicians and other practitioners. It is generally associated with tissue damage.

The musculoskeletal system is no doubt the most common site of pain. In general, the causes are the mechanical, repetitious microtraumas of daily living. These are the diseases of civilization. Our advanced technology promotes a sedentary life-style, which leads to shortening of muscles, tendons, ligaments, and joint capsules, as well as weakness in these structures. We are able to carry on with this limited capacity until an unexpected movement exceeds our limit, and then strains and sprains result. These problems theoretically should heal uneventfully. The treatment includes rest during the acute phase, and as pain decreases over the next few days, a gradual increase in activity is encouraged. Most people with minor strains and sprains should be able to return to nonstrenuous ac-tivity in 7 to 10 days, but full healing usually requires 6 to 8 weeks.

Unfortunately, many women continue to have pain. In fact, pain related to the musculoskeletal system causes more lost work days and disability for women than any other disease category. One reason for this is the unrealistic expectation of success from treatment, hoping that it will provide permanent relief of pain. If discomfort continues, additional treatment is aggressively pursued by some individuals, and this may even be encouraged by some practitioners. Various medications are prescribed or purchased over-the-counter. Endless sessions of manipulation and other questionable methods are sought, and usually a woman can find someone who will provide questionable treatments. Countless new gadgets are invented and promoted to take advantage of musuloskeletal pain problems, and new specialty clinics and centers are created. All of these activities are good for the economy and extremely lucrative for the entrepreneurs and the inventors, but it is doubtful that any of this has helped women manage their pain.

treatments of musculoskeletal pain

Few problems can frustrate both the woman and her physician as much as chronic musculoskeletal pain. There are no specific or effective treatments, and, therefore, tranquilizers, muscle relaxants, and pain medications are prescribed. The side effects are often more spectacular than the relief. Surgery is also of no benefit in many of these cases. It is not unusual for a woman with chronic back pain to have had her uterus suspended, then removed, her urinary bladder repaired, her gallbladder removed, her hiatus hernia repaired, her disks removed, and her back fused. Some have had their nerves cut, then have had them stimulated!

What then can we do? Most importantly, the first step is to stop searching for an easy solution and a life free of any discomfort. It is important to rule out any serious underlying pathology. If you feel well, have no fever, no unexplained weight loss or excessive weakness, pain in the musculoskeletal system seldom indicates a serious disease. A thorough examination is most important. A succinct history that you provide to the physician or nurse practitioner is indispensable. Learn to localize the pain accurately, its spread, intensity, and characteristics. Also, when does it bother you most—its relation to time of the day and activity? What makes it worse or better, especially the effect of tension?

Blood tests are helpful to confirm the impression from both the history and the clinical examination. However, blood tests almost never make the diagnosis. This is also true for X-rays and other special studies, such as arthrograms, diskograms, or myelograms. Laboratory studies and X-rays may be completely normal in a proven abnormality. More importantly, they can be abnormal in a woman who is perfectly normal—an incidental finding that has led to many unnecessary treatments and resulting complications. Unless the studies match the examination, treatment directed toward these abnormalities invariably fails.

Many women with musculoskeletal pain who do not have signs of local inflammation (redness, heat, and swelling) or other signs of systemic disease (fever, weight loss, weakness) will have no abnormality on examination, and their laboratory studies are also usually normal. A woman may ask, "How can I have so much pain, and yet you can't find anything wrong with me? Are you accusing me of lying or faking?" Not at all. What the physician has done so far is to make sure that your pain is not caused by a tumor, an infection, or a metabolic abnormality that may be life-threatening or require a specific treatment.

Now, further and more detailed explorations of your problem are needed. Could this pain be due to the way you live? Are you rushing and under constant tension? Muscles are made to contract and relax. Constant muscle tension will cause pain by putting trac-

tion on the bony attachments and by interfering with the blood supply to body parts. We all have experienced a charley horse, and it is very painful. Constant muscle tension is a less severe but chronic form of a charley horse.

Are you happy? Most depressed individuals have decreased muscle tone and poor posture, which puts stress on the joints and ligaments continuously.

Are you overweight? Supportive structures such as the back, hips, knees, ankles, and feet are particularly affected by this increased load.

Are you unwisely trying to avoid aging? We all get older! Degenerative changes occur with advancing age. The degree of degeneration varies in individuals. With degenerative changes, our cartilages, ligaments, muscles, and tendons become less resilient, and they fray more easily. Are we expecting too much out of our body parts—thinking that we are still teenagers, the age group that is strong, flexible, and almost indestructible?

Are you keeping fit? Regular exercise is important to maintain the resiliency and strength of the musculoskeletal system. It is also an excellent way to decrease tension. Physical activity including exercise must be started slowly and increased gradually to avoid strains and sprains, especially in women who have been sedentary.

Are you using proper body mechanics in your everyday activities? This is probably the most common cause of musculoskeletal pain. Injuries usually occur when we are tense, rushed, and not paying attention to what we are doing and how we are bending, lifting, or reaching.

Has the fashion industry gotten the best of you? Do your high-fashion clothes restrict your movements and prevent you from following proper body mechanics in your daily activities? Your high-heeled and platform shoes not only make you unstable, but put an excessive stress on your lower back. Your extra-narrow dainty shoes with pointed toes are excellent creators of bunions and many other foot problems.

What do you gain from having the pain? This may be a rather peculiar question to ask yourself. Did you ever wonder why football and basketball players want and continue to play in spite of obvious injuries? Their answers may be "money" or even love of the game, but the point is that the gain is worth the pain. More significantly, why do some people recover faster if they hurt their back lifting at home, but much more slowly if the injury occurred at work? We must be aware of the secondary gains of illness and the politics of pain. Unfortunately, many of us are unhappy with certain tasks. Having pain may relieve you of tasks you do not like, such as vacuuming and window washing. Or if you can't stand your boss, the injury at work allows you to stay at home and perhaps also to collect compensation. Isn't it easier to complain of pain and use that as a way to avoid the boss? This is usually not a flagrant or conscious effort, but it is believed to be one of the most important contributing factors to continuation of chronic musculoskeletal pain.

It is also difficult to actively involve a woman in resolving a pain problem if she is being lured into "keeping her pain" so that she will receive a lucrative financial settlement. This is a significant problem in automobile and work-related injuries. Women have to choose between recovery from pain or living with chronic pain for financial reward. This complex situation is made more difficult by the way our legal and medical systems are structured, and the most serious outcome is that significant numbers of women continue to live in pain, unable to find fulfillment because they are constrained by the politics of pain.

special situations relating to musculoskeletal pain

pregnancy

Low back pain is common during pregnancy. It is due to increased extensibility of the ligaments in the back and pelvis, which allows the birth canal to adapt to the passage of the child. Also, as the abdomen becomes enlarged, the center of gravity changes, and as a result, a woman has to arch her back to balance herself. Doing so puts more stress on her lower back, and this can cause pain. Abdominal muscles are also weakened due to stretching and lack of use. It is advisable that a woman participate in prenatal classes that include abdominal exercises and proper body mechanics. Exercises continued after delivery not only help to decrease back problems, but also help to regain the prepregnancy weight and muscle tone.

developmental musculoskeletal problems

Alteration in the curvature of the spine is quite common in young women during puberty. This may be due to being conscious of breast development and may result in becoming round-shouldered. Around the time of menarche, an abnormal lateral deviation of the spine called *scoliosis* can be accelerated. Although it may be due to leg length discrepancy, asymmetrical weakness of back muscles, or very rare congenital bony abnormalities, most scolioses have no known cause, thus the name idiopathic scoliosis. All young women should be screened for this condition, since early detection will stop or reverse the abnormality. Early cases may be difficult to detect, but the abnormality will become more evident when you observe the back while the person bends forward. X-rays can confirm the presence of scoliosis. Treatment for cases detected early is exercise. Sometimes bracing will be necessary and if used conscientiously, this will eliminate the need for major surgical correction, which may ultimately be necessary. The brace is only needed until the young woman's bones stop growing but exercises must be continued.

A word of caution: One misconception is that the body is in perfect alignment and must be maintained in that stance. Amazing as the body is, it is not created perfectly. More hours and money have been spent to put joints back in place because they looked crooked to someone on an X-ray. Remember, any neck and back can be positioned to look crooked when an X-ray is taken. More importantly, the crookedness does not mean that it causes pain, or that it needs to be manipulated.

X-rays of the lower back not uncommonly reveal other actual imperfections. *Spina bifida occulta* is a condition in which the arch of the backbone is not completely fused. It has no clinical significance, nor does it cause any problems whatsoever.

Sometimes a portion of the bone (called pars interarticulalis) is not calcified, and this produces the condition called *spondylolysis*. If this is not weakened enough to allow a vertebral body to slip forward, a condition called *spondylolisthesis*, it does not cause any problem. Spondylolisthesis, however, can cause low back pain, and some practitioners will attempt the impossibility of manipulating it back into place. A few cases may continue to cause unbearable pain and may need to be fused, although the result of the fusion is not predictable. Some with solid fusions continue to have pain; others, whose fusions fail, do not have pain.

TRANSITIONAL VERTEBRA. The normal spinal column (backbone) consists of 7 cervical (neck), 12 thoracic (chest), and 5 lumbar (lower back) vertebrae and the sacrum. Sacralization occurs when the fifth (lowest) lumbar vertebra is fused into the sacrum and a person may then have been told they have "one less bone" in their back. If the top part of the sacrum is separated from the sacrum, lumbarization occurs and a person may in this case have been told that they have "one too many bones" in their back. If the fusion or the separation occurs symmetrically, it does not cause a problem; but if it occurs asymmetrically it may predispose the woman to mechanical strain and back pain. The most important treatment for back pain due to asymmetrical transitional vertebra is learning to use your back properly. Some vulnerable women will be subjected to surgery, which may, but usually does not, help their pain.

noisy joints

It is not unusual for people to seek help because their joints crack. Noisy joints are normal and although the mechanism is not definitely understood it is probably due to a sudden separation of joint surfaces that were in contact with one another. A grating sensation is also felt in a joint that has deteriorated due to the rubbing of roughened joint surfaces. Noisy or cracking joints are not a cause for worry or alarm.

extremity pain

Women are prone to *carpal tunnel syndrome*. It is a condition that causes pain in the hand, which usually worsens at night and is relieved by shaking your hand. There may be numbness in the thumb, index, and middle fingers, as well as weakness. It is caused by compression of the median nerve as it goes through a tunnel formed by the bones of the wrist (carpal bones). This condition is easily confirmed by a nerve conduction study. During this procedure, the median nerve is stimulated at the wrist and the time to record muscle response will indicate whether the nerve is compressed. The treatment consists of resting the hand in a splint to support and immobilize the wrist. Women who have a tendency to collect fluid are more prone to this condition, and diuretics may help. Surgery is needed if all else fails.

Arm pain is not uncommon. It can be due to nerve root compression in the neck. More commonly, it is due to muscle tension in the neck and upper back. Unfortunately, too many women have the muscles in the neck (scalene muscles) cut or their first rib removed because they supposedly have something called *thoracic outlet syndrome*. The existence of this syndrome is questioned by many physicians. It may exist, but not as commonly as it seems. The diagnosis should be confirmed by detailed electrodiagnostic studies, and if involvement of blood vessels is suspected, an arteriogram will provide a diagnosis. Many women are relieved of their symptoms by proper exercises and correction of posture. Stubborn cases may need surgery if a lesion is confirmed.

When women experience pain in the elbow, this is usually due to strain. The most common area is over the origin of the wrist extensor muscles, and strain here results in the so-called *tennis elbow*. Treatment is rest, anti-inflammatory medications, ice during the acute stage, and heat in the chronic stage. These measures should be followed by gentle stretching and strengthening exercises to improve strength and endurance as the pain subsides. Most important treatment is to avoid strain from excessive, inappropriate use.

Chondromalacia patella is a cause of knee pain that is especially common in growing female teen-agers. This is due to improper tracking of the knee cap (patella) over the femur, which may lead to roughening of the underlying cartilage. The treatment is rest and aspirin as well as strengthening the quadriceps muscles, which control the movement of the patella. In some severe protracted problems, surgery may be needed.

Women who kneel a lot may develop inflammation of the bursa in the knee area. In years past this was called "housemaid's knee."

Foot pain in women invariably is due to poorly fit shoes that are too tight or have too high a heel. When the foot is crammed into a tight shoe, muscles cannot work to relieve the weight borne by the bones and ligaments. The toes are pinched together and may cause nerve irritation or a benign tumor called *Morton's neuroma*. High-heeled shoes force women to stand on their toes, causing pain over the metatarsal heads (metatarsalgia). Too short a shoe also forces the toes to flex excessively, causing *claw toes* or *hammer toes*. Excessive pressure from pointed shoes promotes the formation of bunions. Excessive pressure areas are easily detected by callus formation (corns). Being overweight aggravates any foot pain, and a weight reduction program is an important part of treatment.

torso pain

Shoulder pain is a very common problem. The most common cause is inflammation of the bursa (bursitis) or tendon (tendinitis). This is an impingement syndrome that occurs because every time we elevate the arm above the shoulder, the tendon or bursa is pinched between the shoulder bones. These kinds of pain problems usually respond to rest and anti-inflammatory medication such as phenylbutazone. As the pain decreases, passive range of motion must be carried out to prevent a frozen joint. Some physicians inject steroids into this inflamed tissue, and often dramatic relief follows. However, frequent joint injection with steroids will hasten degenerative changes in that structure.

Sometimes there is calcium in the tendon on X-ray, a condition called *calcific tendinitis*. The presence of calcium does not imply that this is what is causing the shoulder pain. It is not uncommon to find it in the other shoulder of the same individual, but causing no pain. Its presence merely indicates degenerative changes in that structure. It may be, but is not necessarily, the cause of the problem. Moreover, removal of the calcium usually is not indicated. Disappearance at times occurs spontaneously.

Neck and upper back pain are usually due to chronic strain from tension and poor posture—*muscle tension syndrome*, *fibrositis*, and *myofascial syndrome*. Treatment is directed toward elimination of physical, emotional, or other causes of tension and correction of posture. Exercises to maintain the normal movement, strength, and endurance of these muscles are important.

Back pain can be due to a nerve root lesion, *ruptured disk*, or *pinched nerve*, but if the nerve root is irritated, there is a definite pattern of pain, and when it is compressed, there is a specific pattern of weakness. Treatment of nerve root irritation in the neck consists of immobilization with a collar and neck traction. As symptoms subside, neck motion and muscle strength should be restored by a gentle range of motion and strengthening exercises. More importantly, the woman must learn to avoid activities that aggravate her problem.

Most hip pain that women complain of is actually buttock pain. This kind of pain is invariably referred from the lower back and is due to chronic strain. True hip pain is usually manifested as pain in the groin that radiates toward the knee. At times there is tenderness over the lateral aspect of the hip, and this leads to the overdiagnosed, thus overtreated, condition called *trochanteric bursitis*. A groin pull is usually due to stretching of the muscles attached to the bones in the groin region. A once-common condition due to inflammation caused by excessive sitting on hard surfaces, called "weaver's bottom," is rarely seen now that most chairs are well padded.

As aging occurs, the most common cause of hip, knee, ankle, and foot pain is degenerative joint changes. This problem can be managed by weight reduction and strengthening of the muscles, which stabilize the joints to improve control and decrease excessive motion. The movement of the joints should be maintained and pressure on the joints can be reduced by proper use of a cane, crutches, or a walker.

surgical intervention

When do you need surgery? Hopefully never. The prudent surgeon will exhaust all nonoperative treatments prior to subjecting a woman to surgery. Beware of health care providers who exclaim "you have a disk and you need manipulation," or a surgeon who immediately recommends an operation. You certainly have a disk, in fact, you have 23 of them in your back. The disk is subjected to pressure. It does deteriorate with age—in fact, deterioration starts in your late teens or early twenties. It can rupture and cause pain. If a fragment from a lumbar disk extrudes and impinges on the ligament, it can cause pain down the legs. Pain may radiate down the arm if a cervical disk is involved. If it compresses the nerve root, numbness, weakness, and reflex changes occur depending on which nerve root is being pinched.

Sciatica is a common term used to describe the pain that occurs when one of the nerve roots forming the large nerve going down the back of your leg, called the sciatic nerve, is involved. Sciatica is diagnosed by a careful history and physical examination. Seventy-five percent of patients will recover with rest. Heat and massage help decrease muscle spasm and pain. Pain medication and muscle relaxants may be needed. Traction for a lumbar disk herniation only serves to keep you in bed. It does not distract the disk space. If the pain continues or increases, and weakness progresses, a laminectomy is indicated to remove the fragment that is putting pressure on the nerve root. A myelogram is a special X-ray procedure during which dye is injected into the spinal canal. This is done preoperatively to make certain that there are no other conditions that may be causing the problem. This procedure also confirms the location of the herniated disk.

Women who continue to have back pain without evidence of nerve root compression challenge the physician. Some will end up with a myelogram "to clear the air." If it is normal, we are back to first base. If it is abnormal, the patient invariably has surgery, which usually does not help to eliminate the pain.

Be careful and be extremely certain that everything else possible is done for you before you subject yourself to back surgery. If it is properly done for well-selected cases with definite evidence of nerve root compression, it is extremely effective. In less clear cases, it usually fails.

Surgery for pain problems related to degenerative changes is very effective. Practically any joint in the arm and leg can be replaced. Total hip replacement has been done for years and is the most successful of all joint replacements. The replacement of other joints has not achieved as much success.

Musculoskeletal pain is usually the result of the minor trauma of everyday living. This kind of pain usually will respond to conservative treatment—rest during the acute stage, exercise and gradual increase in activity as pain subsides. Women must know this so that they do not allow unnecessary manipulation or tragic mutilation of their bodies under the guise of care. Seeking a second opinion from physicians in different specialties is especially wise if something other than conservative treatment is the first recommendation for a musculoskeletal pain problem. Knowing the causes and treatment options for the aches and pains in your muscles, joints, tendons, and ligaments allows you to take an active part in your care. It is one of the best ways to protect and maintain the health of this important body system. Remember—you ultimately are responsible for your own health.

For additional reading in this area, refer to the following books:

Bonica, J., & Ventafridda, V. *Advances in pain research and therapy* (vol. 1). New York: Raven Press, 1976.

Cailliet, R. *Soft tissue pain and disability*. Philadelphia: Davis, 1977.

Fagerhaugh, S. Y., & Strauss, A. *Politics of pain man-agement*. Menlo Park: Calif.: Addison-Wesley, 1977.

McCaffery, M. *Nursing management of the patient with pain* (2nd ed.). Philadelphia: Lippincott, 1979.

TY HONGLADAROM, M.D. and
GAIL HONGLADAROM, R.N., Ph.D.

osteoporosis:
a special problem for women

There are several health problems that bother women more than men. *Osteoporosis* (a condition in which bone becomes spongelike) is definitely found more often among women. The osteoporoses constitute an ancient group of metabolic bone disorders. Long before X-ray was discovered in 1895, physicians had recognized that the bones of older people often became thin and fragile. As early as the sixth century A.D., Paulus Aeginata described a bone disease that is typical of osteoporosis.

Modern-day anthropologists have studied skeletons from ancient Nubia and found that osteoporosis was much more common in Nubian women than in men. This earlier and more severe bone loss noted in Nubian women was also found to occur more frequently in American Indian women than in men. Studies of contemporary populations support these ancient findings; women still lose more bone than men and this bone loss occurs noticeably earlier in the life of females.

definition

Osteoporosis is defined as a generalized decrease in bone mass as shown graphically in Figure 21.1. Bone mass is made up of bone matrix and minerals. In osteoporosis, both components are decreased.

261

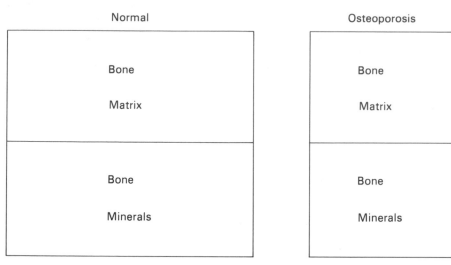

figure 21-1

The term *osteoporosis* means increased porosity of the bone (see Fig. 21-2).

In Figure 21.2, we see that osteoporosis is characterized by a loss of bone mass. It is a disease of "too little bone tissue," not a disease of mineral metabolism.

pathogenesis

Bone is an active tissue. It is constantly being remodeled to adapt to the stress put upon it. During the process of remodeling, if bone resorption (the removal of bone tissue) exceeds bone formation, osteoporosis will occur.

etiology

Osteoporosis may result from many causes (shown in Table 21.1). In 4 out of 5 people with osteoporosis, it is associated with being postmenopausal; in the remainder, it is associated with a variety of diseases. Since other causes have more specific direct treatments, it is essential that women request that the physician conduct a thorough assessment to establish an accurate diagnosis. This is accomplished by taking a detailed history, followed by a thorough physical examination, laboratory studies, and X-rays. A bone scan, bone biopsy, or even more elaborate and sophisticated procedures may be required. Once a correctable cause that would require a specific treatment has been excluded, the diagnosis of postmenopausal osteoporosis can be accepted. Detailed attention to this unique condition that has great significance for women's health is covered in the remainder of this chapter.

incidence

Postmenopausal osteoporosis is one of the most common causes of morbidity in older women today. After age 45, the incidence of femoral neck (hip) fractures in women doubles with each five years of age. By the time a woman reaches the age of 80, she has a 20 percent chance of having had a fractured hip and a 20 percent chance of having had one or more vertebral compression fractures.

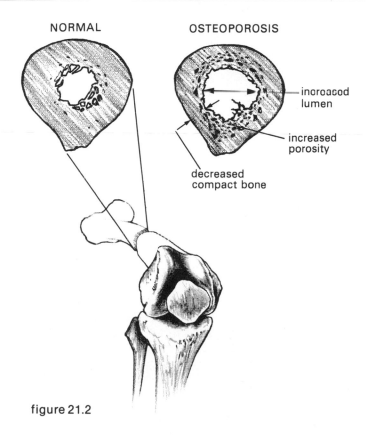

NORMAL   OSTEOPOROSIS

— inoroaοod
lumen

— increased
porosity

decreased
compact bone

figure 21.2

factors affecting osteoporosis

AGE AND SEX. People of all ages and sexes lose a certain amount of bone mass with aging. Maximum bone mass is reached at about 20 years of age. This peak level of total bone mass is greater in men than in women and also greater in blacks than in whites. After age 30, there is normally a 1 to 2 percent loss of bone mass per year. Since women have less bone to start with, the incidence of osteoporosis at all ages is higher in women than in men. It increases sharply in the fifth decade in women, but in men this happens about a decade later. By age 60, about 20 percent of women and 5 percent of men have osteoporosis. Bone mass decreases constantly between age 35 and 75. When a woman reaches 75 years of age, she has lost half of the bone mass in the bones of her spine and between 20 to 30 percent of the bone mass in the long bones of her arms and legs.

One researcher showed that the greatest loss of bone occurs in the first six months after a woman has undergone bilateral oophorectomy (removal of ovaries). A hysterectomy (removal of the uterus or womb) by itself does not alter the hormonal system and, therefore,

table 21.1
etiology of osteoporosis

1. Deficient sex hormone
   A. Estrogen
      1. Postsurgical removal of ovaries
      2. Postmenopausal
      3. Gonadal dysgenesis
   B. Androgen
      1. Aging
      2. Postsurgical removal of testes
   C. Hypopituitarism
II. Hormonal excess
   A. Hyperthyroidism
   B. Hyperparathyroidism
   C. Hypercortisonism
      1. Steroid usage
      2. Cushing's syndrome
III. Immobilization
   A. Decreased physical activities
   B. Paralysis
   C. Casting or bracing
IV. Nutritional lack
   A. Inadequate diet
      1. Protein
      2. Calcium
      3. Vitamins, esp. vitamins C & D
   B. Malabsorption, e.g., postgastrectomy syndrome
   C. Chronic wasting diseases, e.g., malignant tumors
   D. Renal loss, e.g., tubular disorders
V. Others
   A. Metastatic cancer
   B. Bone marrow disorders, e.g., multiple myeloma
   C. Bone matrix structural disorders, e.g., osteogenesis imperfecta
   D. Hepatic osteoporosis
   E. Heparin osteoporosis
   F. Excessive radiation
   G. Poisoning from certain chemicals
   H. Transient osteoporosis

has no effect on bone loss. It is the removal of the ovaries that effects bone loss. Parity (meaning to have borne children) increases a woman's bone mass. The mechanism of this phenomenon is not known. Perhaps the high estrogen levels women have during pregnancy exert a protective effect on bone.

PHYSICAL ACTIVITY. Bone is a dynamic tissue and undergoes constant remodeling. Activity, particularly vigorous exercise, plays a significant role in bone formation. Increased stress on bone stimulates new bone formation and lack of stress results in decreased formation and increases resorption. The rate of remodeling varies widely among individuals and with age. The majority of remodeling occurs during childhood and this process slows down considerably once a person has reached 21 years of age. After age 45, bone remodeling is very slow in both sexes. Although the process continues for life, it does so at a slower rate as we age. Moderate activity, if constant, does play an important role in maintaining bone mass. Adult women however, cannot augment their bone mass by short-term exercise programs.

Pronounced inactivity from any cause—bed rest, paralysis, or being in a cast—accelerates bone loss. However, although it has been suggested by some, it is incorrect to assume that postmenopausal osteoporosis occurs in women because they lead a sedentary life. Most women with symptomatic osteoporosis have been very active physically, and many return to a fully active life after the pain from osteoporosis is alleviated.

HORMONES. The endocrine system that produces hormones is intimately involved in bone formation and resorption. Estrogen (female sex hormone) and androgen (male sex hormone) are both anticatabolic (against the breaking down). In recent years, we have learned that estrogen therapy normalizes both the formation and resorption of bone, and thus prevents osteoporosis.

Corticosteroids (any steroid that has certain chemical or biological properties characteristic of the hormones secreted by the adrenal cortex) have an osteolytic (degeneration of bone) effect, which often produces severe osteoporosis. This side effect curtails its usefulness in various common diseases such as arthritis and lung disease. Prolonged use of corticosteroids is known to result in symptomatic osteoporosis in both women and men.

The catabolic (breaking down) effect of excess thyroid hormone on bones is almost as severe as that of the corticosteroids. The most potent bone-eroding agent, however, is parathyroid hormone, which is essential in maintaining serum calcium in the narrow physiological range. When a person's serum calcium level falls, the parathyroid glands increase the secretion of their hormone, which causes resorption of bone, releasing calcium into the blood. This hormone also acts on the kidneys to increase reabsorption of calcium as well as to change vitamin D into a more active form, which in turn increases the absorption of calcium from the bowel.

CALCIUM. A number of people doing research in this field have suggested that the major cause of osteoporosis in older women is a long-standing calcium deficiency. Calcium is obtained through absorption from several dietary sources. The most important source of calcium in the diet of North Americans is dairy products. Other foods containing calcium are green leafy vegetables and ground bone, which is used as "filler" in some meat products. How much calcium each person absorbs varies widely. We also know that the capacity to absorb calcium declines progressively after the age of 60 in both sexes, but more particularly in women.

While calcium is obtained only through absorption from dietary sources, it is lost from the body by several processes, which function whether or not calcium is being taken into the body. Losses through the kidneys account for 100 to 200 mg a day. A fixed amount of calcium, 125 to 180 mg a day, is continually secreted into our digestive juices. This calcium remains unabsorbed and is then excreted in feces. Calcium is also lost through the skin, but under normal conditions this does not exceed 20 mg a day. In women, there are two other possible ways that calcium is lost. During the last trimester of pregnancy, 25 to 30 grams of calcium are deposited in the skeleton of the baby that is being formed. In addition, during lactation 500 to 700 mg of calcium a day may be excreted in the breast milk.

The recommended daily dietary allowance of 800 mg of calcium for adults is based on what is needed for the ongoing normal calcium losses and absorption, which occurs at a rate of 40 percent. While this amount may be sufficient for some individuals, it may be inadequate for those whose absorption is lower.

When looking for sources of calcium, remember that 8 ounces of nonfat milk contains approximately 300 mg of calcium, and 1 cup of yogurt yields about the same amount of calcium. Cheese, of course, is also a good dietary source of calcium; 1 cup of cottage cheese will give you 200 mg of calcium, and 1 cup of grated cheddar cheese contains 850 mg. Other dietary sources high in calcium are whole wheat products, raisins, rhubarb, turnip greens, spinach, and cabbage. Some fish such as oysters, mackerel, and sardines are especially good sources of calcium. To know the exact calcium content of all foods, you may obtain free from your local Department of Agriculture office a very useful booklet entitled "The Nutritive Value of Foods."

Recent studies have shown that a daily intake of less than 1 gram of calcium in premenopausal women will result in loss of bone, while postmenopausal women require 1½ grams of calcium a day. If sufficient calcium is not available from a woman's diet, the body will take it from the body's bones. The long-term effect of an inadequate dietary intake of calcium relative to normal body losses is demineralization of bone, which is a factor in osteoporosis.

VITAMINS. In humans, vitamin D in physiological doses, that is, 500 International Units a day, promotes the intestinal absorption of calcium, but in higher doses, it enhances bone breakdown.

NUTRITION. Protein is also essential for bone formation. In the absence of alcoholism or dietary fads, protein deficiency is not common in the Western world. It is sometimes found in the elderly, particularly those who live alone, and in these cases it is often as much related to being poor as it is to apathy and poor eating habits.

Several researchers found that children suffering from acute and chronic protein-calorie malnutrition had less dense bones. Women should know this so that they will more readily get assistance from government food programs when necessary. It is important to prevent girls from having fragile bones because if they have less dense bones in early life, they will be much more vulnerable as older women..

Our protein needs are based on body size. For example, a woman weighing 128 pounds should have 45 grams (1½ oz.) of mixed protein daily, half animal and half vegetable. Not only beef, but fish, poultry, eggs, and dairy products are good sources of animal protein. Peanuts, lentils, and beans are good sources of vegetable protein. In vegetarian diets, grains should always be used with legumes, such as beans with rice or wheat with peas, to provide a sufficient amount of high-quality proteins.

diagnosis

There is no specific test or X-ray finding that is diagnostic of postmenopausal osteoporosis. The diagnosis is made after the causes that are listed in Table 21.1 have been excluded. Women do not have symptoms from osteoporosis itself, but from the fractures that occur because of the fragility of their osteoporotic bones. The women who do have symptoms are often petite and fair-skinned, and are 10 or more years older than usual at the time of their menopause, or have had their ovaries removed.

The most common symptom that a woman with osteoporosis has is back pain. This is usually a mild, chronic, low back pain, which is due to the slow deformation of a bone in her spine, or a sudden acute back pain accompanying a spontaneous compression fracture of one of the bones in her spine. The lower part of the spine is an area where a small volume of bone supports the upper half of the body. The stress on a unit of bone in this area is, therefore, very high. The neck of the femur (the long bone in the thigh) is also an area where a small volume of bone supports a large amount of weight. What might seem like just a little trauma can easily result in a femoral neck (hip) fracture. Fractures of the wrist can also result from the bones in the wrist being subjected to a great deal of stress. For example, when a woman with osteoporosis puts out her arm to save herself in a fall, she may very likely break her wrist.

In postmenopausal osteoporosis, all laboratory studies are usually normal. But X-ray examination will in most cases show a generalized decrease in bone density, and this occurs more severely in the spine than in the long bones of the arms and legs. The earliest osteoporotic change that can be discovered with conventional X-ray is the loss of trabecular bone (area occupying center of the bone). This trabecular loss in the upper femur correlates well with subsequent fractures.

In addition to the changes that can be seen when an X-ray is taken, changes are also found when a biopsy of the bone is looked at through a microscope. When the bone sample is viewed, the pathologist's findings usually state that there is a decreased volume of mineralized bone tissue.

treatment

"An ounce of prevention is worth a pound of cure." The most important treatment is prevention, but this is difficult because most people do not follow preventive measures when they are not suffering from symptoms. It is hoped that with the growing emphasis on positive health maintenance, this will change and women will understand that good nutrition and sufficient physical exercise will help prevent osteoporosis. Other treatments that have been used are hormones, calcium, and vitamins. However, women need to know that osteoporosis cannot be reversed, but merely slowed down; therefore, the preventive rather than the curative therapies should be emphasized.

The most persuasive argument that what is being done for osteoporosis is effective is whether the treatment prevents fractures with a minimal amount of side effects. Following is a summary of treatments currently being used for osteoporosis in postmenopausal women.

1. ESTROGEN. Although this kind of treatment does not restore bone that is already lost, estrogens have proven effective because they prevent further fractures. A cyclic kind of therapy is usually recommended that is 25 days on and five days off. In one study of 220 osteoporotic women, 24 had their estrogen therapy discontinued. Nine of 24 developed fractures, seven had their estrogens started again, and the fractures did not continue to occur. The two women who could not have their estrogen therapy restarted because of other health problems continued to sustain fractures. Therefore, many recommend that postmenopausal women with osteoporosis continue small-dose estrogen therapy throughout their lives. There is a question, however, of whether this treatment exposes women to an increased risk of endometrial cancer (cancer of the lining cells of the uterus), cancer of the breast, and thromboembolic disease and strokes, especially in women who smoke and who also have high blood pressure. A woman taking estrogens for any reason including osteoporosis should be informed about the potential risks, discuss this with the physician, and report any health changes or symptoms promptly.

2. CALCIUM. When taken in sufficiently high doses, it will stop osteolysis (bone breakdown), but only at the expense of producing dangerously high levels of calcium in the blood (hypercalcemia) and urine (hypercalciurea), which can cause kidney and bladder stones.

3. FLUORIDE. When taken in doses large enough to increase bone density, it can be toxic to the nervous system as well as the kidneys.

4. VITAMIN D. It is used in the treatment of osteoporosis because it increases the intestinal absorption of calcium. Again, too much Vitamin D may lead to hypercalcemia and hypercalciurea, with the associated dangers of developing kidney or bladder stones.

5. VITAMIN C. It promotes the formation of osteoid (the protein matrix of bone). Since Vitamin C is water-soluble, there are no harmful results from this substance because the body excretes excess amounts in the urine.

Some researchers have suggested a daily regimen of 50 mg of fluoride and 1 gram of calcium, combined with 50,000 IU of Vitamin D taken twice a week. This regimen is based on the assumption that the fluoride will stimulate bone matrix formation and the simultaneous administration of calcium and vitamin D will mineralize this new bone. Women must understand that these high doses of fluoride, calcium, and vitamin D can produce hypercalciurea (high levels of calcium in the urine) and kidney stones, hypercalcemia (high levels of calcium in the blood), and a painful condition resulting from generalized increased density of the skeleton called fluorosis.

Unfortunately, fragile osteoporotic bones will sustain fractures. At the time of the fracture, very severe pain may occur, requiring potent pain-relieving medication and perhaps even temporary immobilization for two or three weeks, the length of time that the acute pain usually lasts. Being immobilized, however, may predispose a woman to further bone loss and, in effect, worsen the process of osteoporosis. As the fractured vertebra begins to heal, the pain usually tapers off, but the deformed vertebra very often leads to a stooped-over look in women, and some readers have probably heard this referred to as the "dowager's hump." A loss of height usually results from this type of osteoporotic fracture. The deformed vertebra that usually remains may also cause pain from mechanical or nerve root irritation. The latter causes of pain may be misinterpreted as additional fractures, but this can be decided by an X-ray examination, which can be compared to the X-rays that were taken when the first fracture occurred. It is very important that a woman's height is measured when she is first seen regarding her osteoporosis, because when your height is maintained you can be quite certain that additional vertebra have not collapsed.

The fractures in osteoporotic bones usually heal normally and the process takes about 3 to 4 months. However, additional fractures usually do occur if appropriate preventive measures are not taken. The most acute pain associated with osteoporotic fractures usually subsides in two or three weeks. At this time a physical therapy program should be planned so that there is a gradual increase in activity that is within the woman's limit of tolerance. A dorsolumbar corset may be prescribed to support the body and to restrict the movement of the fractured spine. Women with osteoporosis should be advised to support their weight with their arms while sitting and also when standing by using a walker or crutches. If a woman is overweight, this is an extra burden on her already fragile bones and a weight reduction program should be suggested. Swimming is an excellent exercise, and women are encouraged to participate in this activity for the purpose of slowing down osteoporosis as well as for other health benefits. Many organizations, such as the YWCA, have early morning and late afternoon swims for working women so that the nine-to-five day need not preclude an exercise program. Walking and bicycling, in addition to ordinary general activity, are all ways to slow down osteoporosis. Proper isometric exercise will strengthen the muscles that support the spine, and posture exercise programs will eliminate the poor posture that puts additional stresses on the bone.

When your back feels tired, take a few minutes and rest, stretched out on your back. Also take time to analyze your work and try to simplify what is needed. Good safety precautions should be employed in the home as well as in your workplace to prevent fractures.

Proper body mechanics prevent injuries and if you have not had instructions in proper lifting and bending, classes are also available for these purposes, and many good pamphlets on the topic are available.

Few health problems are so specifically related to women as osteoporosis and few are so bothersome for such a long period of time. Unfortunately, most women know very little about this condition and few are involved in preventive health programs. This overview of the necessary background information about osteoporosis should be a stimulus for women to become actively involved in preventive health programs.

Aitken, J. M., Hart, D. M., & Lindsay, R. Oestrogen replacement therapy for prevention of osteoporosis after oophorectomy, *British Medical Journal*, September 1973, *3(5879)*, 515–518.

Barzel, U. S. Osteoporosis II. New York: Grune & Stratton, 1979.

Dalen, N., & Olsson, K. E. Bone mineral content and physical activity. *Acta Orthopedica Scandinavica*, 1974, *45*, FASC 2, 170–174.

Dalen, N., Halberg, D., & Lamke, B. Bone mass in obese subjects. *Acta Medica Scandinavica*, May 1975, *197(5)*, 353–355.

Goldsmith, N. P., & Johnston, J. O. Bone mineral: effects of oral contraceptives, pregnancy, and lactation. *Journal of Bone and Joint Surgery*, July 1975, *57A(5)*, 657–668.

Gordon, Gilbert S., Vaughan, C. *Clinical management of the osteoporoses*. Acton, Mass.: Publishing Sciences, 1976.

Heaney, R. P., & Recker, R. P. Estrogen effects of bone remodeling at menopause, *Clinical Research*, October 1975, *23(4)*, 535.

Hongladarom, T., & Anderson, D. Transient Osteoporosis. *Contemporary Orthopedics*, April 1980, *2(2)*, 148–154.

Jowsey, J. Osteoporosis: its nature and the role of diet. *Postgraduate Medicine*, August 1976, *60(2)*, 75–79.

Meema, S., & Meema, H. E. Menopausal bone loss and estrogen replacement *Israel Journal of Medical Science* (July 1976), *12(7)*, 601–606.

Nilsson, B. E., & Westlin, N. E. Changes in bone mass in alcoholics. *Clinical Orthopedics*, January–February 1973, *90*, 229–232.

Riggs, B. L., Hodgson, S. F., Hoffman, D. L., Kelly, P. J., Johnson, K. A., & Taves, D. Treatment of primary osteoporosis with fluoride and calcium. *Journal of the American Medical Association, February 1980, 243(5)*, 446–449.

Trotter, M., & Hixon, B. B. Sequential changes in weight, density, and percentage ash weight of human skeletons from an early fetal period through old age. *Anatomical Record, May 1974, 179(1)*, 1–18.

Urist, M. R., Orthopedic management of osteoporosis in postmenopausal women. *Clinics in Endocrinology and Metabolism, July 1973, 262*, 159–176.

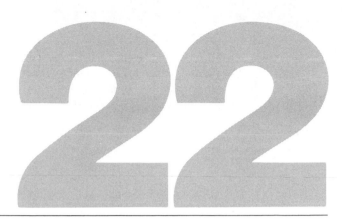

RUTH McCORKLE, R.N., Ph.D. and
BARBARA GERMINO, R.N., Ph.C.

women and cancer

Cancer occurs in one of every four persons in the United States, most of whom believe that its diagnosis means death. However, for some, advances in modern detection techniques and early treatment mean that they become free of the disease once treated. But for others in whom the disease progresses beyond the possibilities of treatment, the uncertainties of what to expect and how to manage what is happening to them and their families continue to grow more poignant. This chapter presents an overview of what is known about cancer, its psychological impact, and how it is diagnosed, treated, and managed.

psychological impact

Cancer is not one disease but many. The different forms of cancer are slowly being recognized as chronic diseases, since people with some types are living longer. A diagnosis of cancer is dreaded not only because it symbolizes death, but because of the fears associated with adapting to an enforced, unwanted lifestyle until death. Fears include those of uncontrollable pain, helplessness, wasting of the body, increased physical and social dependency, and abandonment by other people (Feder, 1966). Thus, when a diagnosis of cancer is made, an unusually stressful experience follows, which can disrupt a person's established lifelong patterns of behavior (Caplan, 1956).

The majority of people who develop cancer are encountering a new experience. Even if they have known someone with cancer, chances are that the type of cancer and the treatment recommended for that other person will be different from what they will receive. Many cancers require a variety of combination therapies, and treatments change over time. As a result, the price paid for comprehensive cancer care can be emotionally and financially draining.

One of the major difficulties associated with cancer is the lack of a specific test to determine its presence or absence. Consequently, patients may be subjected to numerous procedures and consultations to rule out a number of specific diseases. As one can imagine, this process is time-consuming and expensive for the patients, their families, and the health care professionals.

the incidence of cancer

Cancers are diseases that are not discriminatory of race, sex, age, or economic and social class. The incidence of cancer increases as people get older, and yet it affects the young at unpredictable times. Most often it occurs when least expected. It is not uncommon that the victimized person has never previously been ill or hospitalized. Even at the time of diagnosis, many people cannot imagine that they have cancer because their tumors have remained "silent" and unnoticeable.

Physicians classify cancers according to location within the body. In women, locations in which cancer most frequently occurs are breast, colon and rectum, uterus (corpus and cervix), lungs, and ovaries (Silverberg, 1980). Breast cancer is thought to occur only in women, and yet, infrequently, it does occur in men.

The rise in the incidence of cancer is to a large extent a reflection of the medical progress that has sharply reduced mortality from other diseases, such as tuberculosis and pneumonia. As people live longer, an increase in the incidence of certain cancers is likely to occur. The most notable increase has been that of lung cancer in both sexes. In contrast, there has been a remarkable reduction in the incidence of cervical cancer for women. There has also been a decrease in stomach cancer for both men and women. Nevertheless, the incidence of cancer of all types is expected to continue to rise because of the growing number of older people in the United States. This is likely regardless of whether substantial improvements of cure rates for certain cancers are made. In other words, cancer mortality will inevitably increase unless new means of controlling cancers are found, taught to physicians, and accepted by the public.

development of cancer

what cancers are

The word cancer comes from Latin, and means "crab." In medical terminology, cancer is used to mean a large group of different diseases, all of which have in common a process called malignant neoplasia. Neoplasia means new tissue growth and is a process in which abnormal cells multiply rapidly, uncontrolled by normal body functions. Neoplasia can mean either benign (relatively harmless) or malignant (potentially dangerous) tissue growth, but is usually used to mean the latter. Cancers are malignant neoplasms that are specifically named according to the body site where they originate or the type of body tissue they involve. They can take the form of a solid mass, circulating cells, or abnormalities of a particular type of body tissue (see table 22.1).

Whatever form cancers take, they are different from benign neoplasms in several ways. Tissue cells in benign neoplasms are usually more typical or normal in appearance when viewed under a microscope. Malignant cells are abnormal and grow in a disorderly rather than an organized way. Benign neoplasms are usually surrounded by a kind of tissue capsule, or at least their edges are clearly defined. Malignant neoplasms rarely have such a capsule or clear definition. Although benign neoplasms are usually not life-threatening, they

table 22.1
examples of malignant neoplasms and their classification

	NAME AND DEFINITION	TYPE OF NEOPLASM	LOCATION
I.	Sarcomas: Arise in connective tissue (such as bone, cartilage, & fatty tissue) and muscles.		
	A. Fibrosarcoma	Solid Tumor	Fibrous tissue
	B. Chondrosarcoma	Solid Tumor	Cartilage
	C. Angiosarcoma	Solid Tumor	Endothelium of blood vessels
	D. Leukemia	Circulating abnormal cells	Blood, lymph nodes, spleen, bone marrow
	E. Hodgkin's disease	Lymphomas Circulating abnormal cells	Lymph nodes
	F. Multiple myeloma	Plasmacytomas Circulating abnormal plasma cells	Blood, bone marrow, spleen
II.	Carcinomas: Arise in tissues that cover or line such organs of the body as skin, intestines, uterus, lung, breast.		
	A. Squamous cell carcinoma	Solid Tumor	Epithelium tissue
	B. Basal cell carcinoma	Solid Tumor	Basal cells of the skin
	C. Adenocarcinoma	Solid Tumor	Gland cells (parenchyma)
	D. Bronchogenic carcinoma	Solid Tumor	Lung (bronchi)
	E. Choriocarcinoma	Solid Tumor	Placenta

do grow and expand and can be dangerous by causing abnormal pressure or taking up limited space. They usually grow slowly and remain in one place. Malignant neoplasms occassionally are slow-growing, but, more often, they grow rapidly and spread through the body in several different ways. Cancers can spread or metastasize by invading adjacent tissues directly or by malignant cells that travel through the body via the lymph or blood to another site (see Table 22.2).

factors
that may cause cancer

Although all cells in the body are able to divide and multiply to produce new cells, this process is controlled and occurs in response to the body's need for new tissue for normal maintenance or regeneration. For example, a wound stimulates formation of new cells, which help to close and heal it. Newly formed cells are the same in structure and function as the old cells from which they came. The process produces differentiated or clearly defined cells.

Malignant neoplasms violate all these rules of cell growth and reproduction by growing and multiplying uncontrollably—not in response to the body's needs and often to the detriment of those needs. They use oxygen, food, and energy that would otherwise nourish normal cells. If this process is prolonged and extensive, it may leave the person malnourished and weak.

Although the specific etiologies of cancers are not yet known, a large body of research indicates that there are probably at least two general mechanisms involved in this complex multifactorial process. The first is a stimulus of some kind that causes a normal cell to change into a malignant neoplastic cell. The

table 22.2
characteristics of benign and malignant neoplasms

BENIGN NEOPLASMS	MALIGNANT NEOPLASMS
Grow slowly	Usually grow fast
Grow by expanding and can cause pressure, but do not invade nearby tissue	Invade nearby tissue, grow in all directions
Are usually surrounded by tissue capsule or have clearly defined margins	Are rarely encapsulated and often poorly differentiated from normal tissues
Remain in one site— do not spread throughout the body	Spread (metastasize) in other parts of the body via the blood or lymphatics and set up secondary tumors
Are solid tumors only	May be solid tumors or circulating abnormal cells
Are made up of tissue often similar to tissue of origin	Are made up of abnormal tissue and atypical cells, not well differentiated
Cause minimal tissue destruction—usually the result of pressure	Cause much tissue destruction because of invasion and metastasis

second is the body's ability to destroy or overcome these newly formed malignant cells before they proliferate too widely. Normally, the body's immune system protects against infections and many diseases by reacting to and destroying invading bacteria, viruses, or other harmful invaders.

carcinogens

The federal government, many organizations, and private foundations are supporting research that explores the relationship of carcinogens to the development of cancers. "Carcinogens are physical, chemical or biologic factors that increase the likelihood of cancers in humans or animals" (Burkhalter, 1978, p. 29). Carcinogens can act in various ways and at many sites in the body. They are not always associated with the occurrence of cancer unless the exposed person is susceptible or unable to overcome the abnormal changes stimulated by the carcinogen. In many instances, exposure must be over long periods of time or at concentrated levels for the carcinogens to have their effect. Occupational, environmental, nutritional, and viral carcinogens have been identified and are being studied.

signs and symptoms
of cancer

PRIMARY TUMOR. The signs and symptoms associated with solid tumor cancers and with benign neoplasms are often similar. They are caused by the mechanical effects of the primary tumor or a secondary growth in a distant part of the body. The solid neoplasm occupies space and, as a result, can obstruct the lumen of a duct or tube and exert pressure on the surrounding mucous membranes and nerve endings. The person's awareness of the symptoms depends on the location of the neoplasm and its nature, that is, how fast it grows and how likely it is to spread. As a cancer grows, it occupies an increasing amount of space. The growing mass of abnormal cells can interfere with the blood supply of the surrounding tissue, interfere with the function of an organ, press against nerve endings, and activate the body's defense mechanisms.

Frequently, a cancer begins in the body without any signs or symptoms, as in the case of most breast cancers. As the cancer grows, the woman may find it herself if she practices self-breast examination, her partner may find it during sexual activity, or her doctor may find it during a physical examination. The point is that in order for it to be felt, it must have reached a substantial size. The larger the breast cancer, the more likely it is that it will not be localized in the breast. In either event (local or distant disease), there are recommended treatments to help the woman with what is happening to her. It is extremely difficult for a person who is feeling perfectly healthy to understand the need for extensive and prolonged treatment that will temporarily interfere with her life-style so she can live a longer life, and yet, in fact, this is frequently the case.

Conversely, women with symptoms may have difficulty in getting the help they need. For example, a woman who does not feel well and has become increasingly tired, depressed, and unable to work may go from one physician to another because no doctor is able to find anything wrong with her. This woman is frequently labeled by physicians and other health care professionals as "neurotic," and she begins to doubt her own ability to perceive what is happening to her body. Some time later, it is not uncommon for this woman to be given the diagnosis of cancer of an unknown primary site. This example illustrates the additional technological advances that are needed to diagnose the many different forms of cancer. Although there have been some major discoveries to help diagnose cancer early, other methods are needed. With the present limited tests and procedures, many patients are subjected unnecessarily to verbal accusations that imply that the problem is in their "head" rather than in their "body." The person with a feeling that things are not right with her is the best judge that something is amiss.

The most important symptoms to be aware of are changes from the person's usual pattern of functioning, such as eating, sleeping, and walking. A thorough assessment of the change needs to be reported: its onset, whether gradual or sudden, and its duration, whether prolonged or intermittent. If changes are gradual, they may go unnoticed until a marked alteration is apparent. This frequently occurs with weight loss. A person may lose a few pounds each week, and suddenly it becomes obvious that she has lost 20 pounds.

GENERALIZED DISEASE. There are some neoplastic diseases such as leukemia that are manifested as a generalized disease (nonsolid tumors) from their onset. A woman may notice that she is tired, has a tendency to bleed or bruise easily, has lost weight, is pale, short of breath, and has a fever. These are all symptoms of leukemia, but can just as easily be symptoms of other diseases. The physician must test for various disorders that need to be ruled out; in some instances, the tests are not as sophisticated as they should be, and although leukemia may be suspected, the tests are inconclusive.

METASTATIC DISEASE. One of the characteristics that distinguish cancerous cells from normal cells is their ability to break away from the primary cancer mass and move to other parts of the body. The process whereby a malignant tumor disseminates throughout the body and establishes secondary growths is known as metastasis. The spread of the cancer can take place by several routes throughout the body. The two most common are by the lymphatic system and the bloodstream. As the cancer grows, cells can penetrate into the blood or lymphatic systems and become lodged there or move along the channels of these two systems to distant parts. For example, a woman may have a primary tumor in her left breast and the cancer may be surgically removed. Prior to surgery, several cancer cells may have broken away and invaded the lymph nodes in the axilla and along the breast bone. From there, the cancer can travel to other lymph nodes in the body, such as those in the neck and spread from lymph nodes to veins by the lymphaticovenous system. Spread and growth of cancer depends to a great extent on the venous pathways involved. It is not uncommon for the bones of the vertebral column to be invaded by small cancer cells circulating in the veins surrounding the vertebra.

The cancer cells can also enter the bloodstream, as the lymphatic system drains into the thoracic duct and the lymph spreads directly throughout the body to other parts such as the lungs and skeleton (see Fig. 22.1). It is important for the woman who elects to have her breast removed to understand that a small circulating or lodged cluster of cancer cells along the vertebrae or other parts of the body may be undetectable at the time of the original breast surgery. It may take a period of months or years before the cancer growth becomes large enough to make its presence known by symptoms such as nagging back pain, difficulty in lifting heavy objects, or changes in gait. To prevent the spread of the cancer from the breast when surgery is performed, the recommended treatment is adjuvant chemotherapy. (This is discussed in detail in the section on treatments.)

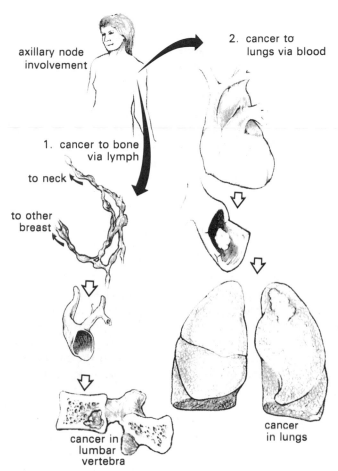

axillary node
involvement

2. cancer to
lungs via blood

1. cancer to bone
via lymph

to neck

to other
breast

cancer in
lumbar
vertebra

cancer
in lungs

figure 22.1
two common pathways in which cancer metastasize

diagnosis of cancers

Cancers vary greatly in the ease with which they can be diagnosed. The particular point in the disease course at which symptoms appear also varies with the kind of cancer. A definitive diagnosis of most cancers requires some combination of health history, physical examination, laboratory tests, cytologic evaluations, biopsy specimens, and radiological studies. All of the procedures are important, but the latter three are often necessary in or-

der to positively confirm a cancer diagnosis.

cytology

Cytologic evaluation (cell studies done under high-powered microscopes) can identify malignant cells, sometimes very early in the neoplastic process, and often before there are any noticeable symptoms. Since cells of the epithelium, or lining, of organs are constantly and rapidly replacing themselves with old cells sloughing off, it is easy to obtain a cell specimen for cytologic study by aspirating mucous secretions or gently scraping mucous membranes with a blunt wooden scraper. The Pap smear requires a special staining technique, which is used to differentiate normal from abnormal mucosal cells of the uterus and cervix (see chapter 26). Abnormalities of the sputum (mucus) coughed up from the lungs and of specimens washed out of the bronchi (breathing passages leading to the lungs) are also detected cytologically.

histological specimens

A definitive diagnosis of cancer can be made when the pathologist examines a specimen of malignant tissue. Since there are vast differences among cancers and cancer treatments, most physicians prefer that the specific kind of malignancy be documented from a tissue specimen so that treatment can be equally specific. A tissue specimen can often be obtained by simple biopsy, a procedure whereby a very small section of abnormal tissue is excised with a surgical tool—usually quickly and with a minimum of discomfort. Skin lesions can be easily biopsied on an outpatient visit, as can cervical lesions or rectal polyps. Biopsies of internal organs require hospitalization and surgery or endoscopy, a procedure in which a flexible instrument is inserted into the esophagus, bronchus, or rectum to visualize a lesion, using mirrors or fiber optics to obtain a tissue specimen.

radiological studies

Routine X-ray studies may or may not help in the diagnosis of cancers, depending on their location. Some malignancies, like cancer of the lung, can be detected with regular X-ray studies, but many require more specialized radiological studies.

Contrast studies are those in which some kind of radiopaque substance is swallowed, instilled, or injected in order to permit visualization of internal body structures and spaces. The simplest and best-known type of contrast study is the G.I. (gastrointestinal) series, in which radiopaque barium may be swallowed or instilled as an enema to outline the various portions of the gastrointestinal tract.

Air contrast studies are sometimes used in diagnosis of brain tumors. In these procedures, a small amount of spinal fluid is removed through a needle and replaced with the same amount of air. The air serves as a contrast medium to highlight abnormalities.

Radiopaque dye can be injected into an artery (arteriogram) or vein (venogram) to outline a portion of the circulatory system and to look for abnormalities. Dye can also be injected into the circulation to visualize specific organs such as the liver, gallbladder, and the kidneys.

Tomography is a method of visualizing layers of body tissue by using a special narrow X-ray beam and computer equipment to obtain a three-dimensional picture. Both the presence and size of tumors may be estimated in this way. A CAT scan (computerized axial tomography) is a special kind of tomography which allows the printing of pictures of "slices" of tissue for close examination with minimal discomfort and without a surgical incision.

Radioisotope scanning is a way of examining the density of tissue in particular organs. The swallowing or injection of a liquid radioisotope, which is drawn to a particular type of body tissue, enables its concentration in that tissue. Measurement of radioactivity emerging from that area may be used to help detect tumors or metastases.

Ultrasonography is a technique for visualizing internal body structures by directing ultrasonic waves (those sounds beyond the range of human hearing) into body tissues and recording their reflection. Varying the frequency of ultrasonic waves enables examination of both deep and superficial body structures.

treatment goals

prevention

One of the most important efforts in cancer treatment is in prevention—the application of knowledge about factors that seem to cause cancers, in an effort to prevent malignancies from occurring. Major attempts to educate the public are part of the American Cancer Society's ongoing program and include intensive efforts to warn about hazards such as cigarette smoking. The "Seven Safeguards" against cancer, as suggested by the American Cancer Society, are:

1. LUNG. Reduction and ultimate elimination of cigarette smoking.
2. COLON-RECTUM. Proctoscopic exam as routine in annual checkup for those over 40.
3. BREAST. Self-examination as a monthly female practice.
4. UTERUS. Pap test for all adult and high-risk women.
5. SKIN. Avoidance of excessive sun.
6. ORAL. Wider practice of early detection measures.
7. BASIC. Regular physical examination for all adults.

In addition, prevention should include avoidance of prolonged exposure to radiation and known carcinogens. Since our knowledge of factors that cause cancers is incomplete, prevention is only one of the goals to which efforts are being directed.

early detection

Early detection is the next priority, since several types of cancers, particularly skin and cervical cancers, are likely to be curable in the early stages (see chapter 26 for information on cervical screening). Efforts to find one simple, inexpensive screening test to detect the presence of cancers in the body have, to date, been unsuccessful. There are, however, specific screening techniques for several of the common types of cancer. Breast cancer is still most effectively detected by women who conscientiously and carefully examine their own breasts once a month. Thermography, mammography, and xerography (see chapter 28) are all radiologic techniques available for screening for breast cancer. However, these are not recommended for all women on a regular basis.

Screening for colon and rectal cancer by rectal examination and a proctosigmoidoscopic exam for those over 40 to 45 years of age are recommended by the American Cancer Society. The proctosigmoidoscopic exam is done with a flexible scope and system of fiberoptics to examine the interior of the rectum and lower colon. The procedure is uncomfortable, both physically and psychologically, but is considered to be well worth the person's tolerance because it increases the chance of early detection and treatment of colon cancer.

There is current disagreement among the experts about the need for annual chest X-rays and cytologic analysis of the sputum as a screening test for lung cancer. The conservative opinion appears to be that cigarette smokers and people with a family history of lung cancer or heavy exposure to asbestos or other air pollutants should have an annual physical examination and chest X-ray.

Cancers of the mouth and pharynx can be detected early by routine medical and dental examinations. Skin cancers are also highly visible and, therefore, detectable by examination at an early stage. It is vitally important that each individual be aware of unusual or changing skin lesions such as sores that do not heal or changing warts and moles. Familiarity with the normal appearance of such lesions will help to determine when they are changing or not healing normally, so that medical consultation may be sought.

cure

The term "definitive treatment" is often used by health professionals in discussing the goals of cancer therapy. Definitive treatment means treatment intended to produce a cure or a significantly prolonged survival time. "Palliative treatment" is designed to relieve distressing symptoms, such as pain, and to improve the person's quality of life. It is not directed toward a cure.

Once a cancer has been diagnosed, the diagnostic process will include staging to ascertain the extent of growth of a cancer so that treatment goals can be determined. The goals of treatment will vary with the extent of the malignancy, the presence of metastasis, and the growth pattern of the particular type of tumor. A cure in the treatment of most cancers is defined in terms of 5- or 10-year survival from the time of diagnosis. This criterion has been the traditional one used in clinical research of cancer treatments and has been considered a relatively significant point beyond which the rates of recurrence for many cancers drop drastically. Consequently, the chances of cure in the traditional sense are greatly enhanced. It is important to remember, however, that prognosis in cancer is based on statistics describing large populations and that there are often exceptions.

treatments

There are three major treatment modalities used to treat cancer: surgery, radiation, and chemotherapy. An additional one is immunotherapy. Depending on the type of cancer and how extensive it is throughout the body, one or more types of therapy can be used. The plan of treatment is based on the condition of the patient, on the nature, extent, and location of the cancer, and what the expectations are of a specific tumor response to a given therapeutic approach. The initiation and confirmation of a plan of therapy should be contingent on the person's abilities to understand and participate in the treatment options.

The purpose of all three methods of treatment is to remove or destroy all cancer cells in the body. To date, no method has been developed that is completely successful. The term "cure" is used cautiously. Although the physician may be reasonably certain that all the cancer cells have been surgically removed from a person or destroyed by radiation, there is no way to be positive. Often the physician measures the person's successful response to treatment in years of survival rather than in terms of absolute cure. Thus, the patients who are alive and well at the end of five years are said to have a five-year cure.

surgery

Surgery is the oldest form of treatment for cancers. In the past, surgery was recommended primarily to cure the patient, because the surgeon believed the malignant change in a tissue remained localized at the primary site long enough to be diagnosed and removed. This approach was based on the assumption that cancer was confined to one part of the body as a solid tumor. This is an oversimplified explanation of a complex process. It is now accepted that most cancers that are large enough to be diagnosed have had the time and opportunity to travel to distant parts of the body, forming secondary cancers (metastases). Therefore, the treatment of cancers by surgery to cure a person needs to be redefined. Surgery remains an important treatment, and the diagnostic and palliative aspects of surgery may be of greater benefit to the patient than some of the recommended radical operations of the past in situations that could in no circumstances be curative (White, 1978, 169–186).

DIAGNOSTIC SURGERY. Surgeons are frequently asked by a person's primary physician to provide a diagnostic service in the treatment and management of cancer. A biopsy specimen is usually taken to establish a definite tissue diagnosis, which identifies the nature of the cancer. It is important that the physician know the type of cancer because certain types of carcinomas and sarcomas behave and respond differently to specific treatments.

STAGING. It is also important for the physician to know the extent of a cancer in order to select the most appropriate form of treatment. In other words, the surgeon establishes not only the type of cancer, but also how much cancer there is throughout the body and where it is located. The stage or extent of the disease process is used to determine the best treatment plan for each patient and also to establish the prognosis or estimated time that the person may survive from the cancer.

If the physician suspects metastasis or wants to eliminate doubt that it has occurred, the biopsy specimen of a gland from a regional node or distant site will be taken to establish if cancer from the primary site has spread. For example, frequently, lung cancer spreads to the lymph nodes in the neck. If this is suspected by the appearance of a mass on the chest X-ray, and an enlarged or swollen lymph node in the neck, the surgeon would surgically remove the node in the neck and determine its tissue type before attempting to remove the mass in the lung. If the neck node is positive for cancer, the recommended primary treatment would not be surgery but, instead, radiation therapy or combination therapy.

Occasionally, staging requires biopsy specimens from several sites such as the liver and bone marrow. In Hodgkin's disease, it has become routine practice for the patient to undergo a diagnostic laporatomy (abdominal operation). During the procedure, the surgeon takes biopsy specimens from the liver and abdominal lymph nodes and removes the spleen. If the specimens are negative, the patient most likely will be treated locally at the primary cancer site with radiation. If the specimens are positive, treatment will include combination chemotherapy and radiation.

CURE. If the primary cancer is thought to be confined to a specific organ or body part, the cancer is surgically removed. When removing a primary cancer, it is preferred that the surgeon perform a wide excision in order to remove the entire tumor and a proportion of normal tissue surrounding the cancer. This frequently implies that entire organs and limbs are removed.

PALLIATION. Palliative surgical treatment may

be indicated when there is no likelihood of curing or removing all of the patient's cancer, and when distressing symptoms cannot be managed by radiation or medication. The primary purpose of palliative surgery is to improve the quality of the patient's remaining life and not to perpetuate an already difficult situation. If the surgical intervention will not relieve or lessen the person's distressing symptoms, the patient should be made aware of this and be given the opportunity to refuse the procedure. Few preventive procedures are warranted, particularly if the patient is free of distressing symptoms (see chapter 3 on Information Exchange). But in the presence of distressing symptoms, there are times when palliative surgery is indicated and will improve the patient's life. A woman who has developed an ulceration of the breast due to cancer can be relieved of its bleeding and infection if a simple mastectomy is performed. Although the surgery is not curative, it affords the patient relief of symptoms. However, the symptoms may be equally relieved by the use of radiation therapy; therefore, it is important that the patient be evaluated by a team of specialists to determine her ability to tolerate and survive the surgical procedure versus the radiation treatments.

HORMONAL MANIPULATION. Surgical intervention of cancers that are dependent on hormones constitutes a special area of cancer surgery. In other words, some cancers grow as a result of specific hormones available in the body. For example, breast cancers in some premenopausal women are dependent on a supply of estrogen. The most common operation to reduce the estrogen supply is an oophorectomy (removal of the ovaries). This procedure has reduced the amount of metastatic tumor in the bones and soft tissues of women with breast cancer and has extended their length of survival from months to years.

Other surgical procedures include bilateral adrenalectomy (removal of the adrenal glands) and hypophysectomy (removal of the pituitary gland).

RECONSTRUCTIVE SURGERY. Since the late 1960s, the combined treatments of mastectomy (surgical removal of a breast) and adjuvant chemotherapy have increased the length of survival of women with breast cancer. As a result, many women are requesting breast reconstructive surgery after their incisional area has healed. Since the plastic surgery techniques are extremely sophisticated and the results quite satisfactory to both the patient and her partner, this additional procedure offers some women who might refuse surgery, or delay it unnecessarily, a more acceptable treatment choice than an amputated breast.

PREVENTIVE SURGERY. With the public's increased awareness on cancer prevention, there are some patients who will elect to undergo preventive surgery. There are some lesions that are suspected of being precancerous. Examples are polyps of the colon and rectum, leukoplakia of the oral cavity following chronic irritation, and certain pigmented moles. Also, some women may elect to have bilateral prophylactic mastectomies with silicone implants five days after surgery, if one or more of their immediate family members has had breast cancer and if they have multiple cysts or lumps in their breasts that are painful and have been biopsied. Women who are contemplating surgery to prevent various forms of cancer should always obtain a second opinion from a physician before consenting to an operation whose effects are irreversible.

radiation

There are two approaches to radiation treatment—external and internal.

EXTERNAL RADIATION. External radiation therapy consists of treatment that uses machines to produce X-rays or gamma rays. Most machines are electrical, but some use radioactive substances such as cobalt 60. These machines are either orthovoltage or megavoltage. The machines are classified according to their penetrating power, which, in turn, depends on the wavelengths of the rays they produce. Orthovoltage machines are used primarily for skin cancers or lesions in which the maximum effects are obtained close to the skin surface. Megavoltage machines are used for cancers that are deep within the organs surrounding structures of the body.

Special machines are located on the ground floor or basement of hospitals. Generally, people receive treatment as outpatients and go to the radiation therapy unit at a designated time five days a week. The number of days a person is treated depends on the purpose of the treatment and the recommended course

for that particular cancer and its location. Radiation therapy can be given during a person's hospitalization in combination with other procedures or treatments such as surgery.

Treatments are administered in private rooms by a large radiation machine that can be directed to a specific area of the body (see Figure 22.2). One person is treated at a time in the room alone for a specific amount of time each day. The person is placed on a hard-surfaced table and is instructed to lie still during the timed radiation dose. The site where the treatment is administered to the body is marked so that the exact same area can be treated each day. It is important for a person to understand that the treatments are most effective if they are given in the exact same location each time and are given for the specified length of time needed to either destroy or control the cancer. Generally, treatments only last a few minutes, but for the patient the time may seem unusually long, especially since the

figure 22.2.
woman receiving radiation therapy from a large megavoltage machine in a private room monitored by a closed circuit television system

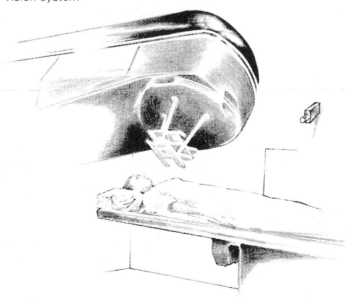

door to the room is closed during each treatment. No one is allowed in the room with the patient because the radiation can have harmful and cumulative effects on anyone exposed to it. These effects are tolerated by the patient because the exposure is limited. Although no one is in the room with the patient, each person is monitored by closed television and open intercom systems. If the person becomes distressed during an individual treatment, the person can tell the radiation technician immediately and the therapy will be stopped. This is especially helpful for children to know who are receiving treatment.

INTERNAL RADIATION. Internal radiation therapy consists of various radioactive substances and application techniques to treat cancers directly inside the body rather than from the outside. There are three categories of internal radiation treatments: (1) systemic, (2) interstitial, and (3) intracavitary. Systemic therapy can be administered either orally or intravenously. A radioactive chemical is given to the patient and the chemical enters the person's bloodstream and has a preference for a particular place in the body. For example, radioactive iodine (I^{131}) is used to treat hyperthyroidism or certain kinds of thyroid cancer. The iodine travels to the thyroid gland, and in some cases of thyroid cancer it is possible for the radioactive iodine to destroy the gland and the cancer along with it.

Interstitial therapy consists of the placement of an applicator directly into the cancer where localized radiation is administered to the cancer cells with very little radiation reaching healthy tissues. For example, long thin needlelike containers filled with a radioactive substance such as radium, cobalt, iridium, or gold can be inserted directly into the cancer. The technique is especially useful for cancers in the mouth or neck where the tumor is surgically inaccessible or where surgery would be too extensive to warrant the disfigurement associated with it.

Intracavitary therapy is the placement of a radioactive substance into a body cavity such as the chest, abdomen, or vagina. One of the most common forms used is for the treatment of cancer of the cervix, usually with radium or cesium.

GOALS OF RADIATION. It is not uncommon for people to be extremely frightened when the physician suggests their primary treatment be radiation therapy. In the past, large numbers of patients were treated with radiation in the hope that it would extend their life or ease their discomfort. Shortly thereafter, they would die as a result of their disease, but many related their premature death to the treatment. Today, radiation therapy is recognized as a primary mode of treatment for some cancers and as an important adjuvant therapy for others. It also remains an important palliative therapy for cancers that are no longer curable.

CURE. There are at least four considerations that must be taken into account to determine if radiation is to be the physician's first-line defense against the cancer or whether it is to be used as a secondary attack in conjunction with other treatments. First, the radiotherapist must know what type of cancer the person has, whether it is sensitive to radiation, and its expected pattern of spread. Some cancers are more radiosensitive than others. Second, the physician needs to know where the cancer is located and its dimensions. Some cancers may be located in an area that is difficult to reach surgically without destroying important surrounding tissues, in which case radiation may be a more effective treatment. Third, the physician must know what volume of the body needs to be treated. In radiation therapy, it is usually wise to include a margin of healthy tissue around the cancer to be assured of eliminating or controlling the growth. If the volume of cancer is too large, a systemic treatment such as chemotherapy would be more appropriate. And, four, the physician needs to know what normal structures are located adjacent to the cancer. Radiation therapy destroys cancer cells *and* normal cells. Therapeutic doses of radiation usually do not kill cells immediately, but rather they work by damaging the cells so they are unable to proliferate. This process occurs for all cells within the radiation field; therefore, the physician wants to limit the number of normal cells affected, especially if major structures are involved such as the spinal cord. Radiation therapy used to cure the person's cancer is recommended because it has been proven to destroy cancers in a localized area of the body. It may be used in combination with surgery preoperatively since radiation can shrink the cancer and make it surgically resectable or it can reduce the spread by destroying the peripheral cells of the cancer. It has also been used in combination with surgery postoperatively as a prophylactic measure such as in the case of breast cancer.

PALLIATION. Palliative radiation therapy is given primarily to relieve distressing symptoms and prevent complications. When the goal of therapy is palliation, the patient may have widespread disease, but have a localized area in the body that has become bothersome, such as an active cancer that has spread to the head of the femur (see Figure 22.3). Radiation therapy to this area will destroy the cancer in the bone, relieve the person's pain, and allow the bone to bear more weight so that the person can continue to walk.

RADIATION REACTIONS. Reactions from radiation therapy can be systemic or localized. Local reactions depend on the area of the body

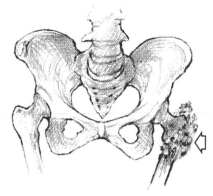

figure 22.3.
a secondary cancer metastasized to the head of the left femur from a primary breast cancer

being treated and usually are associated with a disturbance of function of that body part. A local reaction is called a side effect. For example, a person with cancer of the neck who is receiving daily radiation treatments will develop the side effects of a sore throat and have difficulty in swallowing. She subsequently will have difficulty in eating solid foods because the throat is included in the treatment field for neck cancers. These side effects are temporary and will gradually subside after the treatments are finished. Often patients are unaware that the side effects are actually brought about by the therapy and can become depressed because they think their cancer is becoming worse as a result of the increased symptoms.

A particularly bothersome side effect to women may be a local skin reaction at the site of the therapy. The characteristic skin reaction is called erythema (reddening of the skin). Erythema usually occurs after the second week of treatment and the reaction may be acute or chronic. An acute reaction occurs when a person has received a large dose of radiation in a short time. Often, sweat glands are affected and may be permanently destroyed. The person loses her hair and it may or may not grow back. When the tissues heal, there is usually a permanent discoloration of the skin that resembles a suntan. The skin area may itch and remain flaky for several weeks. A medicated ointment can be applied to the skin to relieve these symptoms.

Systemic reactions can affect the entire body, and they can be characterized as a general change in the body, such as malaise, fatigue, anorexia (lack of appetite), or depression. Patients report that they have little energy to do the things that they would like while they are on treatment, and they find that they are resting at unexpected times. This need for rest frustrates many people. Not all patients experience systemic reactions, and it is not clear why some people have a reaction and others do not. Patients with an optimistic attitude regarding the effects of their treatment seem to manage the experience better than do patients with a negative outlook.

Extensive and prolonged radiation treatments to areas in the body that include a large amount of bone can cause reactions that warrant special monitoring by the physician or nurse. Radiation treatments to the bone suppress the bone marrow and the production of cells that protect patients against infection (leukocyctes) and bleeding (platelets). Patients need to be taught the signs and symptoms of these reactions so that complications can be prevented rather than becoming a crisis.

chemotherapy

Chemotherapy technically is all drug therapy, but it is a term used increasingly only for cancer drug therapy. Drugs have been used to treat cancers since the time of the ancient Egyptians, when arsenical ointments were applied to skin lesions. The drugs used today be-

gan with mustard gas, a "poison gas" used during World War I. This gas caused suffering and death for thousands of soldiers. During World War II, large quantities of gas were shipped to Europe for possible use against the Germans. During one of the shipments, a ship was sunk. Victims who survived the sinking later died, and autopsies revealed that the gas had severely damaged their bone marrow and lymphatic systems, the tissues that form and harbor white blood cells. The potential usefulness of this agent against cancers that involve a proliferation of leukocytes was recognized. The discovery led to the development of the mustard-gas derivative nitrogen mustard, which became one of the first agents for treating cancers no longer considered curable.

Initially, its use was determined by trial and error for people with cancer, but this practice is no longer allowed. Today, a drug's use is dictated by its effects on animals. No cancer drug may be used for humans that has not been tested on animals first. The tests are usually performed on mice under specified conditions.

The treatment of cancer with drugs is not an exact science, nor can it be until the cause of individual cancers can be identified. Some people feel that a single drug in the future will cure cancer, but this notion is unrealistic because cancer is not a single disease but hundreds. In other words, no single substance can be effective for all manifestations of cancers. The state of the art and science of chemotherapy are relatively undeveloped and certainly far from definitive.

Treatment of a specific cancer by chemotherapy is indicated when the cancer is not confined to a single area or organ of the body. The control of the cancer requires a systemic treatment, which means that the whole body is treated. Chemotherapy is administered to the person with cancer in pill form taken orally or by an injection or infusion into the bloodstream. A single drug or combination of drugs may be given. Usually, the drugs can be taken only in limited doses, since they produce undesirable and potentially harmful side effects if the effects of the drug are not carefully monitored. When reactions are expected, the patient may be admitted to the hospital and may receive the chemotherapy under controlled conditions, such as in the treatment of advanced Hodgkin's disease where the primary cancer is not confined to a single area or region of the body (see Figure 22.4). The patient can spend one or two nights in the hospital, receive her chemotherapy and have limited side effects, since they can be managed with other medications such as antinausea

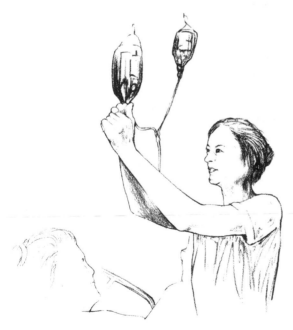

figure 22.4.
woman hospitalized overnight to receive her chemotherapy intravenously

drugs. With this approach, bone marrow depression is not severe and the need for blood replacements and antibiotics is lessened.

The purpose of chemotherapy is to do the maximum amount of damage to the cancer cells with a minimum amount of harm to the patient. Researchers have shown that a person has the greatest likelihood of cure when the number of malignant cells present is smallest. From a biological perspective, this poses a problem because most early cancers are not large enough to find with the present methods of detection. Therefore, it is likely that many patients with an apparent local tumor at the time of diagnosis have formed secondary micro-metastases in other parts of the body. These patients are ideal candidates for adjuvant chemotherapy. The purpose is to increase the person's chance of a cure when the risk of recurrence is high. The best results have been obtained by using full-dose intensive chemotherapy simultaneously with or immediately following surgery or radiation. This approach is frequently used for breast cancer.

In the presence of known metastasis of solid tumors, drugs are considered effective if they produce a reduction in disease of 20 percent or more when given as a single drug. At present, several drugs are usually given together since the response rate can often be improved by combining drugs (Price & Hill, 1978, pp. 265–276).

LIMITATIONS. The use of chemotherapy is limited by the drug's decreased effectiveness over time and its toxicity. Drugs gradually lose their effectiveness because of the body's increasing ability to resist them. In that event, another drug may be tried. Chemotherapy attacks both cancer and healthy cells. The toxic reactions may be extremely unpleasant. The normal cells most vulnerable to destruction are those that grow and divide rapidly, such as cells of the hair follicles, the lining of the gastrointestinal tract, and the bone marrow where blood cells are produced. Common symptoms reported are temporary loss of hair, painful sores in the mouth, nausea, vomiting, and diarrhea. Since the drugs can cause a decreasing supply of crucial blood cells, patients may become anemic, have a reduced ability to form blood clots, and be more prone to develop infection. Because of these side effects, patients need regular blood tests to be sure that their blood cells do not fall to dangerously low levels. There are many nursing care measures for lessening the side effects of these drugs. Patients need an ongoing relationship with their health care providers and should be encouraged to share their reactions and experiences so that appropriate interventions can reduce the side effects. It may be necessary for the physician to stop treatment if the side effects become too disturbing and unpleasant. Once the reactions have subsided, treatments can be instituted again.

Immunotherapy

In addition to the three major treatment approaches to cancer management, immunotherapy is sometimes used. Immunotherapy is the treatment of cancer by stimulating the body's own defense mechanism against the disease. It dates back to ancient times when it was used in India and China to treat smallpox. Live smallpox virus derived from pustules was injected at full strength into people free of the disease in an effort to keep them from getting it. Consequently, the shots caused as much disease as they prevented, but the curative potential was recognized.

Immunotherapy is not a conventional form of cancer treatment, but is the subject of intensive research at major medical centers. It is usually administered as an adjunct to surgery, radiation, or chemotherapy. The treatment is recommended after the bulk of the cancer cells have been removed or destroyed. Reduction of the tumor size allows the immune response maximal expression. Thus far, the positive results obtained from the use of immunotherapy have been limited. A major advance has been that patients with acute myelogenous leukemia have had the natural history of the disease altered by applying immunotherapy during remission; the length of their survival has been extended.

role of research in cancer treatment

Efforts are continually being made through research to increase a person's chances of survival by various treatments used alone or in combination. Individuals who qualify and are selected to participate in research studies to test the effects of treatment protocols must be informed by the physician of what is to be done, what the alternative treatments are, and what side effects will result from participating in the treatment. Patients who agree to participate must sign a consent form and a copy must become a permanent part of their medical record. It is important that people who decide to participate in a research protocol understand that they can stop treatment at any time without jeopardizing their right to have medical care that is available to the general public.

Research plays a major role in the future management of cancer. It is being done not only on the effects of new and combined treatments, but also on understanding the causes of cancers at the cellular level and the discovery of new technological advances to aid in early diagnosis and prevention.

cancer as a chronic illness

Cancer is often a chronic illness both because of the length of its physical course and because of its impact on the individual and family involved. Chronic illness poses particular problems of daily living with which individuals and families cope in differing ways and with differing degrees of success. Individual and family adaptation to the changes imposed by cancer takes time, energy, courage, and caring. Personal accounts of those who have learned to live with cancer's ups and downs give credence to the observations of health professionals that many families come through the illness experience with increased strength and personal growth.

For those people who would like to read about the personal accounts of persons with cancer, the following books are recommended:

Kohn, J. B., & Kohn, W. K. *The widower.* Boston: Beacon Press, 1978.

Kushner, R. *Breast cancer: A personal history and an investigative report.* New York: Harcourt, 1975.

Lee, L. *Walking through the fire.* New York: Dutton, 1977.

Parker, J. H., & Parker, R. B. *Three weeks in spring.* New York: Berkeley, 1978.

West, J. *The woman said yes.* New York: Harcourt, 1976.

recommendations

Most women sometime during their lifetimes will either develop cancer themselves or know someone with cancer. In either event, people with the disease or those who come in contact with them may feel frightened, ashamed, awkward, isolated, and/or unsupported. Following are some general guidelines that may be useful in helping people to manage during these times.

If you think you have cancer:

1. See a physician. If your concerns are not heard, find a physician who will hear what you have to say and what you want done about it.
2. Ask questions about various treatment choices. Try to understand why the treatment recommended is best for you.
3. Obtain a second opinion, especially if a treatment choice involves major irreversible changes in your life.
4. Try not to make a rash decision. Weigh care-

fully the consequences of treatment alternatives. Be clear on the treatment effects and what consequences are reversible and what are irreversible.

If you know someone with cancer:

1. Try not to treat the person in a way different from that before the diagnosis. People with cancer do not want to infer from other people's behavior that they are different. Generally, because people do not know how to behave, they convey a range of behaviors that are awkward and unintentional, such as pity and avoidance.
2. Inquire about the person's welfare, but do not ask questions that require a lot of detail about the person's physical condition. It is difficult for the ill person and family members to handle numerous inquiries and repeat the same answers a number of times.
3. Offer help to the person by assisting with concrete tasks such as shopping, meal prepa-

ration, lawn care, pickup of medications, or transportation.

4. Limit the amount of direct contacts with the ill person if that individual has limited energy to interact with you. If you want to be with the person, learn to be comfortable being there without talking.

5. Inquire about the person's family. Often, family members need an opportunity to express their feelings and concerns to someone who will listen; but do not pry.

6. Try not to react to the person and their family's concerns, but listen. Many times people need to share their feelings and frustrations with someone, and yet they do not want anything done about the situation.

7. Validate with the person what you are feeling, especially if you feel the person is becoming more distant from you. Often, extensive treatments cause changes in a person that neither individual may be aware of. A diagnosis of cancer is a very important time for people to share feelings, thoughts, and parts of themselves with one another.

8. If the person needs help, encourage her to call the American Cancer Society or the Cancer Information Line in your Community.

Burkhalter, P. K. Theories of causation, in P. Burkhalter & D. Donley (Eds.), *Dynamics of oncology nursing.* New York: McGraw-Hill, 1978.

Caplan, G. An approach to the study of family mental health. *U. S. Public Health Reports,* 1956, *71,*10

Feder, S. Psychological considerations in the care of patients with cancer, *Annals New York Academy of Sciences, 1966, 125,* 1020–1027.

Price, L. A., & Hill, B. T. The role of chemotherapy. In R. Tiffany (Ed.), *Oncology for nurses and health care professionals.* London: Allen & Unwin, 1978.

Silverberg, E. Cancer statistics, 1980. *Ca–A Cancer Journal for Clinicians,* January/February, 1980, *30,* 23–38.

White, H. Surgical oncology, in R. Tiffany (Ed.), *Oncology for nurses and health care professionals.* London: Allen & Unwin, 1978.

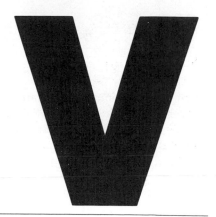

GAIL HONGLADAROM, R.N., Ph.D.

HEALTH RESOURCES

Informed women, interested in their health status, are probably the best health resource. Unless we have information, interest, and motivation, the finest clinics, hospitals, and physicians cannot give us wellness. How can we promote our own health? In this final section, you will discover how and why we, ourselves, are vital to achieving and maintaining our own health state.

This book began with encouraging women to reorient their thinking toward managing their own health. The other chapters provide many of the "how to" options for women's health and are given to the reader from the unifying perspective of self-care and self-help. It is very important for women to understand that self-care and self-health interest should not compromise the care they give themselves or obtain for themselves. Self-care in collaboration with health care from professionals can help women obtain the best possible health outcomes. Understanding ourselves, knowing when it is necessary to be assertive or aggressive, and also understanding when we might want to examine these feelings with a therapist are essential. Self-examination of our bodies is as important as examining our feelings, and breast self-exam should be a routine part of our lives to protect our longevity.

Many programs—governmental and community-sponsored—promote and try to maintain women's health. They do little good if we do not know about them or know how to use them properly. We must assess the power we have to change not only our own health status, but the health status of our families, friends, and community. Many women have never considered the positive attributes of power; many bemoan their "powerlessness." Women need to understand that power can be a positive force for their health and their lives. We can change the prospects for our health, and through new knowledge, new self-care practices, and self-awareness, we can assure positive health prospects for our future.

CATHERINE M. NORRIS, R.N., ED. D.

women and the self-care movement

Health professionals, in their theories of care, practice of care, research about care, and in their tremendous impact on public policy, have assumed that the only resource for health care is professional service controlled by professionals. But more and more people are challenging this paternalistic, authoritarian, self-serving concept. People are beginning to think of themselves as reliable sources for primary health care. The vast potential of health expertise that exists in individuals, mothers, and families can no longer be ignored. Nor can a person's prerogative to increase her technical capability and her right to full participation in her own health care be ignored. The potential health effect for millions of women on the health of our people is mindboggling to contemplate.

Almost any woman in the community today knows more about health, disease, and medical care than the average physician did at the turn of the century. She is demanding recognition as a primary health caretaker, independent of or in some kind of partnership with professionals, and if this does not occur, she may choose to function independently of the health care system. Women, men, husbands, wives, and families are beginning to define their rights for developing their own definitions of health, their own priorities, and their own options. They want to develop their own abilities for living the good and healthful life, for preventing and managing disease and dis-ease, for assessing and treating health and illness problems. They want an open health care system that they are free to use and leave.

293

They do not want to be labeled neurotic or uncooperative for not using the single route through a closed system. This is the essence of the self-care movement—control, responsibility, freedom, increasing options—improving the quality of life.

history of self-care

People have always provided health care. Family members have cared for themselves and each other, and there were folk and granny caretakers to call upon in most communities. But mothers have been the basic health providers throughout the history of the civilized world. Today, mothers still treat poison ivy, upper respiratory infections, fever, diarrhea, vomiting, headache, blisters, boils, warts, backaches, sore feet, constipation, indigestion, and earaches, to name a few. They dispense pain remedies, cough medicines, nose drops, suppositories, cathartics, vitamins, sleep medications, soaks, enemas, and other treatments based on their own knowledge, folk remedies, or a neighbor's advice. People have always "doctored" themselves.

Self-care has a literature that is more than 100 years old, and most old cookbooks provided self-care information. Pioneer housewives also kept diaries or some kind of household account book and recorded how they treated illness—things that seemed to help—as well as the discovery and use of new herbs. By placing treatment and cure information in cookbooks, the mandate for health care was placed squarely on women's shoulders. In the *White House Cookbook* published in 1901, there are remedies for boils, ringworm, pain with teething, bad breath, pimples, diarrhea, constipation, fever, weak stomach, chills, diphtheria, flatulence, growing pains, foot arch pain, toothache, earache, stings, croup, hemorrhage, asthma, prevention of colds, and antidotes for poisons. Recipes for treatments include broths, teas, gruels, puddings, poultices, cordials, soaks, and cough syrups. In the 1940s, when "anxiety" finally reached the United States from Europe, there was a significant increase in mental health self-care books. In this same period, there was an increasing number of books on how to sleep and what to eat.

With the advent of early diagnosis, elective surgery, scientific pharmacotherapy, and complex technology, medical science took and society gave away much of the monitoring and self-care that people had performed. The definition of disease remained unchanged, but people's perception of their own competence in wellness and illness care was undermined. Freedom and control were given to others.

In the 1960s, people were often perplexed and amused by youth's commitment to natural foods, folk remedies, herb teas, *Good Earth* catalogues, and home delivery of babies. A basketful of plastic vaginal instruments, marked 35 cents each in a health food store, produced quite a jolt about the extent of the self-care movement. Youth was portraying disillusionment and pessimism with the medical establishment. Today, many people and some professionals are ready for change in the health care delivery system. Various fronts are moving to regain control and freedom of choice in health matters. Where women have become accustomed to being cared for, health professionals in many instances are ready to help them take responsibility for their health care. Where women's confidence is so undermined that they belong to the

group called the "worried well," the task may be difficult.

one perspective of the self-care movement

If revolution means vigorous dissent, refusal to accept, and radical change, the self-care movement is a revolution. It began as an antiprofessional movement emphasizing self-care, caring for each other within the commune, family, or neighborhood, employing indigenous health care workers and using volunteers. Care was often based on knowledge from a variety of written materials and old remedies or common sense ideas about health care. The most important part of the revolution was changing the focus from illness care to health care. Diet, including health-promoting herbs, tonic teas, natural foods, activity, and emotional serenity had high priority. Traditional structures, formalities, and systematization were avoided and replaced by present-oriented, informal, interpersonal networks. Often storefront centers, runaway houses, and drug centers kept no records. Youths examined themselves and each other, fathers or non-nurse midwives delivered babies, gurus taught relaxation techniques, and lay volunteers talked down people on bad drug trips.

In addition to seeming antiprofessional, the movement appeared anti-intellectual. The emphasis was on being human, warm, respecting, and giving. But whether this was anti-intellectual or a reaction to extreme materialism, mechanistic practices, and inhuman treatment needs consideration. Only recently has the revolution provided the perspective we need to look at the health care delivery system and to locate the function and responsibility of the individual.

what is self-care?

Self-care has come to mean those processes that permit people and families to take initiative, to take responsibility, and to function effectively in developing their own potential for health. This includes preventing illness and detecting, assessing, or treating deviations from health. At the federal level, this movement is generally referred to as the health education or patient education movement, but the concept of self-care is preferred because it stresses people being responsible for their own health. Health education and patient education also suggest that someone is going to develop a program to control the education of patients. This systematization or bureaucratization appears to have been one area of client-professional conflict.

Although professionals since about the 1960s have given clients more power in administering health care and in determining to some degree who should give health care, no one previously challenged the power of clinical practice. To do self-care women (and men) will have to challenge this power. To become educated to do what professionals claim as their prerogatives in maintaining health and treating illness is quite a change in the concept of health care. Already, professionals writing about health and patient education programs emphasize organization for the activities (federal, health care system, hospital). Compliance is of great concern. There is concern that some people are going to go off "half-cocked."

There is concern about imposing sanctions on people who do not learn to do their own care, who do not practice health, and who use up more than their share of the health resources. While recognizing the need for organization and program, the basic premises of self-care must be formulated with client consensus.

why self-care?

Self-care appears to be an idea whose time has come, and many forces have contributed to this rapidly growing movement: (1) wide dissatisfaction with health and medical care; (2) personal need to manage one's own health care; and (3) prohibitive costs of health care. Scientists say that putting more money into health care will not improve the nation's health to an appreciable extent. Personal behavior, genetics, and environment are the keys to health promotion and disease reduction.

Self-care is a more viable option now that we are moving away from an acute to a chronic disease orientation. Medicalizing many nonphysical, social, educational, and formerly criminal problems has put physi-

cians into the trap of trying to be all things to all people. Physicians cannot do all the divorce, sex, rape, and family planning care and counseling. They cannot treat all criminals or all people with learning problems. If medicine is to do its job, solutions to many recently medicalized problems must come back to the people. The civil rights movement has given impetus to the people's right to know and to control their own bodies. Blue Cross-Blue Shield has published a white paper endorsing patient education. Coverage for costs of self-care may not be far behind. At the federal level, there is interest in reimbursing for the costs of patient education. Where there is money, programs develop.

activity related to self-care

In 1974, the Bureau of Health Education was established at the Center for Disease Control in Atlanta. Even though all Public Health Service agencies have educational responsibilities, health education has not been any agency's primary concern. The main function of the bureau is to identify ideas, programs, and models that would be useful to other people and applicable to other problems. The Bureau contracted with the National Health Council to conduct a study to determine the

need for a national health center in the private sector. The American Hospital Association received a contract to survey hospital activity in the area of patient education. The Bureau will build, test, and document health education models. It will also attempt to foster communication among the professions involved in health education.

The National Center for Health Education, founded at about the same time that the Bureau was established, is a private organization with plans to develop national strategies to carry out the advocacy function for the discipline, to improve the discipline through research, and to provide consultation or other assistance to the health field. Priorities in order of importance are health education in industry, interpretation of the Health Planning and Health Resources Development Act (P.L.93–641) to health education programs and communities, and encouragement of patient education supported by third-party payers.

The American Hospital Association in 1975 began its survey of 5,770 member hospitals' inpatient education programs. A preliminary report indicated that nurses are the most frequent participants in patient education programs. In August 1975, 29 scholars met in Copenhagen to give particular and exclusive attention to the role of individuals and families in the primary health care process.

The National Health Information and Promotion Act of 1976, signed into law as Title I of P.L. 94–317, is significant for the future of "health information, health promotion, health preventive services and education." The three volume "Little Report" (1976) was presented to HEW's Assistant Secretary for Planning and Education/Health. This report addresses three issues—evaluation studies and impact data, self-care, and system utilization. The third volume also includes recommendations for federal action.

When Nelson Rockefeller was chairman of the commission on Critical Choices for Americans, he invited Dr. John Knowles to organize a group to study problems of health care. The report of this group (Knowles, 1977) puts considerable emphasis on individual responsibility for health care.

At least 16 universities now offer formal programs in consumer health education. This is in addition to self-care courses offered under the aegis of continuing education. One of the best-known programs is sponsored by Georgetown University, entitled the "Activated Patient Program," operated in Reston, Virginia, with the goal of teaching people basic skills in preventive care.

Self-care has grown rapidly and at the present time, it is hard to see the whole or even all the parts. Let us take a look at its seven areas of activity.

monitoring, assessing, diagnosing

Probably the oldest means of self-care has to do with monitoring, assessing, and diagnosing health and illness in self and others. These activities include listening and talking, seeing, smelling, and feeling. Instruments have come into general use slowly. Only recently has the public begun to use the sphygomomanometer (blood pressure apparatus) along with the clinical thermometer and watch with a second hand. Listening to one's self has, to some extent, replaced the annual physical. Breast self-examination and monitoring for the seven warning signs of cancer continue to receive emphasis.

Mothers and others diagnose minor illnesses, especially communicable diseases. Although they usually do not make formal diagnoses, they collect and analyze data and make a determination about the severity of the illness. We are only at the beginning of what is possible in this area. Lewis (1974) reports a study in which elementary school children were able to decide when they needed care, could help decide what their health problems were, and what should be done about them. Women are enrolled in increasing numbers in similar courses all across the country and, as a result, are more active participants in their self-care.

Physicians writing newspaper columns and magazine articles are telling people how to make differential diagnoses; for example, the difference between an upper respiratory infection and an allergy. They identify the side effects of drugs and advise people to question their physicians. They place half the responsibility on the patients to ask critical questions. "Women's Health—Questions and Answers" may soon be seen in some of the major newspapers, and these columns will be written by women's health consultants.

Televison is moving into health education and self-care. Physicians discuss health-related topics from care of dandruff to the management of kidney dialysis at home. Program names include "House Call," "Feeling Fine," and "Ounce of Prevention." Dr. Art Ulean is known to "Today" (NBC) viewers across the nation. Nurses also conduct these kinds of programs in some local areas. Women could help these women-directed programs get into their local programming by writing to their television stations.

A large self-care literature is developing. Some of it is gimmicky, but most of it is written with the serious assumption that people will be doing careful assessments and accurate monitoring of their health status, followed by effective intervention. *Go To Health* (Savitz, 1976) and the *Well Body Book* (Samuels and Bennett, 1973) describe how to do self-health examination, but in quite different ways. *Symptoms: The Complete Home Medical Encyclopedia* (Miller, 1976) is more expensive and is written for the educated lay reader. It deals, in ways that promote intelligent self-care, with many symptoms and normal changes throughout the life cycle. Frank and Frank's (1972) *The People's Handbook of Medical Care* is written at less depth, more cautiously, and more from a medical perspective, but may be a place for beginners in self-

care. *The People's Pharmacy: A Guide to Prescription Drugs, Home Remedies and Over-the-Counter Medications* (Graedon, 1976) should be in everyone's home whether or not they are doing self-care. At a time when the intelligent choice of drugs is almost impossible, this is an invaluable guide. It is timely that two reference libraries for medical consumers have been opened in New York City by the Center for Medical Consumers and Health Care Information. A Health Care Book Club is now offering charter memberships.

supporting life processes

Some of the activities that support life processes are built into the habits we learn while growing up. The routines of teeth-brushing, handwashing, using Kleenex, bathing, regular meals, sleep patterns, activity preferences, elimination, and play are ritualistic, done without much thought or planning, because they have become habitual. With habituation comes commitment—a feeling one must act in certain ways, that there is no choice. Most parents want to be good parents so this avenue to self-care may have high payoff and may need to be expanded. The more healthy practices that can be ritualized to become ingrained habits, the better self-care will be. For example, both salt and sugar reduction in children's diets could be ritualized.

Self-care in growth and development means monitoring and assessing maturational processes and progress toward the potential for wellness. It means acting in ways that motivate, support, and provide resources or experiences that move people in the direction of positive health. Mothers have become more sophisticated in doing this for their children. Pediatric nurse practitioners, family nurse practitioners, and school nurse practitioners work with mothers and families toward these ends. Adults are concerned about growth, too. Recent developments in the women's movement have fostered and greatly changed the ways that women think about their life-long potential for health. The search for freedom, control of one's body, relief from boredom or loneliness, and the search for peace and tranquility or self-understanding has promoted much self-care activity.

therapeutic and corrective self-care

People treat themselves and others for hundreds of discomforts and minor illnesses. But people with hemophilia, metastatic cancer, and end-stage renal disease are doing self-care, too. Their self-therapy is not a poor substitute for medicine, but, for them, it is more therapeutically successful and more satisfying. The demedicalization of pregnancy and delivery is also taking place on a small scale for a very satisfied clientele.

People are asking for the right to die on their terms, particularly the horribly maimed and the terminally ill. In a concept of self-care, this becomes a reasonable option. We are only at the beginning of looking at self-care in this area, but people want the information upon which to base decision-making and intervention. Self-care has the potential to make informed technicians out of many, if not most, people.

prevention of disease and maladjustment states

Women are generally aware that they will live longer if they keep themselves at low risk for cardiovascular disease, emphysema, diabetes, and cancer. But what women do not generally know is that early life experience and life-style

choices are additive. The effect of a child eating a poor diet cannot be eliminated by eating an adequate diet later on. Scars from malnutrition and other organ changes caused by malnutrition persist throughout life. Stress in early life may not be erased by counseling or therapy years later. In elementary and high schools, our future hypertension patients are being identified. And while some organs like the lungs have considerable recuperative powers, full function never returns. We have data about the later effects of drug taking in the case of dicthylstilbesteral and amphetamines, but not in the use of the "pill" and a myriad of other drugs. Women for themselves and women as mothers need to keep informed and to share the best information they can get. This does not mean that one takes personal blame or chides one's children with threats of what will happen if! Women should learn and mothers should teach their children to select experiences that in most instances are useful and with the knowledge that these useful experiences have prestige and are enjoyable. Even learning self-control has tremendous status attached as well as satisfaction.

Women want to know about aging, and they want to know if they must become senile or whether senility can be prevented. People of all ages want to know how to be successful interpersonally, how to be productive, how to cope with stress, particularly desertion, failure, and grief. In terms of aging, women are considered to be middle-aged and old before men. At a national invitational conference of endocrinologists (in other words, a prestigious, mostly male group), middle age for women was defined as 35 to 55, and for men, 55 to 65 years of age!

Women live longer than men and so must face the grief and loneliness of widowhood much more frequently. Women are deserted, in a sense, by their children as they leave home. This leaves women as a group searching for new ways to be creative and productive. As divorce becomes more frequent, more women find themselves alone with or without children. All of these situations—aging, grief, loneliness, loss, and desertion—are fraught with pathological outcomes of depression, chronic illness, and personality disorganization unless there is a good interpersonal support system and opportunities for growth. We also need a coalition of women to redefine healthy living for women, including definitions of the ages of women. Senior citizen groups, women's commissions, church groups, industrial health programs, and universities are moving to deal with some of these problems, and women can enter the movement through membership in one of these groups.

Most public schools offer health and fitness courses, but they are often boring to the students. Courses in self-care are not offered and so responsibility is placed on the students and parents. Student progress is not monitored or evaluated in terms of either health practice or progress. Exhortation, advice, and simplistic explanation often take the place of scientific knowledge. Along with lack of evaluation of practice and progress, there is no testing of knowledge.

specifying health needs and care requirements

The validity of one's perception of one's own needs was a lesson of the 1960s when youth brought the health establishment to task. Not only did a single norm give way to a variety of norms, but each individual's right to self-definition was established. The widest possible options based on inner direction were demanded. Conforming to health professional and other closed-system choices was rejected by many. Once the validity of personal needs assessment is accepted, it follows that treatment as defined by professionals will be questioned. Resources requesting client input would be expected to evolve. Definitions of optimum health for a particular person, options selected, and risks taken would be negotiated rather than decreed. Some nurses are doing this kind of care, and most professional nurses are ready to do it.

Using this concept, the whole health care system must be open. It must be open not only to self-care, but must open up opportunities for new caretakers and new roles for old caretakers. We need to allow or invite nurses, gurus, podiatrists, hypnotists, ministers, acupuncturists, and others to join the mainstream of health care to do what they can to promote self-health care. The old hierarchy must give way. Operating on the periphery of the system or outside it is not appropriate for those who have a contribution to make.

Health needs sound different when women list and describe them. They may not sound right at first to the professional, but with more women expressing them in this fashion the professionals will very likely overcome these semantic problems. It may be more effective to meet one's own health goals no matter how much this falls short of goals set by professionals than to meet only the goal of successful rebellion against professionals.

This aspect of self-care is also in its infancy, but is beginning to have more appeal, especially to women and youth. It also has appeal to the elderly who want to stay in their own homes. Many elderly women have self-care sessions in their retirement houses or settlements.

evaluating and monitoring
health care

It is becoming common practice for physicians who write medical advice columns to indicate that people have the right to reasons for treatment, the right to informed consent, the right to confidentiality, and the right to privacy. Mendelsohn, the "People's Doctor" writing in the *Tucson Daily Citizen*, said, "I am surprised that parents of any child placed on dilantin would not be informed in advance about the drug's obvious and common effects on the gums." In another column he warns about contraindications, precautions, adverse reactions, and dosage instructions for thorazine and compazine.

Minorities, especially minority women, are demanding better care. Women are asking that their complaints be considered seriously and fully investigated. The elderly are also demanding better care. They are not satisfied with a two- or three-minute visit for which a physician collects a sizeable fee from their Medicare insurance. They are asking for the help they need so that remaining in their homes is an option. Implicit in their criticism, complaints, and demands is the idea that peo-ple must learn how to better evaluate their own health care.

grass roots
or self-initiated health care

Some models of self-care are not open or not fully open to professionals. Some are operated as commercial or proprietary ventures, while some are operated and controlled by the clientele themselves. They include all levels of self-care, but are considered separately here because in most of these models primary therapeutic concepts include admitting that one has a health deficit and that someone with a similar problem can help. Intervention strategies include emotional support and those that have been helpful to the people involved. Professionals generally do not have large groups of people with the same health problems so they would not use these methods. Professionals also are not peers, and a peer as therapist may be a basic tenet of the program. Since programs like Weight Watchers and stop smoking groups have been quite successful, women might want to develop and study more group models in which the client is the therapist.

nurses and self-care

Disease prevention, health promotion, and the nation's health have had high priority beginning with Florence Nightingale. A woman literally invented these concepts to meet the needs she saw, and women, as nurses, have been at the forefront of health (not medical) care since the last century. Nurses originated the concept of self-care at the beginning of the twentieth century. Public health nursing built and refined its discipline on certain self-care concepts. Nursing was among the early professions to anticipate an ambulatory client future with clients fully responsible for much of their health care and fully participating in all aspects of their care. But as sick care developed in hospitals, priorities changed and professional nurses no longer had the freedom or the time to do patient education or teach self care.

Today, 1,250,000 women nurses have the opportunity to make health care really health care. The tasks involved are herculean. Work is required at several levels—political, health care policy, professional, and program development. Individual commitment and individual expertise need to be incorporated into women's thinking as they negotiate for their health. In most reports about patient education research, health educators direct the work of nurses and, in some cases, do health and self-care teaching (Little, 1976). Health educators are interning in nursing areas and learning such things as colostomy care, preoperative care, and postoperative care. Here is another instance of the "cookie dough" approach to nursing where emerging disciplines have cut out substantive areas of practice and developed them, leaving nursing with only the scraps between the cutouts. Nurses may have to confront laying claim to what is nursing. Nurses need to ask whether directing patient education and self-care programs ought to be a step on the promotional ladder for nurses or whether other disciplines should have these positions. The next few years may be critical for nurses as women in maintaining and articulating their scope of practice within the total field of the health disciplines. Today's health problems are solved by competing in the political area both for existence and for the right to contribute to health care programs.

Self-care will require a complete change of focus for the health care system and for society. Nurses, who for more than half a century have been in on the ground floor of self-care, are in a strategic and obvious position to help reorient the focus of health care delivery. Nurses can also work to make the health care system more open for more people. Women need to be free to enter, free to learn, free to use or reject what is offered, free to ask for help, free to have all information about themselves, and free to leave without derogation. This concept of nursing care includes patient advocacy. Nurses can support the inclusion of health care workers who have functioned on the periphery of the system or outside it altogether. This includes nurses themselves who need to be accepted as members of the team by both medicine and administration. The nurse practitioner movement has provided direct access to patients and greater accountability for care in only a few years' time, but there are many forces at work to maintain an elitist authoritarian framework for health as well as illness care.

Some professional schools have established departments of citizen education. These departments build close relationships with community groups, provide health education services, and test innovations in patient education practice. Some schools of nursing have the resources and are ideally suited to take the leadership in the self-care movement using this kind of model. Nurses using this model would have service areas they control. Practice could progress rapidly without the burden of sick care or the blocks encountered in the sick care model.

All health professionals need to change their concept of "patient." People must be seen as powerful, competent, responsible, and well motivated, rather than as weak, needy, unintelligent, and like bad irresponsible children. People, especially women, must be trusted to act in their own best interests. Nurses are ideally educated and situated for the job of placing the responsibility for health care where it belongs—on the people of this nation. Clients must also change their concept of professionals—nurses, not physicians, are self-care professionals.

There is a great shortage of health education and self-care literature for children. Knowles (1977) said, "Children tire of 'scrub your teeth,' 'don't eat that junk,' 'leave your dingy alone,' 'go to bed,' and 'get some exercise'." Mothers, teachers, and nurses who know growth and development as well as health needs and health risks for the various age groups could collaborate in preparing imaginative and exciting self-care materials and develop ways to test knowledge and changes in practice. Nurses, teachers, and mothers can become the school health care team.

In terms of method, health professionals need to stop "telling" and "preaching." Teachers of health care need to be experts in strategies for motivating, exploring, experiential learning, placing responsibility, facilitating, negotiating health care goals, practices or regimens, persuading, and rewarding successes. Nurses and teachers to some extent have already moved from the traditional dual model of care to a group model. Group models cost less and students learn as much from each other as they do from teachers. Community colleges have developed large group models. The largest group models needing dynamic programs include industrial workers, school children, and members of the women's movement. Nurses as women are prepared to teach and are in a strategic position to lead both in teaching methods and in developing group models so that women, as mothers and as workers, can learn to live the good life and to preserve the one life given to live.

Self-care can open an exciting vista for the future of health care. It provides not only vast new opportunities for improved health care, but a reaffirmation of life's goodness, realness, and worth. It offers new opportunities for women to collaborate and greater opportunities for meaningful function. If women do not take full membership in the self-care movement, it will be medicalized, formalized, and institutionalized into the existing pathological model of care.

Frank, A., and Frank, S. *The people's handbook of medical care.* New York: Vintage, 1972.

Graedon, Joe. *The people's pharmacy: A guide to prescription drugs, home remedies and over-the-counter medications.* New York: St. Martin's, 1976.

Knowles, John (Ed.), Doing better and feeing worse. *Daedalus: Journal of the American Academy of Arts and Sciences,* Winter 1977.

Lewis, M. A. Child-Initiated care. *American Journal of Nursing,* April 1974, 74, 652–655.

Little, A. D. *Appendix of project descriptions for a survey of consumer health programs.* Springfield, Va., U. S. Department of Commerce, National Technical Information Service, P. B., 1976, 251–774.

Little, A. D. *Executive summary: A survey of consumer health education programs.* Springfield, Va., U. S. Department of Commerce, National Technical Information Service, P. B. 1976, 251–773.

Miller, S. *Symptoms: The complete home medical encyclopedia.* New York: Crowell, 1976.

Samuels, M., and Bennett, H. *The well-body book.* New York, Random House, 1973.

Savitz, B., Ed. *Go to health.* New York: Dell, 1976.

DONNA M. MONIZ, R.N., M.N.

women and assertiveness

Assertiveness involves direct action aimed toward getting what you want. At the same time it respects the rights of others. Assertiveness means expressing feelings as you choose and defending your territory when it is attacked. It means all this without feeling anxious or guilty.

Assertiveness is more easily understood when compared to passivity and aggressiveness. Women have been taught to be passive, to put everyone's needs before their own. Passivity is giving in to the will of another, letting others make your choices and interpret your feelings for you (see Figure 24.1). Aggressiveness is another behavioral approach

to situations. Men are often permitted, even encouraged, to express aggression, while expression of aggression is suppressed in women. Aggression means going after what you want at another's expense. It involves transgressing the other's territory and depriving them of their rights.

Another behavioral style is a combination of passivity and aggressiveness. Passive-aggressive behavior appears to be giving in, while actually one is fighting back indirectly. It occurs when a person feels hostile and helpless at the same time. It is a sneaky, manipulative manner of doing things. A person who is passive-aggressive obstructs and fights by *not*

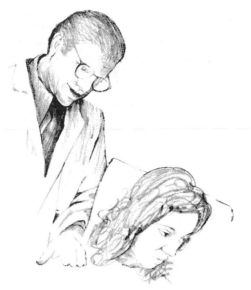

figure 24.1
physician talking with a passive woman about the diagnostic tests and treatments he has planned

doing. Often this was a woman's only way to deal with a domineering male.

A sample situation illustrates the various choices a woman has when coping with a particular problem. A woman is visiting her doctor for a gynecologic problem. She wishes to have a friend remain in the room with her during the examination. Both follow the medical assistant into the room, but the friend is asked to wait outside. An assertive woman would state that she wanted her friend to stay and possibly give a brief explanation of the reason for the request. A passive response would be to say nothing when the friend was asked to leave. An aggressive response might involve a loudly spoken objection and a hostile comment about the medical assistant. A passive-aggressive reaction would be initial submission and later expressing one's anger by not paying the physician's bill.

why a particular problem for women?

Women are not the only ones who can benefit from assertiveness lessons: both men and women exhibit all ranges of behavior. However, society's definition of a woman's role in modern American society has been a passive one. From birth, woman are socialized to defer to others as wives and mothers. In a marriage, the woman is expected to provide support and nurture to her husband and children by sacrificing herself. The woman's stereotyped role is so deeply ingrained that men and women are often unaware that they live out their parents' examples, even while consciously challenging traditional values (Bem, 1970).

Women throughout history have been con-sidered inferior to men in terms of power, intelligence, and ability to do certain types of work. Although this has been true for at least 2,000 years, there is reason to believe that some earlier societies were thoroughly matriarchal (Davis, 1971). It is unrealistic to expect women suddenly to become assertive in their adulthood when they have been taught for 20 years to subjugate their desires.

Assertiveness within the health care system is particularly challenging. First, the system is a hierarchical, male-dominated institution, with power derived from specialized knowledge. Second, women comprise a large majority of the "patients" or consumers of health care. Women seek services for birth control and childbearing in addition to the illnesses and injuries that bring both men and women to health care providers (Frankfort, 1972). Women are also the majority of those treated by mental health facilities (Chesler, 1972).

Although the majority of health care providers are women, they are concentrated at the least powerful levels of the system; male doctors are in control. These factors combine to make women feel like helpless victims of the nonpatients paid to care for them.

why be assertive?

Assertive behavior helps people get what they want. More importantly, a woman and those with whom she has contact generally feel good about the assertive interactions. The goals themselves are as individual as each woman. However, the following is a list of rights for women consumers in the health care system. This list may help you clarify what you really want.

A woman has the right to:

1. Make decisions that affect her health.
2. Obtain the information necessary to choose among various alternatives.
3. Privacy and confidentiality.
4. Safe, dignified care regardless of ability to pay.
5. Maternity care that preserves the mother's control over the birth, while protecting the infant from harm.
6. Considerate, informed counseling about menopause.
7. Choose abortion or sterilization without the signature of her husband or the approval of a physician panel.
8. Sensitive care regardless of sexual preference.

There are other benefits to being assertive besides the specific goals achieved. A woman will experience a sense of power and competence in her personal world. She will gradually learn that she can control a great deal of what happens in her own life. And she can do

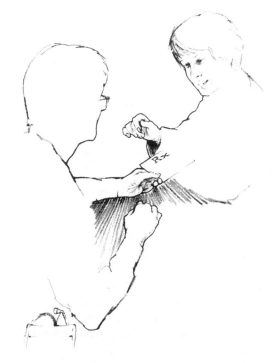

figure 24.2
an assertive woman asking her physician the purpose of the medication he has prescribed and the side effects she might expect

it without being mean and nasty or hurting people's feelings (see Figure 24.2).

Essentially, the advantage of assertive behavior is in improving the odds that one will succeed. But it also involves maintenance of self-respect so that a person feels good about herself whether she wins or loses a particular point. She stays in control and deals on an adult level without insulting others or saying things she will regret later. This is a result of planning and practicing.

Some people think of assertiveness in a superficial way. But it can be a key to making your life go the way you want. It can prevent hostility and violence because people have more effective substitutes and know how to use them.

One caution is in order. Spend some time contemplating what it is you really want or need. Often we think we want or need something that we really don't. Going after it assertively may succeed, but the result may not be satisfying. Ask yourself whether you are responding to the social pressure of friends. Are you playing out a role assigned in your childhood by your parents? Are you doing something just to rebel against them? Assertiveness is a tool that can be used in many situations, but it is more rewarding if what you get is what you truly want or need.

becoming assertive

How assertive are you already? Answer the questions below to find out how you are doing now. Perhaps some situations are easier for you to handle assertively than others. (You might assign number values to the type of situation, depending on how difficult it is for you to handle it.)

- Do you feel guilty when you ask for a change in clinic routine?
- Are you afraid to ask your doctor for a second opinion on a serious problem?
- Do you accept a prescription for medication when you don't know what it is?
- Do you submit to laboratory tests without an understanding of the reason for ordering them?
- Are you worried about taking up the "doctor's valuable time" with your questions?
- Do you give your child medications without finding out from the pharmacist what the side effects are?
- Are you afraid to ask for an estimate of how much a consultation or procedure will cost?

In assessing your own assertiveness, it helps a great deal to keep a journal or log each day. Note the situation, what you said or did, how you are feeling, and what you could have done differently. This can be a wonderful tool to increase self-knowledge.

One of the first steps in becoming assertive is to set goals for yourself. What do you want? It may be only to express an opinion and be heard. But before you speak or act, decide what you want. Try to separate the key issue in your mind from extraneous topics. Often the person with whom you are negotiating will use distraction as a means to keep you from getting your point across. Try to anticipate this. Also, plan your list in order of priority of what you want and try to plan strategies that will get you the thing you want most.

Once you have a clear idea of the issue at hand, use "I" statements to express yourself. Start sentences with "I want . . . ," "I think . . . ," "I feel . . ." rather than "you." This helps to avoid provoking defensiveness on the part of the other person. It signifies that you are taking responsibility for your own feelings. It also exercises your power as a person. The tone of voice and facial expression help convey the message, too. Your tone and expression should reveal self-confidence and firmness. A timid or hostile tone belies an assertive statement. Posture is equally important: sit or stand with your head up and face the person you are addressing. It also helps to look at the person's eyes while you talk. Eye contact makes a statement about your personal power. Often it is necessary to repeat yourself a number of times until you are heard.

To begin your behavior change, pick a situation in which your new behavior is likely to be successful. Practice what you will say in front of a mirror and with a supportive friend. Trying assertive behavior in a low-risk situation will encourage you to go on to more difficult ones.

The ultimate goal is to express your feelings spontaneously and honestly. Initially, however, you may do better with some role-playing in advance. Then pick an appropriate time to give your message. For example, you may choose to give your health care provider feedback in private rather than in front of other clients.

To better understand the suggested techniques, some examples of their application in health care situations are described.

One of the first problems for a woman with a health problem is to select a physician. Ideally this is done when you are feeling well. Then, if you get sick, you will have a physician whom you know and trust. You are in a stronger position to interview physicians and decide on one if you are feeling healthy and powerful. When you call for an appointment, expect to be asked what it is for; give a brief answer. Most clinics or physicians will charge for their time, so you will want to ask about that when you make the appointment. Of course, if you consult on a problem you will be charged for the advice, whether you are examined or not. You pay for the knowledge of health care providers as well as their technical skills.

Judging the clinical competence of a physician can be difficult. If a physician is "board-certified" in a specialty area, he or she has passed certain tests and educational requirements in that area. Usually it means the physician has kept up-to-date concerning new research in the field. Currently, nurse practitioners are also being certified at the national level. Completion of an approved educational program and a passing score on a national test are required for a nurse practitioner to be certified. Another way to evaluate the competence of a clinician is through friends or other health care providers.

Just as important as competence is manner. It is good to have someone you can talk to easily. You want to feel that your concerns are respected, your dignity preserved, and your freedom kept intact. You do not want to have the uncomfortable feeling that your life-style is being condemned by the people you are paying to take care of you. Your own feelings, when talking with the health care provider, are a good gauge of whether this is the right person for you.

The same guidelines apply when you go to a public clinic. The people who work there are paid to take care of you, even if you do not pay the bill directly. You can ask to see someone else in the clinic, although if you change often just to try different ones, you may be suspect. (Some clients change doctors frequently to try to obtain drugs.) A clinic patient has the same rights to quality health care as anyone else.

While you are talking with the practitioner, ask specific questions if you have them. For example, if you are a young woman going to a family doctor, you want to inquire whether she or he delivers babies. Thus, if you think you might become pregnant, you will have the option of going to the same person for your prenatal care. What about natural childbirth? If this interests you, be sure you find out how the physician feels. Ask about breast-feeding. If the physician thinks it is too much trouble, be suspicious. With birth control, is the physician open to a variety of methods or are all his or her clients on birth control pills?

In addition to seeking health care for themselves, women often obtain care for their children, elderly parents, or grandparents. For example, a divorced mother, who was providing most of the support for her four children, moved to a new town. She knew her five-year-old needed weekly allergy shots, but wanted to obtain them at a low price. Initially she went to a clinic that she knew through a friend provided quality care. She found which person in the clinic was responsible for billing. She told this person about her concern and asked directly how much the clinic would charge if she brought the medication with her. After the woman answered appropriate questions about her financial situation (in private), she was told that she would be billed at a special low rate. This mother acted assertively by: (1) stating her concern politely and directly, (2) maintaining eye contact, and (3) asking for what she wanted. She was successful in getting what her child needed and felt competent as a mother.

Another young woman had a grandmother in a nursing home. The institution was part of a chain that was not known for good staffing and high-quality care. The young woman became very upset when she saw that her grandmother was tied into her wheelchair and unable to get out. The older woman was very weak and not always aware of what she was doing. The granddaughter went to the registered nurse on duty and in a loud voice demanded to know why her grandmother was tied up, saying, "I've told them over and over not to do that. Besides being tied in, she has food all over her. Don't you ever wash her up?" She felt mean, but didn't know what else to do.

The young woman would have had better results if she had checked first to see if this was the most appropriate person with whom to discuss the matter. Frequently, in poorly staffed nursing homes, there are temporary nurses "covering" the unit. They have very little power except during the one shift. She could also have shared her concern quietly with the nurse and asked why this was done and whether there were any alternatives. She could have asked what the routines were for bathing, and then requested calmly, but firmly, that her grandmother be washed. If a situation like this recurs and initial requests fail, it is appropriate to speak to the director and/or consider moving the patient to a better home, if possible.

A single young nurse, new in town, needed a Pap test and a refill on her birth control pills. A male gynecologist was recommended by her coworkers. She made an appointment and arrived on time. After a 45-minute wait (with no apology or explanation) she was asked by the office nurse to come in. In the middle of a crowded waiting room, she was asked if she was taking the Pill. She flushed with embarassment, but said yes. The nurse then took her blood pressure. The woman asked what it was, but the nurse did not respond. The woman was angry but said nothing. She met the doctor in a gown sitting on the examination table. Without taking a proper history, he examined her. Without checking with a microscope, he diagnosed a vaginal infection. Without telling her that she would be very sick if she drank alcohol with the medication, he wrote a prescription. After she left, the young woman felt terrible. She was angry that the doctor and nurse were so insensitive and cursory in their procedures. She wished that she had complained about having been kept waiting. She also wished she had insisted on knowing her blood pressure and the reasons he had diagnosed an infection. She decided to write the physician a letter stating why she would never go to him again. Her letter was fair and complete without calling him names. After sending it she felt better. She rehearsed what she might do in a similar situation in the future. Gradually she felt less angry and more capable of coping with future health issues.

At best, assertive behavior will help you obtain the kind of health care you want and need. Using these techniques should result in more feelings of self-satisfaction and fewer feelings of anger and helplessness. If individual assertiveness is not enough, perhaps group actions can achieve the goal. An institution or private practitioner may change quickly when income is at stake.

Remember to practice initially with situations in which you have a good chance of success. Also, remember that the same techniques work outside health care situations; assertiveness can be useful in school, work, and personal relationships.

Bem, D. J. *Beliefs, attitudes and human affairs.* Belmont, Calif.: Brooks/Cole, 1970.

Chesler, P. *Women and madness.* New York: Avon, 1972.

Davis, E. G. *The first sex.* New York: Putnam, 1971.

Frankfort, E. *Vaginal politics.* New York: Quadrangle, 1972.

25

LAURA S. BROWN, Ph.D.

choosing a therapist

For many women in our society today, a "normal" life experience includes a period of time spent in counseling or psychotherapy. There are several possible explanations. Feminist theorists, including Pauline Bart and Phyllis Chesler, have pointed out that the feminine sex role, with its artificial constraints on women's feelings, behaviors, and self-definitions, has led women to experience chronic levels of helplessness, anger, frustration, and depression. Others have suggested that changes in sex roles since the early 1970s have created new stresses for which women were not prepared. Many women may also seek therapy or counseling to gain support and insight during times of life crises, such as parenthood, divorce, career change, illness, or widowhood.

Our culture has become quite therapy-oriented. The idea that a person "needs her head examined" and should be seen by a helping professional is a pervasive one. Before choosing therapy, women should consider the possibility that it is not needed. Self-help groups, counseling, spiritual approaches, and changes in diet or exercise patterns may all have the same outcome as what women want from therapy. Therapy or counseling is often the best choice in instances where there are serious and chronic changes in a person's emotional state. You don't have to be "crazy" to seek therapy. It can serve as a forum in which to examine the choices you have made in your life with the support and aid of another set of eyes and ears.

If you choose therapy, and for whatever reasons, you will probably feel a sense of confusion about what to expect, either from your therapist or from the course of the therapy. Mystery has cloaked therapy with images of a controlling man with a Viennese accent and piercing eyes emerging occasionally from under the fog. This chapter aims to demystify the therapy process and to give women consumers of psychotherapy some data that may be helpful and important to them when selecting a therapist.

The central underlying principle for women in the process of choosing a therapist is that a consumer of psychotherapy *does* have a choice. Often a woman entering therapy does so in the midst of a crisis, feeling badly about herself and her life, and wanting to make changes quickly. Under such internal and external pressures, a person may stay with the initial therapist because that person was there in the crisis, even if that therapist turns out not to be the best choice. The consumer of therapy services who is not in a crisis may also not know the criteria by which to evaluate a therapist whose credentials may carry the intimidating message "I am the expert." This difficulty in evaluating therapists is exacerbated for the consumer because some therapists may believe that a client's desire to exercise the right to evaluate indicates illness. Faced with such obstacles, a woman often gives up her rights without knowing they exist.

Therapy is a transaction similar to the purchase of other consumer services. The criteria for evaluation of success in therapy, however, are a good deal more subjective than those needed to evaluate car repairs or gardening services. Successful therapy often involves risky and painful changes. Even when therapy is working well, a client usually spends some time feeling angry, confused, or uncertain. However, there are some ideas that a consumer can use to make informed choices about the therapist she works with, and some ways to evaluate the progress of therapy.

considerations

If you are seeking therapy from a private practitioner, it is particularly helpful to do some "shopping around." Even in a clinic setting, where you will often have less freedom of choice, it is important to you, as a consumer, to keep in mind and make clear to those working with you those characteristics that you are looking for in a therapist. If you have a strong preference for a therapist of a particular gender, sexual orientation, therapy style, or age group, indicating that preference is the first step to getting the therapist you want, no matter what the setting.

If you are looking for a therapist on your own, there are a number of good places to start your search. Keeping your preferences in mind, you can:

1. Ask friends and others who have been in therapy if they would recommend their therapist to you. Find out why or why not. A strong recommendation from a person whose values you share may be useful, but your best friend's therapist may not be a guaranteed good choice for you.
2. Telephone your community's women's or feminist therapy referral service. A national listing of these resources appears at the end of this chapter. Many therapists who specialize in working with women or who have demonstrated an awareness of women's issues will be listed by those services.

3. Talk with your local mental health association. They will give you the names of three therapists. This will be done randomly, so you will have to carefully investigate to determine if these therapists meet your needs.

Once you have several names, the second step is to schedule initial interviews. Be assertive about asking for a reduced fee or no fee for this interview. Some therapists, particularly those who identify themselves as feminist therapists, will do this as a matter of course. Others may find such a request unusual. Use the feelings and information you get from discussing the no-cost first interview to begin your evaluation of whether you want to enter into a therapy relationship with the person.

Although the questions that you ask in this initial interview will vary with your needs and concerns, you may want to consider some of the factors that follow, which have been identified by other women as helpful when choosing a therapist.

CREDENTIALS.   There are many kinds of therapists and counselors, and they have extremely variable training and formal credentials. Research on therapy outcomes suggests that the type or years of formal training are not the best predictors of a therapist's skills. You may need a therapist with a particular type of training, and it is your right to make that an important part of your choice. Typically, the therapy professions include psychiatry (a medical doctor with speciality training), clinical or counseling psychology (a doctorate and several years of practical training), counseling (a master's degree in a number of fields, including psychology, counseling, sexuality, movement or art therapy, marriage, and family), and psychiatric or psychosocial nursing. A therapist may also be a paraprofessional, a person whose formal education varies, but who has had training in specific, limited helpful skills supplemented by practical experience.

THEORETICAL ORIENTATION.   This affects the way in which your problems are conceptualized, the interventions selected, and the language used during the therapy process. As with credentials, no one theoretical orientation has been clearly shown to be better than others, although behavior therapy approaches have had their outcomes most clearly documented by research. Some of the theoretical orientations that you may encounter include feminist, behaviorist, rational emotive, gestalt, transactional analysis, psychoanalytic, and dynamic. It is your right to ask a prospective therapist about the orientation that will be used, and in terms that you can understand. Also, ask the therapist to explain some of the therapy techniques in which you will be asked to participate.

ATTITUDES TOWARD WOMEN AND WOMEN'S ISSUES. Much recent research and writing has shown that therapists reflect the values of the culture in which they live. When that culture is sexist, and when it holds different standards of mental health for women and men, therapy can act to reinforce the negative effects of sexism. The value-free therapist does not exist; rather, there are therapists who are aware of their values and aware of the ways their values affect their work with clients. In an initial interview, you may want to ask a therapist about value and opinions on those issues that affect you personally. The questions might include: (1) How do you feel about nonmonogamous relationships? (2) Do you believe that it is more important for my marriage to stay together, even when it is harmful to one or both of us, than to facilitate a healthy separation process? (3) Do you think it's all right for women with small children to work outside the home, or for men to work in the home? (4)

What are your feelings about lesbianism or bisexuality? If you are uncomfortable with the ways in which your prospective therapist responds to your questions, you can use that feeling and the information you gather to further refine your choice process. Some therapists have been trained to view such detailed questions with suspicion; you may have to be assertive and persistant, and keep reminding yourself that it is your right to obtain this information in order to make the most informed choice possible.

PERSONAL INFORMATION ABOUT YOUR THERAPIST. Therapy can be an extremely unequal process, where one person (the client) shares much personal information and the other (the therapist) may remain anonymous. You may be comfortable with this; if you are not, you may want to satisfy your curiosity about who your therapist is as a person. This is an extremely sensitive area for many therapists, who may feel that their privacy is invaded by personal questions, or who may feel that it is inappropriate for a client to have this information. If it is important to you to know and important to a prospective therapist that you do not know, you may want to continue the search for a therapist.

As the process of selection continues, you will probably find that a particular therapist seems to be the one with whom you want to work. Before beginning therapy, it is helpful to clarify some issues if they have not been discussed in the initial interview. What about fees? Does the therapist have a sliding scale; what is the payment policy (will you be charged for missed sessions, must you pay at each session, or will a monthly bill be sent)? Is your therapist eligible to receive insurance payment, or can you barter services in exchange for therapy? Does the therapist have a policy about recordkeeping? Who has access to your records, and how is access obtained?

If the therapist tapes sessions, with whom are these tapes shared? How long are tapes kept before they are erased? Some feminist therapists have recommended that clients and therapists make a written contract that clearly specifies the mutual expectations of both people about the course of therapy. Such a contract could include specific agreements made on the above issues, as well as expectations about number of sessions per week, expected length of therapy, and techniques to be used in the course of therapy.

RIGHTS AS A CLIENT. Once you have chosen a therapist and begun to work, you continue to exercise rights as a client. The National Organization for Women (NOW) has developed a Bill of Rights for the Consumer of Psychotherapy,* which outlines issues important to women.

You have the right:

> To ask questions at any point.
> To know if the therapist is available to see you, or if not, how long the waiting period would be.
> To be fully informed of the therapist's qualifications to practice, including training and credentials, years of experience, personal therapy, and the like.
> To be fully informed about the therapist's therapeutic orientation.
> To ask questions about issues relevant to your therapy, such as therapist's values, background, attitude, and life experiences—and to be provided with thoughtful, respectful answers.
> To specify or negotiate therapeutic goals and to renegotiate those goals when necessary.
> To be fully informed of the limits of confidentiality in the therapy setting—with whom will the therapist discuss the case?
> To be fully informed of the extent of recordkeeping regarding the therapy, both in writ-

*Adapted from National Organization for Women's guidelines.

ten or taped forms, and knowledge concerning accessibility of those records.

To be fully informed of your diagnosis (if the therapist uses such categories).

To be fully informed of the therapist's estimation of approximate length of therapy to meet your agreed-upon goals.

To be fully informed regarding specific treatment strategies employed by therapist (talking, body exercises, homework assignments, use of medication).

To be fully informed regarding format of therapy (individual, family, group).

To refuse any intervention or treatment strategy.

To refuse to answer questions at any time.

To request that the therapist evaluate the progress of therapy.

To discuss any aspect of your therapy with others outside of the therapy situation, including consulting with another therapist.

To require the therapist to send a report regarding services rendered to any qualified therapist or organization upon written authorization by the client.

To be provided with copies of written files on the client, at the client's request.

To give or refuse to give permission for the therapist to use aspects of your case for part of a presentation or publication.

To be fully informed about the fees for therapy and the method of payment (including acceptability of insurance).

To be fully informed regarding the therapist's policies on issues such as missed sessions, vacation time, telephone contact outside of therapy, emergency coverage.

To get a written contract regarding conditions for therapy.

To know which ethics code the practitioner subscribes to.

To terminate therapy at any time.

To solicit help from the ethics committee of the appropriate professional organization in the event of doubt or grievance regarding the therapist's conduct.

sex and sexism

Aside from rights, two topics—sex and sexism—often emerge as particularly important to women consumers of psychotherapy.

SEX BETWEEN CLIENT AND THERAPIST. Sexual contact between clients and therapists is considered inappropriate and unethical by all the therapy professions. Such a relationship takes advantage of the power difference between client and therapist, making it difficult for a client to make a free choice of whether to be involved sexually with her therapist. There is evidence that sex between client and therapist is harmful to the client, and little or none to show it is helpful. Unfortunately, a small number of therapists (mostly male) have ignored both ethics and client welfare by engaging in sexual relationships or sexually harassing their mostly female clients. Often such a therapist will justify his behavior to himself and his victims by saying that he is helping you, the client, to deal with "hangups" or "repressions" about your body, touching, or sexuality. In some cases, the therapist will not actually propose intercourse, but may harass clients by engaging in excessive fondling, inappropriate touching, or by making sexually suggestive remarks. If this happens during your therapy, you have the right to refuse to partake in such activities, to refuse to pay for sessions in which such activities took place, and if desired, to report this to another therapist, or to the ethics committee of the appropriate professional association. Reporting such events may prove embarrassing or difficult for you; however, it is helpful to keep in mind that research on this topic has suggested that therapists who violate this ethical issue tend to do so with many clients. Your complaint may interrupt a chain of events that has victimized women other than yourself.

SEXISM IN PSYCHOTHERAPY. As discussed earlier, therapists, like other people, reflect the values and norms of the culture in which they were socialized. A therapist may be unaware of the ways in which therapeutic interventions further the process of discrimination, and a womam therapist is not a guarantee against sexism in the therapy process. As a consumer, you may want to watch for the subtle cues that indicate sexist values at work. Examples of sexism in therapy include: a therapist tells a woman who wears jeans and tee-shirts that she is too masculine-appearing and needs to pay more attention to her dress; a therapist subtly discourages a woman from discussing her career concerns by steering the conversation back to her feelings about her children whenever the career issue comes up; a therapist, working with a heterosexual couple, defers to the man continually, agreeing with his viewpoint and his versions of the couple's conflicts. It is your right, as a client, to confront your therapist about sexism in your therapy and to request that the therapist examine how sexist values are impeding your progress.

The cautions and warnings of this chapter may leave you feeling that you are better off staying out of therapy. But the reality is that most therapists are genuinely caring individuals who hold client welfare high on their list of priorities. Most therapists do not intend to consciously and consistently violate your rights. Awareness of your rights will, however, increase the chance that you get the therapy you want. Such awareness will also add to the active responsibility that you take for your own change and, thus, to your sense of personal accomplishment as you watch yourself grow.

resources for the consumer of psychotherapy

The Association for Women in Psychology maintains a national roster of feminist therapists, with a state-by-state listing of regional and local coordinators. A copy of this list can be obtained by sending $1.00 and a self-addressed stamped envelope to: K.N.O.W. Inc., P.O. B. 86031, Pittsburgh, PA 15221.

A group of feminist therapists associated with the National Feminist Association are in the process of compiling a national register of feminist, radical, and alternative therapists. You can obtain information about this list by writing to: Pat Henry, 1111 W. 10th St., Lawrence, KS 66044. Include a self-addressed stamped envelope.

If you wish to read further on this subject, the following list may be helpful:

Adams, & Orgel, *Through the mental health maze: A consumer's guide to finding a psychotherapist.* Available from Health Research, 2000 P St., N.W., Washington, DC 20036.

Bloom, et al., *Off the couch: A woman's guide to therapy.* Available from Goddard-Cambridge Graduate Program of Local Change, 5 Upland Rd., Cambridge, Mass. 02140.

Chesler, P. *Women & madness.* New York: Avon, 1972

Ehrenberg, O., & Ehrenberg, M. *The psychotherapy maze.* New York: Holt, 1977.

Friedman, S. S., Gams, L., Gotlieb, N., & Nesselson, C. *A woman's guide to therapy.* Englewood Cliffs, N.J.: Prentice-Hall, Inc., 1979.

National Organization for Women (New York Chapter). *A consumer's guide to nonsexist therapy.* Available from NOW.

Tennov. D. *Psychotherapy: The hazardous cure.* New York: Anchor, 1976.

26

ANN BIRNBAUM, Ph.D., M.P.H.

the pap smear: screening for cervical cancer

Cervical cancer is one of the most common forms of cancer occurring in women. Fortunately, this disease can be treated effectively if detected early.

The *Pap smear* is a test that detects changes in the surface cells of the cervix. These changes may be due to cancer or any of a number of other conditions. The majority of the conditions detected are not cancerous. An abnormal Pap smear finding alerts a woman to the need for closer investigation. To make informed decisions regarding her care, a woman needs to understand the Pap smear test and the meaning of its findings.

Unfortunately, many of us learn about the Pap smear's function in a hasty crash course following notification of abnormal smear findings. An abnormal finding, however, does not require an immediate reaction. We can afford to take the time to learn about the anatomy of the cervix and the types of changes that can occur. With this basic knowledge, we can then consider steps to be taken following an abnormal Pap smear finding.

the cervix

Cervix is from the Latin, meaning neck or any necklike part of the body. Since ancient times, the cervix has been described as the "neck" of the uterus. It is the narrow lower part of the

317

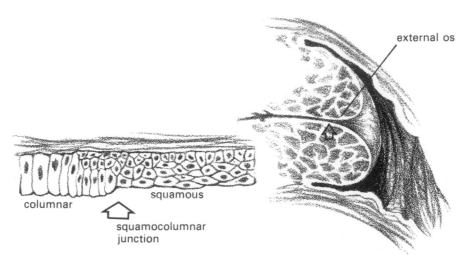

figure 26.1
normal female anatomy

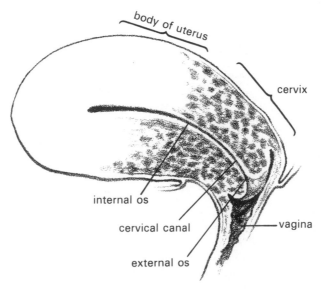

figure 26.2
normal lining of the uterus

uterus and protrudes into the vagina (see Figure 26.1).

The cervix encloses the *cervical canal*, a passage about 2.5 to 3.0 centimeters (or 1 to 1¼ inches) long. This passage extends from the *internal os* (internal opening) in the uterus to the *external os* (external opening) in the vagina. The lining of the cervical canal, the *columnar epithelium*, is a membrane of muc-us-secreting cells. The lining of the vagina, the *squamous epithelium*, is a membrane distinctly different from the lining of the cervical canal. These two membranes, the squamous epithelium and the columnar epithelium, meet at the *squamocolumnar junction* (see Figure 26.2). The majority of abnormal growths in the cervix begin in the squamocolumnar junction.

cervical neoplasia: dysplasia and cancer

When growths occur, the condition, as discussed in earlier chapters, is called *neoplasia*, a term derived from Greek and meaning "new growth." Several kinds of neoplasia can occur in the cervix. Of these, cancer is the most serious. But many neoplasia are *benign* (not cancerous). One kind of neoplasia, *dysplasia* (abnormal growth), is not cancerous, but it may be a precursor of cancer.

Dysplasia is abnormal development of squamous epithelium cells. The condition is confined to defined sites in the vicinity of the squamocolumnar junction and involves only part of the thickness of the epithelium. If all layers of the epithelium are involved, the condition is called *cancer in situ* or *carcinoma in situ*.

Since the discovery of dysplasia and cancer in situ is commonly followed by treatment, we can only make "educated guesses" about the natural course of these conditions. Scientists generally believe that the natural course of dysplasia is related to its severity. Thus, if left untreated, very slight dysplasia will probably regress and disappear. On the other hand, unchecked severe dysplasia will probably persist or progress to cancer in situ. Similarly, cancer in situ may remain unchanged or may progress to *invasive cancer*, spreading to surrounding tissue.

Study of tissue removed by hysterectomy has shown the growth pattern of invasive cervical cancer. In its early phase, the disease spreads beyond the epithelium, but remains within the cervix. Later, it extends to portions of the uterus and vagina, eventually advancing further into adjacent tissue.

Dysplasia, cancer in situ, and early invasive cancer can be treated most effectively. However, these conditions have no obvious symptoms. The absence of symptoms means that we experience no signal that medical care is needed. Therefore, screening by means of the Pap smear is a valuable practice, enabling us to take note of cervical changes that require further attention.

the pap smear

The Pap smear is a technique for studying cells from the surface of the cervix. It was popularized by George Papanicolaou and Herbert Traut in the early 1940s. The term "Pap smear" is short for "Papanicolaou smear."

The Pap smear is a sampling of cells from the region of the squamocolumnar junction. A speculum, a metal or plastic instrument shaped like a duck's bill, is inserted in the vagina. It holds the walls of the vagina apart, permitting examination of the cervix and vagina. The cervix is scraped with a narrow wooden or plastic spatula, usually by inserting one end in the external os and rotating in a full circle (see Figure 26.3). You may feel a twinge or sense of pressure during the scraping, but most women find this procedure quick and painless. The sample is smeared immediately onto a slide, a preservative is applied, and the slide is sent to a laboratory.

Laboratory staff stain the slide and then examine it under a microscope, noting any deviation from normal cell structure and patterns. The laboratory reports its findings to the practitioner who performed the scraping, who then informs the woman of the findings.

Many terms are used in reporting Pap smear findings. Typically, findings are in the following categories:

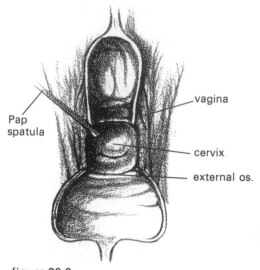

figure 26.3
pap smear procedure

Negative; normal for age and stage of menstrual cycle; no abnormalities.
Benign abnormal cells; irritation or infection present.
Abnormal cells of uncertain origin (might be inflammation or neoplasia).
Mild dysplasia.
Moderate dysplasia.
Severe dysplasia.
Positive; cancer in situ (carcinoma in situ).
Positive; invasive cancer.
Unsatisfactory (inadequate sample, details obscured by blood or infection, spoiled sample or poor preservation).

Every Pap smear report should use descriptive language. Modern practitioners discourage the use of numbered classifications. (Obviously, if a numbered system is used, there must

always be a set of unambiguous definitions for all of the numbers. A report of Class III Pap smear findings, for example, is only meaningful if it is accompanied by a definition of Class III!)

Your practitioner should use clear descriptive words when informing you of your Pap smear findings. Do not hesitate to request explanation of any unfamiliar terms. You may find it helpful to review a copy of your Pap smear report by yourself or with your practitioner. (Pap smear reports are usually less than one page. Findings are described in just a few words.)

The majority of Pap smears are normal and require no additional action. On the other hand, if your smear is unsatisfactory or shows abnormalities, you and your practitioner should plan for further care. Since an unsatisfactory smear does not reflect the state of your cervical tissue, you will want to have another smear taken. You will usually follow benign or uncertain findings with another smear, monitoring to see if the condition continues or changes. Smears showing uncertain findings or dysplasia may also be followed with *biopsy*, examination of surgically removed tissue. Smears detecting severe dysplasia, cancer in situ, or invasive cancer are customarily followed by biopsy.

biopsy

Although a Pap smear can detect the presence of disease, biopsy is necessary for diagnosis. Biopsy, the microscopic study of surgically removed tissue, gives us answers to questions about the extent and severity of the condition, how widespread it is, whether it is cancerous or benign.

Before consenting to a biopsy procedure, be sure you understand its nature and purpose. Ask questions. Request explanations of unfamiliar terms. You will want a description of the proposed biopsy procedure. Where will the procedure take place? Who will perform it? What aftereffects may occur (bleeding? cramping?), and how should these be handled? When will the laboratory work be completed? How and when will the laboratory's findings be explained to you? How will this information help in planning your care?

There are several techniques for removing cervical tissue, three of which are described as follows.

1. PUNCH BIOPSY is the excision of selected specimens, usually from the region of the squamocolumnar junction.
2. In CONIZATION, a cone-shaped wedge of tissue is removed from the region of the external os. (This is also a form of treatment and is discussed later in this chapter under Treatment of Cervical Neoplasia.)
3. ENDOCERVICAL CURETTAGE is the removal of tissue by scraping the cervical canal.

Of these procedures, punch biopsy is the most common and is usually performed in an office or clinic without anesthesia. As some women experience cramping during the procedure, you may want to use relaxation techniques, such as deep breathing, while the tissue is being removed. Also, it may help to have the practitioner narrate the procedure, describing her or his actions while working. If you are more comfortable knowing the details of the procedure, ask for this assistance.

colposcopy

Colposcopy is a technique for examining the cervix and vagina. The colposcope is a binocular microscope. It is equipped with a cool intense light and colored filters. Focused through a speculum on the cervix, the colposcope gives the practitioner a three-dimensional magnified view of the cervix.

A practitioner trained in use of the colposcope will examine and evaluate abnormalities on the surface of the cervix. A colposcopic examination may last as long as 20 minutes, a painless experience, even if tiring. Such an examination often follows abnormal Pap smear findings. In addition to permitting close study of surface abnormalities, colposcopy helps the practitioner identify those areas that should be scraped for a Pap smear or biopsied.

Punch biopsy with colposcopy is more accurate than punch biopsy without this aid. It is also less traumatic than conization, formerly a more common diagnostic procedure. Increasingly, colposcopy or punch biopsy with colposcopy are the preferred approaches for investigating abnormal Pap smear findings.

treatment of cervical neoplasia

Before making a decision about your care, you will want to understand the condition diagnosed. What is it called? How widespread is it? Where is it located in your cervix? What will happen if it is not treated?

Colposcopy and biopsy provide useful information for planning care. You may find it helpful to have your practitioner review your laboratory report with you, explaining any unfamiliar terms. (Biopsy reports are brief. Findings and recommendations take no more than a few sentences.)

Talk with your practitioner about your gynecologic history, life-style, and childbearing plans. Do you have other gynecologic problems? Would you find it easy to have frequent checkups? Do you want to have children? Are you pregnant? Your practitioner needs to consider these matters in helping you choose the most appropriate treatment.

Your practitioner should tell you about the methods of treatment for your condition. You should understand the advantages and disadvantages of each.

In choosing a treatment, principal considerations will be the severity of the neoplasia, location of the neoplasia, childbearing plans, and presence of other gynecologic disorders. Some typical treatment plans are described briefly as follows.

The woman with a diagnosis of dysplasia may find that the biopsy procedure removed all the abnormal tissue. In this case, a plan of care should include Pap smears and colposcopy, monitoring for recurring dysplasia.

If the dysplasia recurs or extends beyond the excised areas, abnormal tissue may be destroyed by *cryotherapy*. Cryotherapy, also called cryosurgery or cold cautery, is a freezing technique used to destroy abnormal tissue on the surface of the cervix. Cryosurgery is usually an office procedure performed without anesthesia. Relaxation techniques should help you handle any cramping during the procedure. Most women have a heavy discharge, which slackens after a week and disappears in three or four weeks. You and your practitioner should agree on a schedule for monitoring changes in your cervix after cryotherapy.

For severe dysplasia and cancer in situ, conization is often the preferred treatment. In conization, a cone-shaped wedge of tissue is removed from the cervix (see Figure 26.4). The wedge includes a portion of the cervical canal that is susceptible to neoplasia, but cannot be reached by cryotherapy. Conization is usually performed under general anesthesia in a hospital. If childbearing is not a concern, you may wish to consider hysterectomy as treatment for cancer in situ, especially if there are other serious gynecologic problems or if neoplasia recur after conization.

In cases of invasive cancer, treatment is by surgery, radiation therapy, or a combination. Your treatment plan must be suited to your situation. Prior to making a decision, you and your practitioner should discuss and schedule any procedures necessary for evaluating your general health and the extent of the cancer. In planning the best treatment for you, the following information should be considered: facts about your general health, facts about

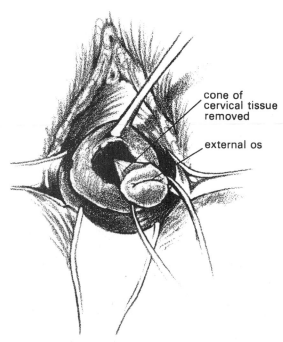

cone of
cervical tissue
removed

external os

figure 26.4
conization of the cervix

the extent of your cancer, available medical facilities and specialists, and your preferences and way of life.

Before giving your consent to a treatment procedure, be sure that your questions about your condition and available treatment methods have been answered completely. What is known about the success and complications of each type of treatment? Where will the treatment procedure take place? Who will perform the procedure? What discomfort or pain is associated with the treatment? How will discomfort or pain be handled? Will the treatment limit your activity afterward and, if so, for how long? What care will be necessary after the procedure?

Don't be reluctant to seek a second opinion in making a decision about your treatment. If you are not ready to make a decision after talking with one practitioner, arrange to discuss your case with another. Reviewing your case anew may give you fresh insight and the opportunity to compare the opinions, knowledge, and behavior of two practitioners.

questions about the pap smear and cervical neoplasia

WHAT CAUSES CERVICAL NEOPLASIA? We do not know the cause, but certain factors seem to increase the risk for this disease—early coitus (during adolescence) and having several sexual partners. Researchers are investigating the possibility that a substance transmitted during coitus causes cervical neoplasia. Researchers are also investigating the possible role of such drugs as birth control pills.

HOW OFTEN SHOULD A WOMAN HAVE A PAP SMEAR? Ideally, a woman should be screened only as often as necessary to assure that harmful neoplasia will be detected while most susceptible to treatment. To screen a woman more fre-

quently is to increase the cost of her health care and to inconvenience her needlessly.

Although it has been customary to recommend that a healthy woman have a Pap smear annually, many practitioners now question this policy. They argue that research is needed to set a schedule for optimum screening. The following general guidelines reflect current thinking, as based on our knowledge about cervical neoplasia and good screening practices.

All women who have had sexual intercourse should have a Pap smear.

All women over 20 years of age should have a Pap smear.

The first two or three Pap smears should be performed at one-year intervals.

If the first two or three smears are normal, subsequent smears should be performed at three-year intervals until age 40.

A woman should talk with her practitioner about her schedule of smears if: (1) she is 40 years of age or older, (2) she has ever had a herpes virus infection, (3) she has ever had gonorrhea, (4) her mother took the hormone diethylstilbestrol (DES), or (5) she is taking birth control pills.

HOW RELIABLE IS THE PAP SMEAR? The majority of Pap smears are taken properly, handled correctly at the laboratory, and reported correctly to practitioners. Nevertheless, women should bear in mind that the Pap smear is not a perfect test. Human error may intervene in the clinic or in the laboratory.

If your smear is unsatisfactory (due to faulty sampling or spoiled or obscured details), your practitioner should recall you for another smear.

To maximize accuracy and minimize error, you should not douche within 24 hours prior to having a Pap smear.

Remember that each Pap smear tests conditions at only one time. Avoid basing a plan of action on the findings of a single smear. In the event of an abnormal smear report, you and your practitioner may wish to schedule one or more smears prior to considering a biopsy procedure. Similarly, not one, but a series of two or three normal smears should assure you that no abnormalities have gone undetected.

WHO SHOULD TAKE THE PAP SMEAR? To be reliable in taking Pap smears, a practitioner must be trained in this procedure. Many types of practitioners receive this training, including midwives, women's health care specialists, and some specialized nurses. There is no evidence that physicians are more reliable than other practitioners.

Bearing in mind that a variety of health care professionals are competent in the Pap smear procedure, consider your impressions and preferences in choosing a practitioner. Does the practitioner seem unhurried and relaxed? Does she or he make it easy for you to ask questions? Do you prefer an informal or businesslike manner? Do you prefer to be examined by a woman?

A good practitioner will help you obtain and understand information necessary for managing your health care and will help you use such information wisely.

SHARON KRUMM, R.N., M.S.N.

breast cancer screening

Breast cancer is the leading cause of death among women between the ages of 45 and 55 and is the most common type of cancer found in women of all ages. The American Cancer Society statistics say that one out of 11 women will develop breast cancer in her lifetime. However, breast cancer can be successfully treated if it is discovered while very small or in its earliest stage. Herein lies the importance of breast cancer screening and detection.

detection methods

Detection refers to the utilization of different techniques and methods to discover cancer of the breast in its earliest stage, when a woman's chances for successful treatment and management are optimal. Screening refers to the process of determining who has the greatest probability or risk of developing breast cancer, and utilizing detection techniques and methods that will discover the cancer in its earliest stage.

In the 1970s, the National Cancer Institute (NCI) and the American Cancer Society initiated 27 Breast Cancer Detection Demonstration Projects (BCDDPs) for the purpose of

325

screening large numbers of women in a diversity of communities. These projects have screened over 280,000 women. Information has been obtained about the medical history and habits of these women and is being interpreted along with the results of the screening examination. This information will very likely lead to a more knowledgeable assessment of a woman's risk of developing breast cancer, from which recommendations of who should be screened and how often can be made.

Being female, along with the woman's age, are the only two factors found consistently to increase the probability of developing breast cancer. Women account for 99 percent of all breast cancers, and the risk of developing it increases with age. There is evidence to suggest a two-to-fivefold increase in risk for the woman whose mother and/or sister has had breast cancer and for the woman with cancer in one breast to develop cancer in the other breast. There appears to be no increased risk for the woman who has not breastfed her babies, or for the woman with fibrocystic disease. However, the woman with fibrocystic disease may have breasts that feel more "lumpy" and, therefore, make the detection of early cancer more difficult by physical examination alone. A number of other factors have also been studied but in many cases the results are contradictory. Unfortunately, publication of these studies in the popular press often presents a confused and fragmentary picture to the woman reader.

Physical examination, mammography, and thermography are used by the BCDDPs and many physicians to detect early breast cancer.

The examination, by a nurse or physician, of a woman's breasts should be included in a yearly physical examination or routine checkup. This includes a visual inspection of the skin overlying the breasts, breast contour, and the nipples. Then the breasts, underarms,

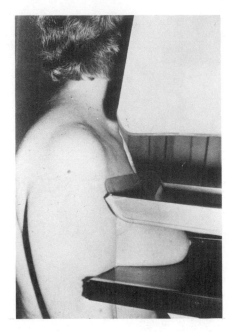

figure 27.1
position of the breast during a mammogram

and nipples are carefully inspected by the examiner's hands while the woman is sitting and again while she is lying down. The woman definitely should be taught how to examine her own breasts at this time if she does not already know how to perform "breast self-examination" (BSE). Such instruction should be requested if it is not offered during the examination.

A breast lump must be at least the size of the head of a thumbtack before it can be felt; therefore, X-rays called *mammograms* are sometimes used to detect early breast cancer (Figure 27.1). Mammograms that are developed and printed on xerox paper are called xeromammograms or xerograms.

The use of mammograms was the subject of much public debate in the 1970s when questions were raised about their value in detecting early cancers in women under the age of

50 and about the possibility of radiation exposure increasing a woman's chance of developing breast cancer. When *mammography* was first used in the early 1960s, the woman was exposed to approximately 15 rads (a measurement of the amount of radiation received) or more, depending on the type and age of equipment used. With today's techniques and equipment, however, a woman receives approximately 1 rad to the skin over the breast and only 0.3 rads to the breast tissue for a two-view examination. Women should inquire about the amount of exposure they can anticipate. The National Cancer Institute now recommends that a woman under 50 years of age not receive yearly mammograms unless she has had cancer in one breast or unless her mother or sister have or had breast cancer, or if the physical examination indicates. Because a woman who has had a cancer in one breast is five times more likely to develop it in the other breast, the additional radiation is less of a danger than failing to detect a second cancer in its earliest stage. This is also true for the woman with a family history of breast cancer. Yearly mammograms for women over 50 have been determined not to cause any significant risk.

The BCDDPs detected 2,700 breast cancers in the 280,000 women screened during the first two years of operation. Of those detected, 70 percent had not spread beyond the breast tissue and 45 percent were so small that they could not have been found on physical examination. They could be found only on X-ray. These findings have led to the concept of minimal breast cancer. Minimal breast cancer refers to a cancer confined to a small segment of the breast or a very small cancer that has invaded the surrounding tissues. A woman with minimal breast cancer stands an excellent chance of being successfully treated. Of women with this early cancer, 4 out of 5 are

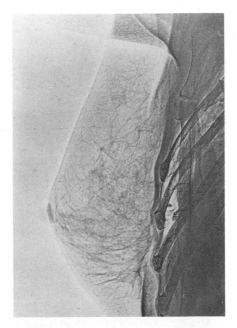

figure 27.2
a thermogram of the breast, with the darker areas representing warmer tissue

free of disease five years after treatment.

Another method of discovering early breast cancer is *thermography*, the study of differences in temperature of normal and abnormal breast tissue. Cancer breast tissue is warmer than normal tissue and this difference can be photographed and transcribed into a graph (Figures 27.2 and 27.3). Experience with thermography has demonstrated that when used alone it is of little value in the detection of early cancer, but it may be of value when used along with physical examination and mammography.

self-examination

Ninety percent of all breast cancers are found by the woman herself or by her sexual partner. The systematic examination of one's own

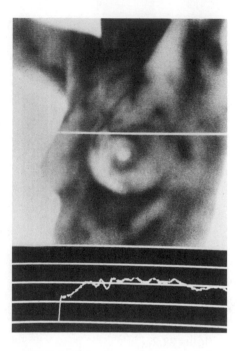

figure 27.3
a graph of breast tissue temperature as measured by thermography, the peaks in the graph represent warmer tissue. breast abnormalities may generate more heat than normal tissue.

breasts should be started when breasts begin to develop at puberty. Although breast cancer is uncommon among girls or young women, breast self-examination should become a health habit that is learned and ingrained early in life and is practiced regularly. Women can assist in this early health habit development by encouraging their school districts to sponsor BSE classes.

A survey tells us that while most women wanted their physicians to teach them how to do BSE, a majority did not receive such instruction. On the other hand, while a majority of the women said they knew how to do BSE, only 25 percent of them did so regularly. One of the common reasons given for not doing BSE was the belief that it was not necessary since their physicians examined their breasts. This assumption is incorrect for two reasons: first, many women do not see a physician regularly, and second, no physician is as knowledgeable about a woman's breasts as the woman who is regularly examining them.

The breasts change during a woman's lifetime. In addition, breast changes occur during the menstrual cycle. Some of these changes are more noticeable the week prior to menstruation, when tender lumps may appear and the breasts swell with fluid. These changes disappear the week following menstruation. Other normal breast changes occur throughout pregnancy, with significant weight loss or gain, at menopause, and if a woman is taking birth control pills. Other hormones and some prescription drugs can cause breast changes. In fact, the breasts are constantly changing throughout life, and knowledge of how your breasts feel during these normal changes enables you to recognize abnormal changes when BSE is done regularly.

An understanding of the basic structure of the breasts is helpful in learning to do breast self-examination. The breasts are composed of mammary glands, fibrous and fat tissues, chains of lymph glands, and muscles (Figure 27.4). The mammary glands produce milk for breast feeding and are connected by tubes, called ducts, that open on the surface of the nipple. Fibrous tissues provide support for the breast. The amount of fatty tissue depends on the woman's age and weight. The lymph glands, or nodes, form chains under the arm and into the chest and act as filters to prevent the spread of diseases. There are muscles that lie directly under the breast bone (sternum) and collarbone (clavicle), which extend under the arm. A woman's breasts quite frequently differ in size and shape.

The only way you will be able to detect very early changes in your breasts is to do breast self-examination regularly and at the

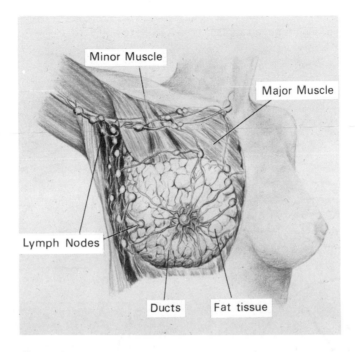

figure 27.4
normal breast tissue showing muscle, lymph nodes, fatty tissue, and milk ducts

same time every month. Women who are still having menstrual periods should examine their breasts during the week following their period. Women who no longer menstruate should select a date that is easily remembered, such as their birthdate or the first day of each month, to do their breast self-examination. It is suggested that breast self-examination be performed more frequently initially in order to become familiar with the consistency of texture in the breasts and to become confident of the technique.

Breast self-examination (Figure 27.5) should be done in three stages: (1) in the shower or tub, (2) in front of a mirror, and (3) lying down. In each stage use the flat part of your fingers, not your fingertips. Be firm but gentle. It is neither necessary nor desirable to press extremely hard to do the examination. Use the right hand to examine the left breast, the left hand to examine the right one. Be sure to feel all of the breast tissue, either in widening circles starting at the nipple and moving outward or in strips from the nipple out and back. The nipples should be squeezed to see if there is any discharge. Most nipple discharges are normal, but if present you should be examined by a physician. The underarm area (axilla) should be included in the examination because breast tissue as well as lymph glands are found in this area.

While examining your breasts in the tub or shower, wet and soap them to reduce friction. Raise your right arm over your head while examining the right breast and the left arm while examining the left breast. By doing this,

figure 27.5
series of drawings showing the seven steps in breast self-examination*

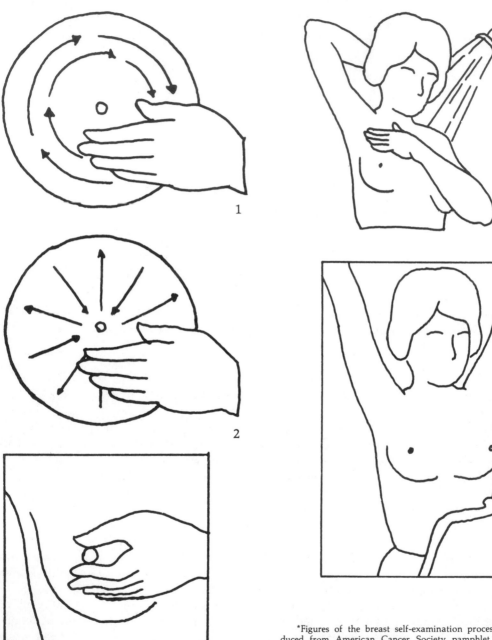

*Figures of the breast self-examination process are reproduced from American Cancer Society pamphlet #77-5000M-11/77-No. 2075-LE. The editors acknowledge the kind permission of the Society to use these materials.

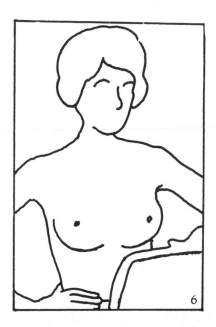

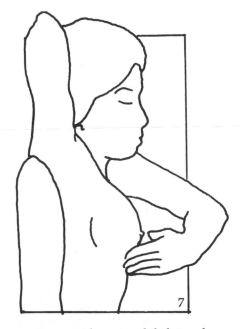

you bring the breast tissue forward and make it more accessible. Some women prefer not to do this part of the examination in the tub or shower, but rather to apply lotion to their hands and breasts to reduce friction while doing the examination.

When examining your breasts in front of a mirror, look for changes in contour and size. Do this first with your hands relaxed at your sides, then raised over your head, and finally with your hands pressing in on your waist. Each position allows you to examine your breasts from a different perspective, which increases the probability of detecting any changes. You should also carefully examine the skin over your breasts for dimpling, puckering, and for reddened areas.

To examine your breasts while lying down, place your hand under your head and a pillow under the shoulder on the side you are going to examine. This causes the breast tissue to flatten out over the chest wall and makes it easier to examine. If you have large breasts, you may need to use a second pillow placed next to the breast for support and to give you a surface against which to press.

Additional information on breast self-examination may be obtained from your local American Cancer Society unit or the American Cancer Society, 219 E. 42nd St., New York, NY 10017, and "The Breast Cancer Digest" is free from the National Cancer Institute, Office of Cancer Communications, Building 31, Bethesda, MD 30305.

biopsy and mastectomy

Although 80 percent of breast changes are not cancer, any abnormal change in your breast should be examined by a physician as soon as

possible. Following the initial examination, your physician may want to re-examine you in a month to determine the effect of the men-

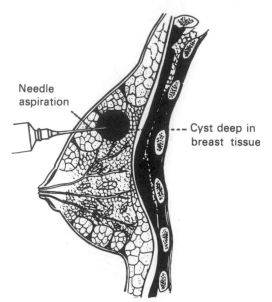

Needle
aspiration

--- Cyst deep in
breast tissue

figure 27.6
a needle aspiration of a cyst deep in breast tissue

strual cycle. You may be asked to stop taking birth control pills or other hormones during this time to see if they could be contributing to the changes. A mammogram may be recommended.

Some breast changes are "lumps" that feel as if they are filled with fluid and are called cysts. Your physician may withdraw the fluid for examination (Figure 27.6). If the withdrawn fluid is clear and the lump disappears, you will probably be instructed to continue breast self-examination and be scheduled to return for periodic examinations. If the fluid is bloody or dark or if the lump remains, your physician will probably recommend that you have a biopsy (see chapter 22).

A biopsy is a procedure in which a sample of the suspicious breast tissue is taken and examined under a microscope. This is the only way that a diagnosis of cancer can be made. In addition to finding bloody or dark aspirated fluid and/or a persistent lump, a biopsy may

be recommended for any of the following reasons: (1) a hard, solid lump that is not fluid-filled, (2) a lump that either increases in size or remains unchanged throughout several menstrual cycles or following the discontinuation of birth control pills or other hormones, (3) a hard, solid lump that is associated with a nipple discharge or skin changes, (4) and an abnormal mammogram. It usually takes several days after a biopsy has been taken before the report or diagnosis is available to the woman.

A biopsy may be done as an office procedure using a special needlelike instrument. The area around the breast change or lump is first deadened with medication and the procedure is quickly done with minimal pain (Figure 27.6).

Frequently, a woman is admitted to a hospital and a biopsy taken while she is asleep under a general anesthetic. This procedure is usually performed by a surgeon. The skin over the lump or breast change is cut open, the lump or sample of tissue is removed, and the skin sewn back together. Many surgeons make the skin opening along the circle of darkened skin surrounding the nipple. This technique allows the skin to be sewn back together in such a way that the resulting scar is barely noticeable. The woman may be discharged from the hospital the following day.

Occasionally, a physician will recommend that a biopsy and mastectomy, or removal of the breast, be done during the same operation. This type of biopsy is called a "frozen section"; and the operation is a one-stage procedure. The sample of tissue is removed while the woman is asleep in the operating room, examined immediately under a microscope, and diagnosis made. If the diagnosis is cancer, the surgeon procedes with the mastectomy. If the diagnosis is not cancer, the skin is sewn together and the woman awakens from the anesthetic. A two-stage procedure refers to the biopsy and mastectomy being done as separate procedures.

Occasionally, women with persistent breast lumps have had to go to three or four physicians before finding one who would recommend a biopsy. Such perseverance is to be applauded. It is unfortunate indeed if any woman follows anyone's advice to go home and stop worrying about herself and then later learns that she has breast cancer.

The fears, uncertainties, and myths surrounding breast cancer and its detection are being openingly addressed by many women, nurses, and physicians, as well as other health care professionals such as health educators and women's health care specialists. It is extremely unwise to underestimate the significance of the emotional and sexual components of breast changes and breast cancer. The encouragement and support of husbands, other family members, and friends is often the most significant factor in a woman's decision to do breast self-examination, have mammograms, or seek medical advice if a breast lump is discovered. In the final analysis, however, it is literally, as well as figuratively, in the hands of every woman to accept this responsibility for herself and to encourage its acceptance by others.

28

HELEN I. MARIESKIND, Dr. P.H.

governmental actions
for women's health

historical background

Early governmental interest in women's health, as opposed to the public's interest, arose in response to the tremendous influx of immigrants into the major U.S. industrial cities during the late nineteenth and early twentieth centuries (Howe, 1976). Social programs to meet the needs of these people, such as Jane Addams's Hull House (Davis, 1973) and Lillian Wald's Henry Street Settlement (Duffus, 1938) were invaluable, but only to relatively few people. They did demonstrate,

This material is drawn from: Helen I. Marieskind, *Women In the Health System: Patients, Providers and Programs* (St. Louis: C. V. Mosby, 1980).

however, the squalid conditions under which most of the new immigrants lived, and the particular hazards these conditions posed to women and children. At the turn of the century, maternal mortality, for example, was estimated at 728 per 100,000. Infant mortality data suggested that 1 in every 10 infants died in the first year of life (*Final Mortality Statistics*, 1979). A study of female factory workers and women who stayed at home showed that among the former there was an infant mortality rate of 199.2 per 1,000 live births as compared with 133.9 among nonemployed women (*Infant Mortality*, 1917).

milk stations—1873–1917

The earliest efforts to improve these appalling statistics came mainly from the private sector through the establishment of milk stations—a place where infants of the poor could receive clean milk either free or for a nominal charge. Classes in child care were also conducted at milk stations, and many nursing mothers attended (Blake, 1977). The first milk station in the United States began in 1873 attached to the New York Diet Kitchen Association and was soon followed by other voluntary efforts (Rosen, 1971). In 1897, the first publicly funded station was opened by the Rochester, New York, Health Department (Goler, 1897). This station offered well-baby checkups in addition to the basic baby care classes and free milk distribution (Blake, 1977).

The success of milk stations in reducing infant mortality, when combined with a program of health visitors who followed up on the babies, led in 1908 to the establishment in New York City of the nation's first Division of Child Hygiene. Under the leadership of Dr. S. Josephine Baker, milk stations grew and soon included a community-center concept in their approach. They were used for "mothers' meetings, sewing classes, Little Mothers' League meetings (education of young girls in maternal care), neighborhood societies, and as general centers where the nurse, through personal efforts, frequently provided food, clothing, medical care, shelter, employment, outings, excursions, etc., for the members of the baby's family" (Blake, 1977).

Other cities expanded their services, including programs encouraging breastfeeding and education on general maternal and child welfare. By 1915, 20 cities had developed child hygiene bureaus as part of their health departments (Goodwin, 1916). Gradually, well-baby clinics with supervision by physicians, visiting nurse programs, and lectures to mothers, replaced the milk stations (Blake, 1977; U.S. Children's Bureau, 1913). The foundation had been laid for subsequent maternal and child health programs.

children's bureau

Issues of maternal and child health were further thrust into the nation's consciousness with the establishment of the Children's Bureau in the Department of Labor on April 9, 1912. Julia Lathrop, the dynamic woman who was the first chief of the Bureau, organized both data collection and surveys of child welfare, as well as the publication and distribution of educational pamphlets designed to encourage maternal and infant well-being. She recognized the tremendous needs of women to know more about their own health and child care. Lathrop resolved that the government should assist in promoting maternal and infant well-being and, with the support of emerging public opinion and of able colleagues such as Grace Abbott, Jeannette Rankin, and Martha Elliott, the opposition to "bureaucratic intervention" was eventually overcome. The pattern of federal interest in the reproductive health of women was set.

early maternal and child health legislation

sheppard-towner act—1921–1929

Numerous efforts on behalf of women and children within both Congress and the Chil-dren's Bureau culminated in 1921 in the passage of the Sheppard-Towner Act (Morris

Sheppard, Texas; Horace Mann Towner, Iowa), known officially as the Maternity and Infancy Act. Opponents to this federal-state program for maternal and infant health had been vocal, sexist, and ignorant of the need for education in good child care practices. The Act was labeled as "socialistic, bolshevistic, and radical."

But Grace Abbott, in late 1921, who was by then the new Children's Bureau chief, determinedly administered this first federal formula grant for health (formula grants allocate money to states on the basis of a formula, generally population times per capita income times need).

By 1927, 45 states and the then Territory of Hawaii had a Sheppard-Towner program for which they met the obligation of matching funds. Abbott summarized the five main areas in which these states had chosen to spend their money as: "promotion of birth registration, cooperation between health authorities and physicians, nurses, dentists, nutrition workers and so forth, establishment of infant welfare centers, establishment of maternity centers, and educational classes for mothers, midwives and household assistants or mother's helpers and 'little mothers.' " After an extension of funding ended in 1929, 19 states and the Territory of Hawaii continued to appropriate monies for maternal and child health programs.

title v
of the social security act

By August 14, 1935, when the Social Security Act was passed, including Title V, which allocated funds for maternal and child health services, it met with little opposition. Providers and patients had come to understand the mutual benefits of giving women funds to seek maternity care. Care, however, was still essentially an expanded version of the Shep-

pard-Towner funding; it did not include delivery coverage. At this time, under Title V, other services were also introduced, for example, benefits for crippled children and well-child care for young children. Services under Title V were generally provided by local health departments, which also received Social Security Act monies through Title VI (*Maternal and Child Health*, 1977). As the states had to match funds provided in order to receive monies, there was no uniform level of coverage or benefits. Nonetheless, despite the limited nature of the funding, Title V was a tremendous boon for women—and for providers. Pre- and postnatal care could be obtained and with the exposure to the medical profession, most women shifted to having their babies in hospitals. By 1940, 55.8 percent of all babies were born in hospitals, a rapid increase from the 30 percent in 1930. Concurrently, but not necessarily causally related, maternal mortality declined from 636.0 per 100,000 live births for the period 1930–1934 to 493.9 per 100,000 live births for the period 1935–1939 (*Final Mortality Statistics*, 1977).

emergency maternity
and infant care

A new effort to provide comprehensive maternity care was developed under the Emergency Maternity and Infant Care (EMIC) program during the period 1941–1946. In August 1941, military personnel in Washington State appealed to the State Health Department for help to meet their obligations to provide maternity services for the wives of the rapidly expanding army. They proposed using special nonmatched project funds from Fund B of Title V of the Social Security Act. The Children's Bureau approved the request, and an emergency program for comprehensive maternity coverage was developed, including for the first time in a federally funded program, coverage for delivery costs, and hospitalization. Response to the program was rapid, and by July 1, 1942, 27 other states had been approved to use B funds for similar programs.

Kathrine F. Lenroot, the chief of the Children's Bureau, and Martha M. Eliot, associate chief, justified use of additional Title V, B funds. Amid much debate, on July 12, 1943, about $4,400,000 was appropriated for fiscal year 1944; after six weeks and surging demand, the Children's Bureau was granted another $18,600,000.

Cries of "socialized medicine" were not heeded, and the program continued to be funded until November 1946; a means test applied in 1943, however, effectively limited the program to wives of servicemen in the lowest pay grades, 4, 5, 6, and 7. Since these grades comprised about 75 percent of the armed forces, many women reaped the benefits of the program. At its peak, EMIC covered the maternity services for 1 in 7 births. By the program's close, 1,200,000 maternity cases had been covered in addition to the care for 230,000 infants (Mulligan, 1976; Sinai & Anderson, 1974; U.S. Congress, 1943). The Act reinforced the use of hospitals as the location for giving birth; minimum standards were also established for hospitals, maternity, and newborn services. Although efforts to revive EMIC during the Korean War failed, CHAMPUS (Comprehensive Health and Medical Plan, United States), the current health program for the armed forces and their dependents, was modeled after it.

contemporary programs

maternal and infant care

Project grants specifically for maternity and infant care were funded as part of the Maternal and Child Health and Mental Retardation Amendments of 1963. They are aimed at providing maternity programs offering "reasonable assurance of satisfactorily helping to reduce the incidence of mental retardation and other handicapping conditions caused by complications associated with childbearing . . . and of reducing infant and maternal morbidity and mortality; they must be established in areas with concentrations of low-income families" (Maternal and Child Health, 1977).

Essentially, these programs are expanded versions of the original maternal and well-baby care provided under Sheppard-Towner. Criticism of the programs has centered on the specialization of the program, however, and in spite of its comprehensive maternity coverage, health care aid is still limited to the event of pregnancy. As soon as the pregnancy terminates, or the mother goes into a higher income bracket, or her child exceeds the age limit, participation ceases (Gold and Stone, 1968; Madison, 1969). On the other hand, numerous women—approximately 740,500 in both 1978 and 1979—have been served, however temporarily, by the programs (Pardee, 1979).

Title V also provides funding for research, more general maternal and child health services, including dental care, and for training personnel for "the health care of and related services for mothers and children, particularly mentally retarded children with multiple handicaps" (*1978 Catalog*, 1978). In general, these programs are administered through the Bureau of Community Health Service, DHEW and, including family planning monies, were allocated $491 million in fiscal year 1979 (Marshall, 1978).

family planning

Parts of Title V of the Social Security Act and Title X of the Public Health Service Act (first passed August 14, 1912) fund family planning programs, which must again be established in areas with large concentrations of low-income persons. Under Title V in 1970, an estimated 2,610,591 (Pardee, 1979) women received contraceptive counseling and services through family planning programs sponsored by health departments or hospital clinics.

Title X, in addition to providing family planning services, specifies that funds should also be used for training programs "to improve utilization and career development of paraprofessional and paramedical manpower in family planning services," for example, the training of women's health care specialists (*1978 Catalog*, 1978). Research monies for the development of "more effective and convenient contraceptives" are allocated under this Act as well (*1978 Catalog*, 1978).

From a national survey in 1976, it was estimated that a total of 4.1 million women received contraceptive services through organized programs, in large part funded by Title V and Title X monies. These were provided through health departments (1,723,000 women), Planned Parenthood (1,108,000), hospital clinic programs (563,000), and other agencies such as free clinics, neighborhood health centers, and community action agencies (689,000). Most women served by these programs had low or marginal incomes, most

were young with low parity, and most had at least graduated from high school (Torres, 1978).

medicare

Medicare, a health insurance program for persons 65 years and older, was introduced by Title XVIII as part of the Social Security Act Amendments of 1965. Part A of Medicare provides basic protection by paying 80 percent of the costs of inpatient hospital care, posthospital extended care, and posthospital home health care. Part B (Medicare Medical Insurance) provides supplemental protection against costs of physicians' services, medical services and supplies, home health care services, outpatient hospital services and therapy, and other miscellaneous services.

Upon introduction of the concept of Medicare, organized medicine railed against it as "creeping socialism," but as with the experience of Sheppard-Towner and EMIC funding of earlier decades, the benefits of a population able to pay for health care and have access to it soon became obvious. After Medicare was initiated, hospitalization among the elderly rapidly increased, although use of ambulatory services did not rise comparably (Somers and Somers, 1967; Donabedian & Thorby, 1969).

In 1976, an estimated 79.2 percent of women (80.1 percent of males) had some form of private insurance and/or Medicare (*Health, United States*, 1978). The requirement of a minimum number of "work quarters" to qualify for Medicare, introduced as an amendment in 1968, is presumably one reason some women were not covered. Medicare is, nonetheless, an invaluable tool for insuring adequate health services for women who may be particularly needy because of their longevity and economic vulnerability.

medicaid

Title XIX of the Social Security Act was also passed in 1965 and amended the Act to provide for the health of the medically indigent through matching federal and state contributions. As with the Sheppard-Towner Act and Title V, states may design their own Medicaid programs within federal guidelines. At a minimum, however, all states must provide inpatient hospital care, outpatient hospital services, physicians' services, screening, diagnosis and treatment of children, and home health care services. In many states, together with matching federal contributions, Medicaid additionally pays for dental care, prescription drugs, eyeglasses, clinic services, and other diagnostic screening and preventive and rehabilitative services.

About 4.6 million women of reproductive age are eligible for Medicaid, and until the recent cuts for abortion funding (discussed later), the program (*Abortion*, 1979) provided them much-needed comprehensive maternity care.

other health-related agencies and programs

Critical to women's health (and obviously also to men's) are the food-related programs offered by the Department of Agriculture. These include the Women, Infants, and Children Program (known as WIC), through which over 1 million participants "identified to be nutritional risks" received benefits in fiscal year 1977–1978; about $550 million was spent on this program in fiscal year 1979 (*1978 Catalog*, 1978; McIntosh, 1979).

Similarly, needy families may be served by the Needy Family Program and can be provided bulk food products such as flour and grains through the Commodities Supplemental Food Program and/or may receive food stamps authorized under P.L. 88–525 of August 30, 1964, with the aim to "improve diets of low-income households by supplementing their food purchasing ability" (*1978 Catalog*, 1978). In fiscal year 1978, an average of 16,043,861 persons participated in the Food Stamp Program and $8,310,918,211 was spent (Younger & Hickman, 1979). Other programs are the Food Donation Program, which specifically mentions "pregnant and lactating women" (*1978 Catalog*, 1978) among its intended participants, the Child Care Food Program for children in nonresidential institutions (*1978 Catalog*, 1978), and numerous school food service programs.

Special populations receive benefits through programs aimed either indirectly at health, for example, employment opportunities for handicapped persons (*1978 Catalog*, 1978), or directly through the provision of health care services to, for example, Native Americans through the Indian Health Services-Health Management Development Program (*1978 Catalog*, 1978), and Appalachians through the Appalachian Health Program (*1978 Catalog*, 1978).

Numerous other programs benefit women and indirectly relate to their health, such as those to combat domestic violence (Domestic Violence Legislation, 1978), to train displaced homemakers (*Comprehensive Employment Training Act*, 1973), child support enforcement (*1978 Catalog*, 1978), and health career opportunity grants for the disadvantaged (Von Borgen et al, 1978).

One agency that has the power particularly to affect women's health is the Food and Drug Administration (FDA). Established in 1906 and essentially in its present form by May 1930, the FDA performs a watchdog function over drugs and medical devices. After 1938, the FDA held drug manufacturers responsible for testing drugs for safety, at least on dogs, prior to marketing, and after 1962, manufacturers had to prove both safety and that a proposed new drug would have the effect it purports to have or is represented to have.

Despite the laws, the FDA has appeared relatively powerless to prevent harmful and/or ineffective drugs from proliferating. It has been plagued by the tremendous influence exerted by manufacturers through drug advertising, lobbying, and political connections. Efforts by the FDA to include informative patient package inserts with, for example, intrauterine devices (Federal Register, 1975), estrogenic drugs (Federal Register, 1976), oral contraceptives (Federal Register, 1976), and progestins (Federal Register, 1978), have been greeted with accusations of interfering with the doctor-patient relationship, of destroying patients' trust in their physicians, of increasing self-diagnosis and self-medication, and, in the case of estrogenic drugs, with a suit by the American College of Obstetricians and Gynecologists (Schmidt, 1977).

current legislative issues

federal funding for sterilization

In response to blatant and tragic examples of sterilization abuse under federally funded programs, specifically the sterilization of the adolescent Relf sisters in Alabama (Relf v. Weinberger, 1974) and cases of coerced sterilization in South Carolina (Federal Register, 1978), DHEW in 1973 proposed guidelines to end these practices. Other examples of abuse, such as those at Los Angeles County University of Southern California Women's Hospital (Madrigal v. Quilligan, 1975), among Native American women (U.S. Gen. Acctg., 1976), and in Puerto Rico (Vazquez-Calzada, 1973), lent support to these DHEW guidelines.

Response was slow to the guidelines that initially established a moratorium on sterilization of people under 21 years of age and of those who could not legally consent. It was found in 1975 that only about 6 percent of the nation's teaching hospitals were in compliance (McGarraugh, 1975). After court challenges against the legitimacy of the guidelines, including an unsuccessful one against a similar proposal in New York City (Gordon v. Holloman, 1976), DHEW prevailed and issued new regulations on November 8, 1978, effective February 6, 1979 (Federal Register, 1978). These regulations try to strike a balance between assuring access to sterilization and preventing coercion or abuse. For an institution to receive federal funding, the guidelines require that a consent form describing the risks, benefits, and contraceptive alternatives to sterilization must be presented both orally and in writing and in a language understood by the patient. Assurances also have to be included stating that no federal benefits will be lost if the patient refuses. Those receiving a federally funded sterilization must be at least 21 years old, mentally competent, and have given consent voluntarily; consent may not have been obtained during labor or an abortion, or when the patient is under the influence of alcohol or drugs. At least 30 days (pre-

artment of Health, New York, 1931, p. 64–65. Cited y Blake, J.B.: 1977 op cit.

dwin, E.R.: *A Tabular Statement of Infant Welfare Vork by Public and Private Agencies in the United tates*. Infant Mortality Series No. 5., U.S. Children's ureau, U.S. Government Printing Office, Washington, D.C., 1916.

Children's Bureau: *Baby-Saving Campaigns: A Preiminary Report on What American Cities are Doing o Prevent Infant Mortality*. Infant Mortality Series No. 1, U.S. Children's Bureau, U.S. Government Printing Office, Washington, D.C. 1913.

e, J.B.: 1977 op cit.

DHEW Health Services Administration, Bureau of Community Health Services. *Maternal and Child Health Programs' Legislative Base*. U.S. Government Printing Office, Washington, D.C., 1977. Source: Rules and Regulations for Title V of the Social Security Act, Subpart A of Part 51a as amended on November 20, 1975. *Federal Register*, Vol. 40, No. 225, November 20, 1975.

urces: *Final Mortality Statistics and Vital Statistics of the U.S. II*, 1915–1977, Division of Vital Statistics, National Center for Health Statistics, DHEW, Washington, D.C. *Vital Statistics of the U.S. I*, 1974. Additional Data from National Center for Health Statistics, Washington, D.C., Personal Communication, 1979.

nai, N. and Anderson, O.W.: *EMIC (Emergency Maternity and Infant Care): A Study of Administrative Experience*. Arno Press, New York, 1974.

ulligan, J.E.: *Three Federal Interventions on Behalf of Childbearing Women. The Sheppard-Towner Act, Emergency Maternity and Infant Care and The Maternal and Child Health and Mental Retardation Amendments of 1963*. Doctoral Dissertation, University of Michigan, Ann Arbor, Michigan, 1976.

.S. Congress, House Subcommittee on Appropriations. Hearings on the First Supplemental National Defense Appropriation Bill, 1944, 78th. Congress, 1st. Session, September 21, 1943.

HEW *Maternal and Child Health Programs' Legislative Base*: 1977 op cit.

Madison, D.L.: Organized Health Care and the Poor. *Medical Care Review*, Vol. 26, No. 8: 783-807, August, 1969.

Gold, E.M. and Stone, M.L.: Total Maternal and Infant Care: A Realistic Appraisal. *American Journal of Public Health*, Vol. 58, No. 7: 1219-1299, July, 1968.

Pardee, R., Deputy Director, Office of Maternal and Child Health, Bureau of Community Health Services, DHEW, Washington, D.C. Personal Communication, April, 1979.

Executive Office of the President, Office of Management and Budget. *1978 Catalog of Federal Domestic Assistance*. U.S. Government Printing Office, Washington, D.C., May, 1978. No. 13.233, p. 161.

Marshall, J.K.: cited in The Role of HEW's Bureau of Community Health Services. *Women's Health Roundtable Report*, Vol. II, No. 5, May/June, 1978.

Pardee, R.: April, 1979 op cit.

Executive Office of the President: 1978 op cit: 13.260, p. 175

Ibid: 13.864, p. 388.

Torres, A.: Organized Family Planning Services in the United States, 1968-1976, *Family Planning Perspectives*, Vol. 10, No. 2:83-88, March-April, 1978.

Donabedian, A. and Thorby, J.A.: The Systemic Impact of Medicare. *Medical Care Review*, Vol. 26, No. 6:567-585, June, 1969.

Somers, H.M. and Somers, A.R.: *Medicare and the Hospitals: Issues and Prospects*. The Brookings Institution, Washington, D.C., 1967.

Department of Health, Education and Welfare: *Health United States, 1978*. DHEW, Washington, D.C., 1978 No. (PHS) 78-1232.

Abortion and the Poor: Private Morality, Public Responsibility. Alan Guttmacher Institute, New York, 1979.

Executive Office of the President: 1978 op cit: 10.557, p. 47.

McIntosh, D., Supplemental Food Programs Division, Department of Agriculture, Washington, D.C. Personal Communication, May 4, 1979.

Executive Office of the President: 1978 op cit: 10.551, p. 42.

Younger, M. and Hickman, P., Food and Nutrition Service, Department of Agriculture, Washington, D.C. Personal Communications, May 11, 1979.

Executive Office of the President: 1978 op cit: 10.550, p. 41

Ibid: 10.558, p. 48.

Ibid: 53.001, p. 754.

Ibid: 13.635, p. 325.

Ibid: 13.228, p. 157.

Ibid: 23.004, p. 632.

See *The Congressional Clearinghouse on Women's Rights. Domestic Violence Legislation*, Vol. 4, No. 8, Washington, D. C., May 22, 1978.

Comprehensive Employment and Training Act, 1973.

Executive Office of the President: 1978 op cit: 13.679, p. 340.

vious regulations stipulated 72 hours), but not more than 180, must elapse between signing the consent and the performance of the operation. This may be reduced to a 72-hour time interval in cases of premature delivery or emergency abdominal surgery. Consent of spouse is not required. Federal funding will not be allowed for sterilization performed on persons in correctional facilities, mental hospitals, or other rehabilitative facilities, or for hysterectomies performed solely for purposes of "rendering the person permanently incapable of reproduction." Adequate records of compliance must be maintained, and in three years DHEW will review the guidelines. DHEW states that a special monitoring program will be conducted to insure compliance, but no sanctions for noncompliance are outlined in the regulations (Federal Register, 1978; Wolcott, 1978).

federal funding for abortions

Although a few states repealed their abortion laws in the late 1960s and early 1970s, it was not until the Supreme Court ruling on January 22, 1973 that abortion became legally available throughout the United States (Roe v. Wade, 1973; Doe et al. v. Bolton, 1973). Medicaid funding for abortions also became available. In 1977, for example, nearly 295,000 Medicaid eligible women obtained abortions although another 133,000 eligible women who wanted them, did not (Abortion, 1979).

In 1976, an active campaign was begun by abortion opponents to prohibit use of Medicaid funds, leading to the introduction by Representative Henry Hyde (Illinois) of an amendment to the Labor-DHEW appropriations bill prohibiting funds for this purpose for the fiscal year 1977. After substantial de-

bate, the House-Senate compromise permitted federal funds for abortion only in those cases where "the life of the mother would be endangered if the fetus were carried to term." An injunction prevented the amendment taking effect until August 4, 1977.

Other campaigns to prohibit funding began at the state level, and suits to overturn these prohibitions were denied by the Supreme Court on June 20, 1977. The Court upheld the right of states to withhold state Medicaid funds for abortion, ruling that "The Equal Protection Clause (of the Constitution) does not require a state participating in the Medicaid program to pay the expenses incident to non-therapeutic abortion for indigent women simply because it has made a policy choice to pay expenses for childbirth (Maher v. Roe, 1977; Beal v. Doe, 1977). The Court also decided that nontherapeutic abortion services did not have to be provided by public hospitals (Poelker v. Doe, 1977). In each year since the Hyde Amendment, similar amendments have been proposed, and each has been progressively more restrictive.

By 1979, the House voted to allow Medicaid funds for abortions only to save the woman's life. Since 1977, Medicaid funding for abortions has decreased by 99 percent (only 2,421 abortions were paid for by Medicaid as compared with about 300,000 in 1977); the 1979 actions by the House reduced even this 1 percent. Funding for abortions for military personnel and dependents through federal health plans was also abolished in 1978, and a similar amendment to the Defense Appropriations Bill was proposed for fiscal year 1979.

State actions have continued to follow the federal trend. As of February, 1979, 18 states still funded abortions, not only according to the 1978 federal criteria for rape or incest victims, to save a woman's life, or to prevent long-lasting physical health damage to a woman, but also for women whose mental health would be endangered if the pregnancy were carried to term, for women who know their children will be born seriously deformed or diseased, for women who know that their child will be so deformed that it will die soon after birth, and for older and young women who are outside appropriate childbearing years. The Hyde Amendment prohibits federal Medicaid funds for all women in these latter categories.

Abortion opponents, in addition to harassment of abortion clinics and women who have had abortions, have also sought to call a Constitutional Convention for the purpose of amending the Constitution to outlaw abortion (Beals, 1979). They have been joined by almost one-third of the states and pose a determined threat to Pro-Choice apathy.

pregnancy disability

In 1976, Congress was asked to clarify the Congressional intent of Title VII of the Civil Rights Act with regard to the inclusion of maternity benefits on company-sponsored disability plans. Congress resolved that employment discrimination does include pregnancy, and by an amendment to the Civil Rights Act, effective October 31, 1978, they required that employers with disability benefit plans must treat pregnancy in the same way as any other disability covered by the plan. The law also stipulated that women affected by pregnancy and related conditions be treated the same as any other employee on the basis of the ability or inability to work. Pregnant women cannot, therefore, be fired or forced to go on sick leave if they can establish ability to work. In addition, pregnancy-related absences would not cause loss of seniority benefits (Bunch, 1979).

By means of a compromise subamendment, employers have the discretion to exclude abortion coverage in their health and disability plans except where the life of the mother would be endangered if the fetus were carried to term. Although abortion costs specifically can be excluded, costs incurred from abortion complications cannot be excluded and disability or sick leave benefits must be paid for the duration of the complications (Beard Amendment). This amendment was the object of a class suit in June 1979, however, by the United States Catholic Conference and the National Conference of Catholic Bishops. They seek to allow employers who have objections to abortion on moral, religious, or ethical grounds exemption from this amendment and to disallow coverage for abortion-related disability (Werner, 1979).

equal rights amendment

Since 1923, basically identical equal rights amendments have been introduced to nearly every Congress. These amendments stipulate that the law cannot treat men and women any differently solely because of their sex (Bonsaro, 1978). Specifically, the current amendment states:

Section 1. Equality of rights under the law shall not be denied or abridged by the United States or any State on account of sex.

Section 2. The Congress shall have the power to enforce, by appropriate legislation, the provisions of this article.

Section 3. This amendment shall take effect two years after the date of ratification (Res. 208, 1971).

Passage of the ERA would particularly benefit

women's job opportunities and security, athletic opportunities, and would mandate recognition of the equal obligations of both parents to support their children. Women's economic rights within the family, the criminal laws, educational opportunities, and eligibility for the armed forces and their benefits would also be affected.

Spurious arguments of coed toilets, homosexual marriage, and forced abortion have been used to cloud the issues of the ERA, with the result that as of 1979, only 35 of the necessary 38 states had ratified it. A 39-month extension for ratification was passed in late 1978.

national health insurance

Since the early 1900s, national health insurance for the United States has been proposed; currently there are several proposals before Congress (Lewis, 1976), and all but one are forms of health insurance plans that would not alter the delivery of health care services, but would, to varying degrees, modify the current methods of payment. The Health Care Service Act (Committee for A National Health Service) is unique in proposing to alter the mode of delivery by nationalizing health care facilities and by making providers employees of the National Health Service.

Women's health issues must be carefully evaluated in national health insurance proposals to insure the inclusion of complete maternity services, including contraception, abortion, genetic counseling, childbirth education, coverage for choice of alternative providers, such as midwives and family practice physicians, coverage for home health services now generally provided by unpaid female relatives, recognition and coverage of women's use of two basic physicians, an internist and an obstetrician-gynecologist, and

adequate mental health s...
support services for sexual a...
abused wives. Most importa...
tive that coverage for wome...
health insurance be indepe...
ment or any marital or livi...
Despite discussions and fanf...
health insurance program a...
as of 1981.

The complex, noncompre...
verse nature of federally funde...
gether with their enormous co...
a more rational means of dist...
health services for women ...
lished. Although the program...
this chapter have benefited m...
en, the maintenance of a dual h...
public and private sectors serve...
nation's health resources rather...
mize them for the common good...

Howe, I.: *World of Our Fathers.* Sim... New York, 1976

Davis, A.: *American Heroine. The Lif...* Jane Addams. Oxford University P... 1973.

Duffus, R.L.: *Lillian Wald: Neighbor...* MacMillan, New York, 1938.

U.S. DHEW: *Final Mortality Statistics an...* of the U.S., II, 1915–1977, Division of... National Center for Health Statistics, ... ington, D.C., 1979.

U.S. Department of Labor. *Infant Mortalit...* ter, New Hampshire. Infant Mortality... Children's Bureau Publication #20,... D.C., 1917.

Blake, J.B.: Origins of Maternal and Child... grams. In *The Health of Women and Chi...* krantz, B.G., Ed. Arno Press, New York,...

Rosen, G.: The First Neighborhood Health C... ment—Its Rise and Fall. *American Journ...* Health, Vol. 61, No. 8:1620–1637, August...

Goler, G.W.: Methods Adopted by the Boar... at Rochester, New York, to Secure Better ... fants. *Archives of Pediatrics,* Vol. XIV:845,...

Blake, J.B.: 1977 op cit.

Blake, J.B.: *Historical Study of the New Yor...*

Von Bargen, P., et al., Eds.: *Health Career Opportunity Grants for the Disadvantaged.* Health Resources Opportunity Programs, Department of Health, Education and Welfare, Washington, D.C., February, 1978. No. (HRA) 78-624.

Effective November 7, 1977. See: Intrauterine Contraceptive Device: Professional and Patient Labeling. *Federal Register*, Vol. 40, No. 127:27796, July, 1975.

Effective October 18, 1977. See: Drugs for Human Use: Estrogens and Other Drugs. *Federal Register*, Vol. 41, No. 190:43108, Sept. 29, 1976.

Effective April 4, 1978. See: Oral Contraceptive Drug Products: Physician and Patient Labeling. *Federal Register*, Vol. 41, No. 236: 53633, Dec. 7, 1976.

Effective December 12, 1978. See: Requirements for Patient Labeling for Progestational Drug Products. *Federal Register*, Vol. 43, No. 199:47181, October 13, 1978.

Schmidt, R.T.F.:ACOG President Explains Suit. *ACOG Newletter*, Vol. 21, No. 9:4, September, 1977.

Relf v. Weinberger, 372 Federal Supplement 1196 (D.D.C., 1974)

Cited in Sterilizations and Abortions: Federal Financial Participation. *Federal Register*, Vol. 43, No. 217, 52146, Wednesday, Nov. 8, 1978.

Madrigal v. Quilligan, CA, No. 75-2057, C.C.D. Cal., 1975

U.S. General Accounting Office Report to Hon. James C. Abourezk, B. 164031 (5), November, 1976.

Vazquez-Calzada, J.: La Esterilizacion Femenina en Puerto Rico, *Revista de Ciencias Sociales*, Vol. 17, No. 3: 281-308, September, 1973.

McGarraugh, R.E.: *Sterilization Without Consent: Teaching Hospital Violation of HEW Regulations.* Public Citizen's Health Research Group, Washington, D.C., January, 1975.

Gordon, W. Douglas, M.D., et al. v. John L.S. Holloman, Jr., et al. Civil Action File No. 76, Cw 6

U.S. District Court, January 5, 1976.

Sterilizations and Abortions. *Federal Register*, Vol. 43:52146, 1978, *op cit.*

Ibid

Wolcott, I., Ed.: Regulations Covering All Federally Funded Sterilizations. *Women & Health Roundtable Report*, Vol. II, No. 11, November, 1978.

Roe v. Wade, No. 70-18, January 22, 1973.

Doe, el al., v. Bolton, No. 70-40, January 22, 1973.

Alan Guttmacher Institute: 1979 *op cit.*

Maher v. Roe, June 20, 1977.

Beal v. Doe, June 20, 1977.

Poelker v. Doe, June 20, 1977.

Beals, J.: Current Issues Facing the Right to Abortion. *Women & Health*, Vol. 4, No. 1: 107-109, Spring, 1979.

Bunch, P.L., et al: The Pregnant Worker—Who Bears the Burden? *Women & Health*, Vol. 4, No. 4:333-344, 1979.

Beard Amendment by Edward Beard, Dem., Rhode Island.

Werner, C.: Pregnancy Disability Law: Round Two. *NARAL Newsletter*. Vol. II, No. 6:6, August, 1979.

Bonsaro, C., Ed.: *Statement on The Equal Rights Amendment.* United States Commission on Civil Rights, U.S. Government Printing House, December, 1978. Clearinghouse Publication 56.

H.R.J. Res. 208, 2nd Congress, 1st. Session, 86 Stat. 1523 (1971).

Lewis, D.: Women and National Health Insurance: Issues and Solutions. *Medical Care*, Vol. XIV, No. 7: 549-558, July, 1976.

Committee for a National Health Service. *A National Health Service—Questions and Answers*, New York, 1975. P.O. Box 2125, New York, New York 10001.

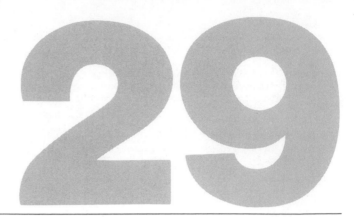

SHERRY L. SHAMANSKY R.N.,
Dr. P.H.

personal power assessment

once upon a parable

The woman refused to put up with her "lemon." It took almost a year, but she succeeded in the struggle to have her money refunded. She suspected that her new car, a $5,500 Volkswagen Rabbit, was a sick creature soon after she drove it home on November 11, 1976. She pushed the horn button and the windshield wipers went on. The radio produced little but static. By the time she reached home, the new car had lost nearly all its power. It had to be towed for service, and the alternator had to be replaced, the first of three replacements. In the next nine months she made some two dozen trips to the dealer for various and sundry repairs. From the begin-

ning, the driver's window would not close completely. The door lock button pulled out of the door on five different occasions. The ever-present vibrations were a symphony of sounds. The catalytic converter was replaced twice, as were the battery, the starter, and the distributor cap. Additionally, there was a leak in the gas line, the snow tires developed tumors, and so it went. She was without the car nine weeks of those nine months. The behavior of the service department was outrageous: "Of course *you* must be doing something wrong—we've never had this problem before!"

The woman initiated action early on. She

confronted the owner of the dealership—to no avail. He clucked conciliatory and patronizing sounds: "Now, dear, we can't have you so upset, can we?" Undaunted, she wrote to the president of Volkswagen Worldwide and sent copies of the letter to the Federal Trade Commission in Washington, D.C.; the state department of consumer protection; the motor vehicles department; AUTOCAP, a national consumers' group; and, finally, to NBC TV's "Action-Line." The numerous responses ranged from overtly hostile to sympathetic; all were unhelpful. As a last resort, the woman consulted a lawyer. It seemed that the conditions set forth in the Magnuson-Moss Warranty Rule governed the manufacture and repair of this car, and in late summer 1977 suit was filed against Volkswagen of America and the local dealership. Within three days, attorneys for Volkswagen proposed an out-of-court settlement. The woman returned her Rabbit and received a check in the amount of $7,500 for the cost of the car and damages that included mental anguish. The woman now drives a Ford.

That woman is the author of this chapter. This is a true story, and I wish I could include it on my resume because I consider it to be one of my most effective uses of personal power— one woman against a corporate giant!

This chapter is about power and, more specifically, about personal power. Why, the reader might ask, is a discussion of personal power included in a book such as this? The literature is replete with lengthy treatises on power and powerlessness among women in today's society. Our feelings of self-worth, pride, guilt, anger, hope, and many other emotions have their roots in the effective use of personal power. Many of us have felt powerless—indeed, victimized—in the face of the health care system. Taking care of ourselves necessitates the exercise of personal power.

It is the intent of this chapter to provide a forum whereby the reader can develop a concept of power that is personally meaningful and useful to her, to explore some of the issues that are believed to contribute to power as a construct, to use the instruments included here (crude and unscientific as they might be) to assess and value one's personal power, and to provide a basis for further thought and discussion. It might be noted that many of these remarks about power are applicable to men as well as women.

The word *power* is highly charged for many people. It connotes dominance and submission, control and acquiescence, or the exertion of one person's will over another. Power may be based on skill, strength, or circumstance. It has been said that power differentiates the "haves" from the "have-nots." One's attainment of power may be at the expense of another. Inherent in this process is conflict. Various theoreticians have suggested that a little conflict is a good thing and that dissonance is a prerequisite for growth.

On the next page is a test with adjectives describing power. Your own score will be of interest as you read through the rest of this chapter.

commonality in thinking

The imposition of rigid definitions is an expression of power on the part of the definer and the acceptance of power by those who choose to use the proposed definitions. The potential conflict inherent during communication that follows without a common under-

test instructions

The purpose of this test is to measure the meanings you associate with the word *power*. You will rate this word on a series of scales. Select your answer on the basis of what the word *power* means *to you*.

This is how to use these scales: If you feel that the word *power* is *very closely related* to one end of the scale, circle as follows:

black (+3) : +2 : +1 : 0 : −1 : −2 : −3 white

black +3 : +2 : +1 : 0 : −1 : −2 : (−3) white

If you feel that the word *power* is *quite closely related* to one end of the scale (but not extremely so), circle as follows:

black +3 : (+2) : +1 : 0 : −1 : −2 : −3 white

black +3 : +2 : +1 : 0 : −1 : (−2) : −3 white

If you feel that the word *power* is *only slightly related* to one side as opposed to the other side (but not really neutral), circle as follows:

black +3 : +2 : (+1) : 0 : −1 : −2 : −3 white

black +3 : +2 : +1 : 0 : (−1) : −2 : −3 white

If you feel that the word *power* is *neutral* on the scale, (that is, both sides of the scale are equally associated with the word), or if the scale is *completely irrelevant* and unrelated to the word, place your circle in the middle space:

black +3 : +2 : +1 : (0) : −1 : −2 : −3 white

---

standing of language may be more harmful than is the restriction of definition. Therefore, some basic terminology may be helpful.

> *Power:* The ability and willingness to affect the behavior of others; such ability is based on a realistic appraisal of one's own strengths and areas for growth. Willingness is based on positive energy. A powerful person seems to radiate an energetic glow, uses her own potential fully, and sees the strengths in others. Power is also based on positive results and actions. Power is one person's degree of influence over another (Claus & Bailey, 1977).

> *Leadership:* The exercise of power, directed through the communication process toward the attainment of a goal.

> *Authority:* The right to take action.

> *Influence:* The capacity or act or power to produce an effect without apparent force. This action implies an acceptance on the part of others.

vious regulations stipulated 72 hours), but not more than 180, must elapse between signing the consent and the performance of the operation. This may be reduced to a 72-hour time interval in cases of premature delivery or emergency abdominal surgery. Consent of spouse is not required. Federal funding will not be allowed for sterilization performed on persons in correctional facilities, mental hospitals, or other rehabilitative facilities, or for hysterectomies performed solely for purposes of "rendering the person permanently incapable of reproduction." Adequate records of compliance must be maintained, and in three years DHEW will review the guidelines. DHEW states that a special monitoring program will be conducted to insure compliance, but no sanctions for noncompliance are outlined in the regulations (Federal Register, 1978; Wolcott, 1978).

federal funding for abortions

Although a few states repealed their abortion laws in the late 1960s and early 1970s, it was not until the Supreme Court ruling on January 22, 1973 that abortion became legally available throughout the United States (Roe v. Wade, 1973; Doe et al. v. Bolton, 1973). Medicaid funding for abortions also became available. In 1977, for example, nearly 295,000 Medicaid eligible women obtained abortions although another 133,000 eligible women who wanted them, did not (Abortion, 1979).

In 1976, an active campaign was begun by abortion opponents to prohibit use of Medicaid funds, leading to the introduction by Representative Henry Hyde (Illinois) of an amendment to the Labor-DHEW appropriations bill prohibiting funds for this purpose for the fiscal year 1977. After substantial de-

bate, the House-Senate compromise permitted federal funds for abortion only in those cases where "the life of the mother would be endangered if the fetus were carried to term." An injunction prevented the amendment taking effect until August 4, 1977.

Other campaigns to prohibit funding began at the state level, and suits to overturn these prohibitions were denied by the Supreme Court on June 20, 1977. The Court upheld the right of states to withhold state Medicaid funds for abortion, ruling that "The Equal Protection Clause (of the Constitution) does not require a state participating in the Medicaid program to pay the expenses incident to non-therapeutic abortion for indigent women simply because it has made a policy choice to pay expenses for childbirth (Maher v. Roe, 1977; Beal v. Doe, 1977). The Court also decided that nontherapeutic abortion services did not have to be provided by public hospitals (Poelker v. Doe, 1977). In each year since the Hyde Amendment, similar amendments have been proposed, and each has been progressively more restrictive.

By 1979, the House voted to allow Medicaid funds for abortions only to save the woman's life. Since 1977, Medicaid funding for abortions has decreased by 99 percent (only 2,421 abortions were paid for by Medicaid as compared with about 300,000 in 1977); the 1979 actions by the House reduced even this 1 percent. Funding for abortions for military personnel and dependents through federal health plans was also abolished in 1978, and a similar amendment to the Defense Appropriations Bill was proposed for fiscal year 1979.

State actions have continued to follow the federal trend. As of February, 1979, 18 states still funded abortions, not only according to the 1978 federal criteria for rape or incest victims, to save a woman's life, or to prevent long-lasting physical health damage to a woman, but also for women whose mental health would be endangered if the pregnancy were carried to term, for women who know their children will be born seriously deformed or diseased, for women who know that their child will be so deformed that it will die soon after birth, and for older and young women who are outside appropriate childbearing years. The Hyde Amendment prohibits federal Medicaid funds for all women in these latter categories.

Abortion opponents, in addition to harassment of abortion clinics and women who have had abortions, have also sought to call a Constitutional Convention for the purpose of amending the Constitution to outlaw abortion (Beals, 1979). They have been joined by almost one-third of the states and pose a determined threat to Pro-Choice apathy.

pregnancy disability

In 1976, Congress was asked to clarify the Congressional intent of Title VII of the Civil Rights Act with regard to the inclusion of maternity benefits on company-sponsored disability plans. Congress resolved that employment discrimination does include pregnancy, and by an amendment to the Civil Rights Act, effective October 31, 1978, they required that employers with disability benefit plans must treat pregnancy in the same way as any other disability covered by the plan. The law also stipulated that women affected by pregnancy and related conditions be treated the same as any other employee on the basis of the ability or inability to work. Pregnant women cannot, therefore, be fired or forced to go on sick leave if they can establish ability to work. In addition, pregnancy-related absences would not cause loss of seniority benefits (Bunch, 1979).

By means of a compromise subamendment, employers have the discretion to exclude abortion coverage in their health and disability plans except where the life of the mother would be endangered if the fetus were carried to term. Although abortion costs specifically can be excluded, costs incurred from abortion complications cannot be excluded and disability or sick leave benefits must be paid for the duration of the complications (Beard Amendment). This amendment was the object of a class suit in June 1979, however, by the United States Catholic Conference and the National Conference of Catholic Bishops. They seek to allow employers who have objections to abortion on moral, religious, or ethical grounds exemption from this amendment and to disallow coverage for abortion-related disability (Werner, 1979).

equal rights amendment

Since 1923, basically identical equal rights amendments have been introduced to nearly every Congress. These amendments stipulate that the law cannot treat men and women any differently solely because of their sex (Bonsaro, 1978). Specifically, the current amendment states:

Section 1. Equality of rights under the law shall not be denied or abridged by the United States or any State on account of sex.

Section 2. The Congress shall have the power to enforce, by appropriate legislation, the provisions of this article.

Section 3. This amendment shall take effect two years after the date of ratification (Res. 208, 1971).

Passage of the ERA would particularly benefit

women's job opportunities and security, athletic opportunities, and would mandate recognition of the equal obligations of both parents to support their children. Women's economic rights within the family, the criminal laws, educational opportunities, and eligibility for the armed forces and their benefits would also be affected.

Spurious arguments of coed toilets, homosexual marriage, and forced abortion have been used to cloud the issues of the ERA, with the result that as of 1979, only 35 of the necessary 38 states had ratified it. A 39-month extension for ratification was passed in late 1978.

national health insurance

Since the early 1900s, national health insurance for the United States has been proposed; currently there are several proposals before Congress (Lewis, 1976), and all but one are forms of health insurance plans that would not alter the delivery of health care services, but would, to varying degrees, modify the current methods of payment. The Health Care Service Act (Committee for A National Health Service) is unique in proposing to alter the mode of delivery by nationalizing health care facilities and by making providers employees of the National Health Service.

Women's health issues must be carefully evaluated in national health insurance proposals to insure the inclusion of complete maternity services, including contraception, abortion, genetic counseling, childbirth education, coverage for choice of alternative providers, such as midwives and family practice physicians, coverage for home health services now generally provided by unpaid female relatives, recognition and coverage of women's use of two basic physicians, an internist and an obstetrician-gynecologist, and

adequate mental health services, including support services for sexual assault victims and abused wives. Most importantly, it is imperative that coverage for women under national health insurance be independent of employment or any marital or living arrangements. Despite discussions and fanfare, no national health insurance program appears imminent as of 1981.

The complex, noncomprehensive, and diverse nature of federally funded programs, together with their enormous costs, suggest that a more rational means of distributing needed health services for women must be established. Although the programs discussed in this chapter have benefited millions of women, the maintenance of a dual health system of public and private sectors serves to divide the nation's health resources rather than to maximize them for the common good.

Howe, I.: *World of Our Fathers.* Simon and Schuster, New York, 1976

Davis, A.: *American Heroine. The Life and Legend of Jane Addams.* Oxford University Press, New York, 1973.

Duffus, R.L.: *Lillian Wald: Neighbor and Crusader.* MacMillan, New York, 1938.

U.S. DHEW: *Final Mortality Statistics and Vital Statistics of the U.S., II, 1915–1977,* Division of Vital Statistics, National Center for Health Statistics, DHEW, Washington, D.C., 1979.

U.S. Department of Labor. *Infant Mortality in Manchester, New Hampshire.* Infant Mortality Series No. 6, Children's Bureau Publication #20, Washington, D.C., 1917.

Blake, J.B.: Origins of Maternal and Child Health Programs. In *The Health of Women and Children,* Rosenkrantz, B.G., Ed. Arno Press, New York, 1977.

Rosen, G.: The First Neighborhood Health Center Movement—Its Rise and Fall. *American Journal of Public Health,* Vol. 61, No. 8:1620–1637, August, 1971.

Goler, G.W.: Methods Adopted by the Board of Health at Rochester, New York, to Secure Better Milk for Infants. *Archives of Pediatrics,* Vol. XIV:845, 1897.

Blake, J.B.: 1977 *op cit.*

Blake, J.B.: *Historical Study of the New York City De-*

partment of Health, New York, 1931, p. 64–65. Cited by Blake, J.B.: 1977 *op cit.*

Goodwin, E.R.: *A Tabular Statement of Infant Welfare Work by Public and Private Agencies in the United States.* Infant Mortality Series No. 5., U.S. Children's Bureau, U.S. Government Printing Office, Washington, D.C., 1916.

U.S. Children's Bureau: *Baby-Saving Campaigns: A Preliminary Report on What American Cities are Doing to Prevent Infant Mortality.* Infant Mortality Series No. 1, U.S. Children's Bureau, U.S. Government Printing Office, Washington, D.C. 1913.

Blake, J.B.: 1977 *op cit.*

U.S. DHEW Health Services Administration, Bureau of Community Health Services. *Maternal and Child Health Programs' Legislative Base.* U.S. Government Printing Office, Washington, D.C., 1977. Source: Rules and Regulations for Title V of the Social Security Act, Subpart A of Part 51a as amended on November 20, 1975. *Federal Register,* Vol. 40, No. 225, November 20, 1975.

Sources: *Final Mortality Statistics and Vital Statistics of the U.S. II,* 1915-1977, Division of Vital Statistics, National Center for Health Statistics, DHEW, Washington, D.C. *Vital Statistics of the U.S. I,* 1974. Additional Data from National Center for Health Statistics, Washington, D.C., Personal Communication, 1979.

Sinai, N. and Anderson, O.W.: *EMIC (Emergency Maternity and Infant Care): A Study of Administrative Experience.* Arno Press, New York, 1974.

Mulligan, J.E.: *Three Federal Interventions on Behalf of Childbearing Women. The Sheppard-Towner Act, Emergency Maternity and Infant Care and The Maternal and Child Health and Mental Retardation Amendments of 1963.* Doctoral Dissertation, University of Michigan, Ann Arbor, Michigan, 1976.

U.S. Congress, House Subcommittee on Appropriations. Hearings on the First Supplemental National Defense Appropriation Bill, 1944, 78th. Congress, 1st. Session, September 21, 1943.

DHEW *Maternal and Child Health Programs' Legislative Base:* 1977 *op cit.*

Madison, D.L.: Organized Health Care and the Poor. *Medical Care Review,* Vol. 26, No. 8: 783-807, August, 1969.

Gold, E.M. and Stone, M.L.: Total Maternal and Infant Care: A Realistic Appraisal. *American Journal of Public Health,* Vol. 58, No. 7: 1219-1299, July, 1968.

Pardee, R., Deputy Director, Office of Maternal and Child Health, Bureau of Community Health Services, DHEW, Washington, D.C. Personal Communication, April, 1979.

Executive Office of the President, Office of Management and Budget. *1978 Catalog of Federal Domestic Assistance.* U.S. Government Printing Office, Washington, D.C., May, 1978. No. 13.233, p. 161.

Marshall, J.K.: cited in The Role of HEW's Bureau of Community Health Services. *Women's Health Roundtable Report,* Vol. II, No. 5, May/June, 1978.

Pardee, R.: April, 1979 *op cit.*

Executive Office of the President: 1978 *op cit:* 13.260, p. 175

Ibid: 13.864, p. 388.

Torres, A.: Organized Family Planning Services in the United States, 1968-1976, *Family Planning Perspectives,* Vol. 10, No. 2:83-88, March-April, 1978.

Donabedian, A. and Thorby, J.A.: The Systemic Impact of Medicare. *Medical Care Review,* Vol. 26, No. 6:567-585, June, 1969.

Somers, H.M. and Somers, A.R.: *Medicare and the Hospitals: Issues and Prospects.* The Brookings Institution, Washington, D.C., 1967.

Department of Health, Education and Welfare: *Health United States, 1978.* DHEW, Washington, D.C., 1978 No. (PHS) 78-1232.

Abortion and the Poor: Private Morality, Public Responsibility. Alan Guttmacher Institute, New York, 1979.

Executive Office of the President: 1978 *op cit:* 10.557, p. 47.

McIntosh, D., Supplemental Food Programs Division, Department of Agriculture, Washington, D.C. Personal Communication, May 4, 1979.

Executive Office of the President: 1978 *op cit:* 10.551, p. 42.

Younger, M. and Hickman, P., Food and Nutrition Service, Department of Agriculture, Washington, D.C. Personal Communications, May 11, 1979.

Executive Office of the President: 1978 *op cit:* 10.550, p. 41

Ibid: 10.558, p. 48.

Ibid: 53.001, p. 754.

Ibid: 13.635, p. 325.

Ibid: 13.228, p. 157.

Ibid: 23.004, p. 632.

See *The Congressional Clearinghouse on Women's Rights. Domestic Violence Legislation,* Vol. 4, No. 8, Washington, D. C., May 22, 1978.

Comprehensive Employment and Training Act, 1973.

Executive Office of the President: 1978 *op cit:* 13.679, p. 340.

Von Bargen, P., et al., Eds.: *Health Career Opportunity Grants for the Disadvantaged.* Health Resources Opportunity Programs, Department of Health, Education and Welfare, Washington, D.C., February, 1978. No. (HRA) 78-624.

Effective November 7, 1977. See: Intrauterine Contraceptive Device: Professional and Patient Labeling. *Federal Register,* Vol. 40, No. 127:27796, July, 1975.

Effective October 18, 1977. See: Drugs for Human Use: Estrogens and Other Drugs. *Federal Register,* Vol. 41, No. 190:43108, Sept. 29, 1976.

Effective April 4, 1978. See: Oral Contraceptive Drug Products: Physician and Patient Labeling. *Federal Register,* Vol. 41, No. 236: 53633, Dec. 7, 1976.

Effective December 12, 1978. See: Requirements for Patient Labeling for Progestational Drug Products. *Federal Register,* Vol. 43, No. 199:47181, October 13, 1978.

Schmidt, R.T.F.:ACOG President Explains Suit. *ACOG Newsletter,* Vol. 21, No. 9:4, September, 1977.

Relf v. Weinberger, 372 Federal Supplement 1196 (D.D.C., 1974)

Cited in Sterilizations and Abortions: Federal Financial Participation. *Federal Register,* Vol. 43, No. 217, 52146, Wednesday, Nov. 8, 1978.

Madrigal v. Quilligan, CA, No. 75-2057, C.C.D. Cal., 1975

U.S. General Accounting Office Report to Hon. James C. Abourezk, B. 164031 (5), November, 1976.

Vazquez-Calzada, J.: La Esterilizacion Femenina en Puerto Rico, *Revista de Ciencias Sociales,* Vol. 17, No. 3: 281-308, September, 1973.

McGarraugh, R.E.: *Sterilization Without Consent: Teaching Hospital Violation of HEW Regulations.* Public Citizen's Health Research Group, Washington, D.C., January, 1975.

Gordon, W. Douglas, M.D., et al. v. John L.S. Holloman, Jr., et al. Civil Action File No. 76, Cw 6

U.S. District Court, January 5, 1976.

Sterilizations and Abortions. *Federal Register,* Vol. 43:52146, 1978, *op cit.*

Ibid

Wolcott, I., Ed.: Regulations Covering All Federally Funded Sterilizations. *Women & Health Roundtable Report,* Vol. II, No. 11, November, 1978.

Roe v. Wade, No. 70-18, January 22, 1973.

Doe, el al., v. Bolton, No. 70-40, January 22, 1973.

Alan Guttmacher Institute: 1979 *op cit.*

Maher v. Roe, June 20, 1977.

Beal v. Doe, June 20, 1977.

Poelker v. Doe, June 20, 1977.

Beals, J.: Current Issues Facing the Right to Abortion. *Women & Health,* Vol. 4, No. 1: 107-109, Spring, 1979.

Bunch, P.L., et al: The Pregnant Worker—Who Bears the Burden? *Women & Health,* Vol. 4, No. 4:333-344, 1979.

Beard Amendment by Edward Beard, Dem., Rhode Island.

Werner, C.: Pregnancy Disability Law: Round Two. *NARAL Newsletter.* Vol. II, No. 6:6, August, 1979.

Bonsaro, C., Ed.: *Statement on The Equal Rights Amendment.* United States Commission on Civil Rights, U.S. Government Printing House, December, 1978. Clearinghouse Publication 56.

H.R.J. Res. 208, 2nd Congress, 1st. Session, 86 Stat. 1523 (1971).

Lewis, D.: Women and National Health Insurance: Issues and Solutions. *Medical Care,* Vol. XIV, No. 7: 549-558, July, 1976.

Committee for a National Health Service. *A National Health Service—Questions and Answers,* New York, 1975. P.O. Box 2125, New York, New York 10001.

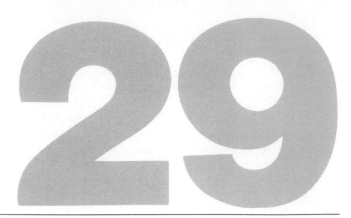

SHERRY L. SHAMANSKY R.N.,
Dr. P.H.

personal power assessment

once upon a parable

The woman refused to put up with her "lemon." It took almost a year, but she succeeded in the struggle to have her money refunded. She suspected that her new car, a $5,500 Volkswagen Rabbit, was a sick creature soon after she drove it home on November 11, 1976. She pushed the horn button and the windshield wipers went on. The radio produced little but static. By the time she reached home, the new car had lost nearly all its power. It had to be towed for service, and the alternator had to be replaced, the first of three replacements. In the next nine months she made some two dozen trips to the dealer for various and sundry repairs. From the begin-

ning, the driver's window would not close completely. The door lock button pulled out of the door on five different occasions. The ever-present vibrations were a symphony of sounds. The catalytic converter was replaced twice, as were the battery, the starter, and the distributor cap. Additionally, there was a leak in the gas line, the snow tires developed tumors, and so it went. She was without the car nine weeks of those nine months. The behavior of the service department was outrageous: "Of course *you* must be doing something wrong—we've never had this problem before!"

The woman initiated action early on. She

IMPORTANT:

1. Place your circles on one space only; do not circle two numbers

black   + 3 : (+ 2): + 1: 0 : − 1 : (− 2 : − 3) white

this (above +2), *not this* (above −2: −3)

2. Be sure to circle every scale—do not omit any.

3. Never put more than one circle on a single scale.

power is:

valuable	+ 3 : + 2: + 1: 0 : − 1: − 2: − 3	worthless
complete	+ 3 : + 2: + 1: 0 : − 1: − 2: − 3	incomplete
harmonious	+ 3 : + 2: + 1: 0 : − 1: − 2: − 3	dissonant
pleasant	+ 3 : + 2: + 1: 0 : − 1: − 2: − 3	unpleasant
beneficial	+ 3 : + 2: + 1: 0 : − 1: − 2: − 3	harmful
clean	+ 3 : + 2: + 1: 0 : − 1: − 2: − 3	dirty
fair	+ 3 : + 2: + 1: 0 : − 1: − 2: − 3	unfair
nice	+ 3 : + 2: + 1: 0 : − 1: − 2: − 3	awful
important	+ 3 : + 2: + 1: 0 : − 1: − 2: − 3	unimportant
comfortable	+ 3 : + 2: + 1: 0 : − 1: − 2: − 3	uncomfortable
kind	+ 3 : + 2: + 1: 0 : − 1: − 2: − 3	cruel
right	+ 3 : + 2: + 1: 0 : − 1: − 2: − 3	wrong

Now total the numerical values from each of the 12 items to find your score.

0–11:   You view power as a negative attribute.

12–24:   You view power as a neutral attribute.

25–36:   You view power as a positive attribute.

Assertiveness: The ability to stand up for one's rights without violating the rights of others or being excessively anxious about the consequences of one's behavior. Assertiveness is a set of skills that can be learned. Assertiveness is thinking and behaving in ways that maximize one's legitimate rights without detracting from the legitimate personal rights of others (Clark, 1979).

Aggressiveness: Aggressive behavior has an element of trying to control or manipulate others. Feelings or opinions often are ex- pressed in an accusatory, punishing, or hostile way. Aggressiveness suggests that one does what one wants regardless of the rights of others (Clark, 1979).

Success: Success is defined in terms of whether people get to do what they perceive as their work. Success can also be defined as the ability to function in a chosen avocation or profession with some measure of peer recognition. Commonly, there is also a sense of accomplishment, of goal attainment.

sources of social power

Where do we find or derive power? Six bases for social power have been identified by French and Raven (1968), social psychologists whose research suggested that the relationship between the person with power and the recipient of power (the one influenced) is of the greatest importance in establishing a power base.

The first basis of power is *reward.* A person perceives that compliance with the wishes of a superior will bring positive sanctions. Hence, reward power is based on the exercise of positive sanctions. Its corollary, and a second source of power, is *coercion,* which is based on fear. A person perceives that failure to comply with the wishes of a superior will lead to punishment. Coercive power involves negative sanctions such as threats of harm, withholding rewards, or other threats of punishment.

Legitimate power, the third basis for social power, stems from the recipient's belief that the person with power has a legitimate "right" to that power and that the recipient has an obligation to accept that person's influence. Legitimate power is often derived from the position of a manager in the organizational hierarchy. For example, a hospital administrator possesses more legitimate power than does the assistant administrator. This type of power is the authority vested in a role of office that is accepted and recognized by the members of the organization. There are internalized values that dictate that the leader has the right to prescribe behavior for the follower in a given domain.

A fourth basis is *referent* power. It is based on a follower's identification with a leader. The leader is admired because of one or more personal traits, and the follower can be influenced because of this admiration or attraction or desire to emulate or to establish a friendly relationship with the leader.

The fifth basis for power, *expert* power, varies with the extent of knowledge the follower attributes to the leader. The leader with this type of power is someone with expertise or special skill or knowledge. The possession of one or more of these characteristics gains the respect and compliance of peers and personnel. However, it is interesting to note that the important factor for this power base is not the actual "extent" of knowledge possessed by the expert, but the amount of knowledge that is "attributed" to her by others. In other words, as far as expert power is concerned, it's not so much what you know, but what people *think* you know.

The sixth kind of power, *informational* power, is based on the content of the communication between the leader and follower. The most important characteristic of informational influence is that it is socially independent of the source. The basis of this power is the information communicated. It is the content of the communication that is important, not the nature of the influencing agent (French & Raven, 1968).

A number of studies have shown that the bases of one person's power over another vary with the individual's relative position in an organizational hierarchy. Those persons in positions of superiority, by virtue of their status, have greater access to legitimate, reward, and coercive power. Their expert and referent power, if they possess any, are power sources brought to the position by the person herself. Legitimate, reward, and coercive power tend to be attributed to people in superior positions, while referent, informational, and sometimes expert power are more common in situations where there is a more equal distribution of power, such as among peers. These six sources of social power might be reclassified into two major categories: (1) power based primarily on organizational factors, and (2) power based on individual factors; or, in other words, personal power coexists with situational power.

Others contend that power based on individual factors may be of two types: one type of power is original or unique and puts the person who has it in a class by herself; the second type of power locates the individual in the context of a group with distinguished abilities. People in positions of political leadership have been of either type, and any one leader is not necessarily both (Deloughery & Gebbie, 1975).

a basis for personal power

A strong, intact self-concept and heightened and ever-growing self-esteem form the foundation for one's personal power. Erich Fromm (1956) described the active element of love as primarily giving, not receiving. Some people interpret "giving" as "giving up"; "it is better to give than to receive" suggests that there is more virtue in suffering deprivation than in experiencing joy. For others, giving is the ultimate expression of power. "In the very act of giving I experience my strength, wealth, and *power.*" Fromm says that "love" involves care, responsibility, respect, and knowledge. These elements are interdependent and are found in the mature person who develops her own power in a productive way, who has given up fantasies of omnipotence, who wants primarily what she has worked for, and who has acquired humility based on inner strength.

That women are socialized not to be self-actualizing people in today's society is an issue that has received much attention in recent years. Women are urged to consider whether they are doing the "right" thing and whether their actions will please others. The act of pleasing others and doing the right thing may happen at the expense of their own growth and personal power. The secondary status of women has caused society to envision them in the roles of helpmate, nurturer, and "beloved imbecile" (Grissum & Spengler, 1976).

Established values govern every society. These cultural norms or behaviors are believed to be appropriate for individuals according to their sex. Every society uses its major institutions to reinforce the behavioral norms it has established and changes them only as the needs of society change. Throughout history, behavior appropriate for women has centered around reproduction, which has been assumed to be central in a woman's life. The health care system with all of its institutions has been used to legitimize societal views of appropriate feminine behavior. In much of psychiatry, women have been viewed as essentially "breeders and bearers—potentially warm-hearted creatures but primarily simple cranky children with uteri, forever mourning the loss of male organs and male identity" (Chesler, 1971).

These attitudes are attributable, in part, to the writings of Sigmund Freud. His theories of personality development tended to deny that women had individual identities; instead, his notions of a castration complex and penis envy assumed that women were biologically inferior to men. Freud's disciples expanded the concept of femininity to include such adjectives as passive, unstable, intuitive, dependent, inconsistent, weak, empathetic, subjective, and sensitive. By contrast, men were seen as independent, aggressive, task-oriented, competitive, self-disciplined, stoic, rational, analytical, objective, confident, and controlled. Witness the following comparative statements that might fall under "sexist semantics":

He is well-travelled	She's been around
He is under pressure	She must be getting her period
He's contemplating an idea	She's indecisive
He's highly organized	She's obsessive-compulsive
He's powerful	She's castrating

It is true that some of the characteristics attributed to women have positive connotations in our society; however, many of these traits are seen as negative. Conversely, those characteristics ascribed to men are ones that are strongly valued in American society—as long as they are held by men. Women who have tried to emulate some of the so-called male attributes, women who have veered from the often passive roles of wife, mother, and noncompetitor and who have attempted to function in roles traditionally considered to be male, have been regarded as suspect, if not outright abnormal. These sex-appropriate behaviors supported by popular scientific thought have been the underpinnings for the development of different educational programs for the sexes, for career counseling, and for determining different areas of employment. Such sex-linked stereotypes are still prevalent and are reinforced in children's books (although not as much as before), textbooks, various communications media, and through advertising. Thus, children learn early on what behaviors are expected of them, and these behaviors are carefully cultivated.

Society seems to support the posture that femininity and achievement are mutually incompatible. Matina Horner (1974) conducted a long-term study that provided evidence that many women have a motive in avoiding success. The college women in her study became anxious about attaining success because they expected negative outcomes if they did, such as social rejection or feelings of being unfeminine. Horner stated that "women still tend to view competition, independence, intellectual achievement and leadership as basically in conflict with femininity." She concluded from her research that higher education for women was believed to be more acceptable if its purpose was to contribute to a more interesting wife, mother, and helpmate.

The anxiety that women experience about success is often costly. Many young women perform at lower levels when they are placed in competitive situations with men. Those who are successful often denigrate their own performance in the presence of males. It is not unusual to note that successful men are often described according to their occupational role; however, women, if and when they are described as successful, are so characterized in terms of their sex role. If women are described as successful according to their avocation, it may sound like this: "She's a good doctor—for a woman" or "She's a remarkable district attorney, and she's pretty, too."

Competition may be problematic in yet another way. Novelist Erica Jong (1977) notes that:

Every woman who has ever excelled in her field knows that the bitterest experience of all is the lack of support, the envy, the bitterness we frequently get from our female colleagues. We are hard on ourselves and hard on each other, and women not only hold support from other women, they openly attack. We have too little charity for each other's work, and are too apt to let the male establishment pit us against each other. [p. 11]

It appears that not only are women's career opportunities narrowed and their aspirations diminished, but many women seem to remove themselves from competition when faced with the conflict between their feminine image and the pursuit of their real potential. The way to success is highly complicated and intricately designed. It contains many elements such as responsibility, respect, power, persistence, and self-determination, among others. We would do well to scrutinize these factors before leaping into action—or inaction.

seeing for yourself

Look hard at the setting in which you work or are being educated. What is the operant value system? Which behaviors are being rewarded? What items appear on the evaluation forms? Are evaluative statements unilateral? Are you being socialized into a dependent, passive role, or does your position demand accountability, independence, and responsibility? In which role do you seem more comfortable? Why?

Now propose 10 strengths you recognize in yourself. Do you use them? Does your educational or work environment support them and help you to grow? Do others in your environment recognize your strengths? Do you share the knowledge of your strengths with others?

Now think about the last time you performed successfully. Did you believe that your success could be attributed to your abilities? When did you last fail at a task? Did you feel that your lack of success was due to your inability? Did you discuss this failure with others? Did others serve as a support system for you?

What is your present salary? Does it reflect your worth? Is it similar to the salaries of others who have the same education, experi-ential qualifications, and levels of responsibility?

Now think about the last time you felt powerless. Who or what seemed more powerful? Why was power important at that time? What militated against your achievement of power?

Now identify the last time someone studying or working with you was successful at something. How did you feel in their presence? Did you congratulate them? Did you support them? When was the last time you were working or studying with someone who failed at something? How did you feel? What did you say? Were you a support? (Brooten, Hayman & Naylor, 1978)

Responses to these questions are undoubtedly a reflection of the extent to which we have been socialized into more or less stereotypical roles. It is hoped that these questions will provide a springboard from which we can continue to explore and enhance our bases for personal power.

supplicant communication

Women can have expert knowledge, but if they can't communicate their ideas to others clearly, forcefully, and fluently, they will have little power or influence. Women can possess expert skill, but if they can't demonstrate their skills to others and facilitate action, they will have little power and influence. Women can have an excellent organization, but if they can't sell their products and services to others, the activities of the organization will be underused and unappreciated.

To say that our educational system has not been highly successful in teaching us the rudiments of effective communication is an understatement. We continue to have difficulty in speaking up and speaking out, in presenting logical, meaningful arguments, in modifying opinions and attitudes through persuasive communication. Ineffectual delivery coupled with poorly selected vocabulary can serve only to weaken the impact of excellent ideas. Many women lack confidence when confronted with public speaking. This state of affairs may be due in part to years of conditioning ("Silence is a women's glory") or a belief that what we have to say is unimportant and therefore not worthy of being heard by others. We have few female role models who are excellent orators. Women also seem to believe that their conversation is trivial. How many of you have noticed that women tend to use more "polite" constructions: "Would it be all right if we . . .?" or "tag" questions: "Won't you please . . .?" Women are more likely to say, "Goodness, the health care system is in a mess, isn't it?" Men are more often heard saying declarative statements and clear commands. Others have found that even when women do use declarative sentences to express opinions, they frequently use intonation patterns that make them sound like questions (LeRoux, 1978). It is no surprise, then, that women seem less confident, more deferential, and in need of approval.

What do we do about supplicant communication? Hereafter, desist from asking permission to speak, to think, or to act. Substitute declaration for supplication. Rather than "Would you mind if I ask a question?" use "I'd like to know if . . ." Prisoners and slaves (and children, sometimes) are required to ask permission, and we all know that stories about well-adjusted prisoners and slaves have no basis in fact.

It seems unnecessary to belabor the point because the facts are well documented, but our communication patterns reflect a great deal of sexism. The apparent marginality of women is recognizable in the dominant "maleness" of the English language. The ordinary person is always male—"man in the street."

Note the stereotypic bias reflected in the following words: "sissy," derived from the word "sister," suggests timidity, while "buddy," from "brother," suggests friendship or closeness. The male gender is associated with high-ranking positions. Witness the fact that the masculine pronoun is applied to physicians, lawyers, diplomats, and others. This linguistic sexism invades our life, and we have accepted it without challenge—until recently. However, an increased awareness—sensitive antennae—of such elements in the communication process may contribute to a more influential, powerful style of oratory among women. Relearning does occur. Attitudes do change.

HOOKERS: HOW TO AVOID USING POWER*

Restrainer
I lead a very stainless life
And have from the beginning.
A pillar, I, of rectitude—
I never think of sinning.

Oh, not for me the wanton sins
That others may parade to.
It's not that I'm a saintly soul
It's just that I'm afraid to.

Georgie Starbuck Galbraith (1971)

That little poem seems to capture the essence of a point that is interesting to ponder—the extent to which women seem to be hooked on avoidance mechanisms that interfere with the effective use of power. The first of these is guilt, that luxurious emotion that absolves us from changing our behavior, taking risks, assuming unpopular stances, or initiating action. It helps us to avoid the anticipated pain of change.

"Catastrophizing" (Donnelly, 1979) is a process through which we avoid taking a positive action by imagining that the very worst is about to happen. When we catastrophize, we

*Reprinted by permission of the author.

feel guilty and continue in our old patterns. Once again, our educational system contributes to this process. And, to some extent, the health care system abets catastrophizing in that we are taught to anticipate the worst. It is a habit that prepares us for possible emergencies and thus is protective. But when this process is carried over into other areas of our lives, it may be detrimental. Anticipating an emergency in our health status is quite different from anticipating a disaster every time we assert our rights or express opinions.

Catastrophizing is the bridge that connects guilt with fear. Fear is internal; it is sustained by a thought system that we prevail on to help us avoid confronting our own self-imposed dread. Wayne Dyer (1979) states: "If you started on a scavenger hunt today and you were told to bring back a bucket full of fear, you could look forever, but you'd always come home empty-handed." Consider the following statements:

> I'll fail.
> I'll appear stupid.
> I'm not certain.
> They might not approve.
> I'd feel guilty.
> That would make them angry.
> I won't get into heaven.
> Something awful will happen if I do that.
> I couldn't stand myself if I did that.

Do those words sound all too familiar? Such statements tend to immobilize us and prevent us from operating from a position of power and influence.

Another avoidance mechanism we invoke from time to time is shame. Shame might be seen as the penalty for not pleasing, and for women, pleasing is often a high priority. No one enjoys feelings of shame, but women are doubly threatened because avoiding public shame has been part of our socialization. Confronting shame necessitates risking disappointment, ridicule, and frustration. Vulnerability is inherent in risking shame. Those women who are frequent risk-takers comment on their sense of extreme vulnerability, both in the positive and negative senses of the word.

If it is a valid assumption that avoidance mechanisms such as guilt, fear, and shame interfere with the effective use of power, then some caveats about avoidance mechanisms are in order: (1) begin to recognize these patterns in yourself and others, (2) stand back, take some distance, and try to maintain perspective and objectivity, (3) simplify things, (4) try to decipher *what* is happening first before puzzling over *why* it is happening, (5) address goals rather than problems, and (6) simplify things if possible.

influence: its use and misuse

In any situation where two people interact, they influence each other in some way. At times the influence we exert is quite deliberate; at other times, unintentional. Influence is a natural consequence of living and interacting. Therefore, while the consequences of influence may be good or bad according to each person's point of view, the fact of influence is very natural and expected. Have you ever considered the ways in which we create that special impact? People's styles of influence tend to cluster within some common dimensions. That is, while we influence one another in our own unique way, at the same time some

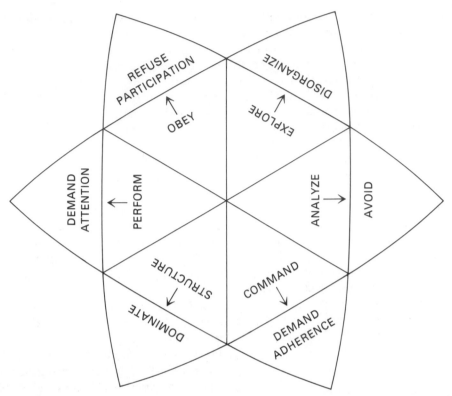

figure 29.1
spheres of influence

recognizable patterns emerge that facilitate the development of a general classification system. Furthermore, these styles can be changed.

Figure 29.1 is an arbitrary model of some of the common styles of influence. It consists of three dimensions: performing vs. analyzing, commanding vs. obeying, and structuring vs. exploring. Although these categorizations may be an oversimplification, they also may be thought-provoking. Several comments must be made before each domain is examined. No one dimension is mutually exclusive of another. An individual can be a com-

mander and an explorer simultaneously. It is reasonable and preferable that people are capable of functioning in more than one sphere. Each sphere or any combination of spheres is value-free. Each of us must decide which we prefer according to our predetermined goals. These spheres reflect our individual preferences, that is, the performer prefers to perform. Most of us behave in a designated way because of the effect it produces.

PERFORMING VS. ANALYZING. Spontaneity and applause are the hallmarks of the performer, while insight and understanding are the hallmarks of the analyzer. This is not to say, however, that the performer is without insight, or vice versa. Rather, it is a continuum of degree and emphasis. The impact of these styles of influence are productive if they are not carried to the extreme. The performer often causes others to experience pleasure, relaxation, and enjoyment, while the analyzer whets the curiosity of others and stimulates respect. However, when either of these styles becomes extreme, the negative effects of these behaviors are felt. The performer comes to demand excessive attention; the analyzer comes to appear aloof and unreachable.

COMMANDING VS. OBEYING.   The commander's style of influence is to encourage others to strive diligently toward a common goal. She seeks allegiance and is characterized by confidence. The obeyer seeks the support of the group and pursues the tasks necessary to achieve success. She seeks affiliation and is characterized by allegiance. She is the loyal member. However, when the commander extends her authority to the extent that she demands all-consuming adherence, others become resentful. Conversely, the loyal member, in the extreme, may become a spectator, a nonparticipant who tends to isolate herself from the group.

STRUCTURING VS. EXPLORING.   The explorer is the creative soul, that reactive person who adopts a serendipity attitude toward life. Each day is a new adventure; life is a mystery to be lived. For the structurer, life is a problem to be solved. Organization and planning are of paramount importance in success. No plan is tantamount to chaos. In the extreme configuration, the explorer is loose, disorganized, and fragmented, qualities that cause others some considerable irritation and frustration. When the structurer's behavior becomes excessive, she becomes perfectionistic, controlling, and others feel limited by her task-orientation (Strickland & Arnn, 1977).

The reader is probably evaluating this section by applying these concepts to herself. In so doing, she might be asking herself some questions. With what style of influence am I most comfortable? What is its impact on others? What is the impact of other's behavior on me? Do I recognize some of these characteristics in me? Am I satisfied with my impact on others? To what extent has our socialization as women contributed to our assuming the more extreme configurations in our styles of influence? To what extent do these extreme configurations impede our effective use of personal power?

model for personal power assessment

What follows (see Figure 29.2) is a somewhat tongue-in-cheek test for the reader to assess her own basis for personal power. The basis for personal power is seen as a triangle, the axes of which are "actions and results," "professional expertise," and "style of influence." Those purists in research methods will undoubtedly feel that the scientific basis for this instrument is suspect. Indeed, that is the case. The items are all everyday occurrences that cause us some consternation. Our responses to these situations are complicated and often reflect elements unrelated to our sense of personal power. Nevertheless, this test is offered as a way to encourage further exploration and perhaps discussion among friends.

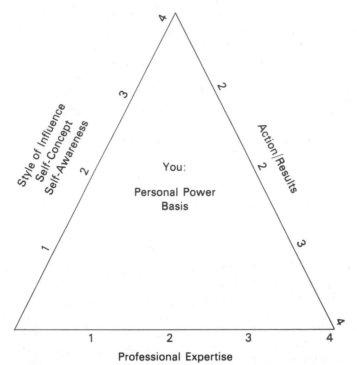

figure 29.2
a model for personal power assessment

	1 Almost Never	2 Seldom	3 Usually	4 Almost Always
Instructions: Circle the number that most closely represents your response.				

ACTION/RESULTS

1. When you receive a well-done steak in a restaurant and you asked for it rare, you eat it well done because you don't want to cause a problem.	1	2	3	4
2. If someone next to you is smoking and the smoke is causing you discomfort, you continue to sit there and say nothing in order not to offend the smoker.	1	2	3	4
3. If someone pushes ahead of you in line, you say nothing and let him stay, but you are furious.	1	2	3	4
4. If you are confronted with the dilemma of sending out greeting cards during the holidays when you'd rather not do it, you buy the cards, address the envelopes, pay the postage, and hate every minute of it.	1	2	3	4

5. If you are rushed for time and you see a long line at a checkout counter in the grocery store, you wait in line and fume over the lack of help and the fact that you are being unnecessarily delayed. 1   2   3   4

6. If you are asked to make arrangements for a party when you would rather not do so, you go ahead and do it and feel upset that you are always the one who does it. 1   2   3   4

7. If a neighbor's dog is barking loudly in the morning and disturbing your sleep, you lie there and get angry. 1   2   3   4

8. If you need three onions at the grocery store, but all the onions are in two-pound bags, you either get no onions or buy the two pounds you don't need. 1   2   3   4

9. If, after having returned home, you notice that you have been overcharged 69 cents on your grocery bill, you do nothing because you don't want to return to the store and because people will think you are cheap to complain about such an insignificant amount. 1   2   3   4

10. If your doctor tells you to return for a second visit for some problem, although your problem has obviously been resolved, you return on schedule, report that you are fine, and pay for the visit. 1   2   3   4

TOTAL THE NUMBER OF POINTS FOR THE FIRST 10 ITEMS AND DIVIDE BY 10:_____

	1 Almost Never	2 Seldom	3 Usually	4 Almost Always
STYLE OF INFLUENCE/SELF-CONCEPT/ SELF-AWARENESS				

1. If you are a stranger at a social gathering, you hang back and hope that someone will invite you to participate in the discussion. You are uneasy. 1   2   3   4

2. If you are late, or if you wish to leave early, you tend to overapologize. 1   2   3   4

3. If people say to you, "How can you do this to me?" or "If you cared about me you would . . . " or "You are really disappointing me . . . " you feel guilty. 1   2   3   4

4. If someone tries to entice you into his own personal gloom, you listen to the person's complaints and eventually feel as sad as the other person. 1   2   3   4

	1 Almost Never	2 Seldom	3 Usually	4 Almost Always
5. If someone makes an unrealistic demand on you, you have difficulty saying "no."	1	2	3	4
6. If you feel that you have been abused, you avoid asking to see supervisors.	1	2	3	4
7. If your doctor or dentist calls you by your first name, it is nonetheless difficult for you to call him/her by his/her first name.	1	2	3	4
8. If your doctor keeps you waiting over an hour for an appointment for which you arrived on time, you say nothing, because you understand how busy and important doctors are.	1	2	3	4
9. If someone compliments you about something, no matter how small, your whole day is "made."	1	2	3	4
10. If someone criticizes you in a negative manner, you are crushed.	1	2	3	4

TOTAL THE NUMBER OF POINTS FOR THESE 10 ITEMS
AND DIVIDE BY 10:_____

PROFESSIONAL EXPERTISE	1 Almost Never	2 Seldom	3 Usually	4 Almost Always
1. If competitive situations arise on the job, you tend to shy away from them.	1	2	3	4
2. If your employer asks you to stay late and you have another important engagement, you break your engagement and work.	1	2	3	4
3. If you have more things going on than you have room to accommodate in your busy calendar, you get tense, irritable, and try to do everything while devoting a minimal amount of time to each and giving nothing your complete attention.	1	2	3	4
4. If you are confronted with red tape and barriers erected by bureaucrats, you are easily befuddled.	1	2	3	4
5. If you feel that you deserve a promotion or a raise, you wait until your superior thinks it is time to do something for you.	1	2	3	4
6. If you are asked, you continue to sit on committees and participate in job-related rituals although it frustrates you.	1	2	3	4

7. If you stay home from work for legitimate reasons, or if you stay home *to* work, you worry about it.   1   2   3   4

8. If someone criticizes your work, you get nervous, explanatory, and upset.   1   2   3   4

9. If you are given an evaluation by your superior with which you disagree, you accept it and say nothing.   1   2   3   4

10. You seldom feel confident that people look up to you, respect you, and like your ideas, although you have received feedback to that effect.   1   2   3   4

TOTAL THE NUMBER OF POINTS FOR THE LAST 10 ITEMS AND DIVIDE BY 10:_____

PLOT YOUR SCORE FROM EACH CATEGORY ON EACH AXIS OF THE "PERSONAL POWER TRIANGLE" TO VISUALIZE YOUR PERSONAL POWER BASIS.

summary

Power is an attitude; it does not exist without a powerholder. No class of people, no minority group, no elite group can achieve or use power without organization. Behind that organization is a person. Power is invariably personal. Power, the ability to influence others to do as you wish in an effort to reach a goal, has two limitations: (1) the extraneous facts (everything else going on in the world), and (2) conscience or intellectual restraint (deciding what you cannot or what you will not do). How the powerholder will react is invariably personal (Berle, 1969).

Power is called a potentiality, that is, power is available if one chooses to use it. That is a loaded statement! The reality of that statement often comes as an "ah-ha" experience; it frequently comes in retrospect—after the precipitating event. My success in the case of the Volkswagen Rabbit was to cause me reverberations for some time to come (to say nothing of some exhilarating cocktail party conversation). I think about that effective exercise of personal power and I still smile, I still feel powerful. It behooves us to recognize the power we have in order to use it fully and wisely. On the other hand, if we overestimate our power and attempt to employ power we do not possess, we set ourselves up to fail. Power, that highly personal commodity, is vested in human beings—knowing, feeling women who are free to choose our courses of action. Power becomes an actuality rather than a potentiality when we decide to exercise it wisely.

Claus, E., & Bailey, J. T. *Power and influence in health care.* St. Louis: C. V. Mosby, 1977, p. 17.

Clark, C. C. Assert yourself! *Journal of Practical Nursing,* January 1979, p. 29.

French, J. R. P., Jr., & Raven, B. H. Bases of social power. In G. Lindzey and E. Aronson (Eds.), *Handbook of social psychology* (Vol. 4, 2nd ed.). Reading, Mass.: Addison-Wesley, 1968, pp. 166–184.

Deloughery, G. L., & Gebbie, K. M. *Political dynamics.* St. Louis: C. V. Mosby, 1975, p. 79.

Fromm, E. *The art of loving.* New York: Harper, 1956, p. 17.

Grissum, M. & Spengler, C. *Womanpower & health care.* Boston: Little, Brown, 1976, p. 246.

Chesler, P. Women as psychiatric and psychotherapeutic patients. *Journal of Marriage and the Family,* November 1971, *33,* p. 753.

Horner, M, and Walsh, M. Psychological barriers to success in women. In R. Kundsin (Ed.), *Women and success: The anatomy of achievement.* New York: Morrow, 1974, pp. 219–237.

Jong, E. Speaking of love. *Newsweek,* February 21, 1977, p. 11.

Brooten, D. A., Hayman, L., & Naylor, M. *Leadership for change: A guide for the frustrated nurse.* Philadelphia: Lippincott, 1978, pp. 56–57.

LeRoux, R. S., Communication and influence in nursing. *Nursing Administration Quarterly,* Spring 1978, *2,* pp. 51–57.

Galbraith, G. S., Restrainer, *Wall Street Journal,* October 5, 1971.

Donnelly, G. F., Frankly, Ms. Scarlett, I Can't Work Another Double. *RN,* January 1979, pp. 79–81.

Dyer, W. W. *Pulling your own strings.* New York: Avon, 1979, p. 32.

Strickland, B., & Arnn, V. Orientation on understanding interpersonal influence. *Journal of the American Dietetic Association,* September 1977, *71,* pp. 229–234.

Berle, A.A. *Power.* New York: Harcourt, 1969, pp. 37–134.

NANCY MILIO, R.N., Ph.D.

women
and the prospects for health

Without some major redirections in national policy, women's health—traditionally better than men's—will decline. The policies that will make the difference in women's vitality and freedom from disability and early death are not only, or even most importantly, those that concern health services. Rather, they are much broader, the ones that affect the things that *make health*.

What will best improve prospects for the health of women will also improve the health of all Americans. This reality should make it possible for women to involve themselves in many decision-making arenas in ways that will serve the health interests of the public—of their sons, husbands, and lovers, of future generations—as well as the interests of their own health as women.

what the future holds

What are the prospects for women's health, and how might they be made better?

By the year 2000, if women continue on their current paths, their health will become more like men's. A recent sophisticated study forecast that women will have higher death rates from heart and respiratory disease than they had in the mid-1970s, while men's rates

363

will decline. Women will almost reach men's high rates of death from cirrhosis. And they will not experience improvements from vascular and digestive conditions as much as men (Mushkin & Wagner, 1978).

This view of the turn-of-the-new-century stems from the social fact that women's lives are becoming increasingly like men's. Until recently, men have been the most vulnerable to modern forms of illness, to most of the serious chronic conditions that bring disability to the prime mid-decades of life and result in biologically early death, or a prolonged, constricted old age. Now, the new ways of women are making them also more vulnerable to ill health, adding to traditionally female health problems.

The warp and woof of new and old ways weave a modern pattern that looks something like this. Most obvious is the ever-growing share of women entering the "men's" world of paid work, and especially those with young children. More women are living alone, before or after marriage, and more are family heads. In other words, women's role in household economics is looking more like the traditional male role (Milio, 1979)

More paid work generally means more discretionary income for women and more freedom to purchase beyond the essentials. Women now buy and use more cigarettes and alcohol, more prescribed drugs, and often more food calories than they need. Women continue to be less physically active than men in work and sports, and so the "average" woman may be almost 20 percent heavier than her "ideal" weight (the weight best suited to long life). These are the habits well known to be linked to chronic lung, liver, and heart disease, as well as cancer, high blood pressure, diabetes, and other lifelong disabling conditions (Milio, 1981). About 70 percent of women's cancers are linked to their eating and

smoking habits (Gori, 1979). There is also evidence that women who both drink and smoke in moderation (less than 20 cigarettes and one or two drinks a day) are apparently far more vulnerable to cancers of the throat and larynx than men who follow the same habits (Schottenfeld, 1979).

But the traditional low-income status of women nevertheless remains. Almost one-third live in poverty. These, of course, are most vulnerable to both inflation and recession, to price rises in food, fuel, and shelter, to unemployment and low-paid jobs. Again, low income and poverty bring higher risk of almost every form of acute and chronic illness, as well as more severe consequences, like greater disability, more complications, and greater likelihood of death.

At the work places where they now spend increasing shares of their lives, women are no less exposed to the same job hazards as men, the chemicals, tars, noise, and injuries long faced in "men's" work. At the same time, they face the risks of more traditionally female employment, such as in hospital work, with its radiations, microorganisms, and rotating workshifts. And since women continue as well their traditional large role in such labor as agricultural field work, they confront the dangers there of pesticides and too-heavy, fatiguing tasks, especially hazardous if they are pregnant.

Yet, growing membership in the work-for-pay world has not reduced the burdens of household work. Women workers, compared with men, still spend an extra six hours in non-paid work each week, leaving that much less time for relaxation and healthful ways of coping with the strains of job and home.

Perhaps as a shortcut to deal with the new responsibilities, chosen or not, of job, career, family, and community, more women seek respite by overeating, drinking, or smoking.

More have elevated blood pressures and blood serum cholesterol, as well as excess body weight and increasing rates of chronic illness (Hayes et al., 1978; Milio, 1977). This is especially so for those in low-paid jobs or in administrative jobs, and those who attempt dual career-household roles.

All of these threats, from the requirements of job and household, the excesses of affluence or deficits from poverty, the short circuits to relief, new or old, compound the potential hazards of that sex-linked potential of women, childbearing or its prevention. It is now well known how overweight or underweight, smoking and alcohol, worksite hazards and fatigue, and previous illness endanger mother and baby, or, when avoiding pregnancy through certain contraceptives, place some women at risk of heart disease and cancer.

This merging of newer "male" economic-related patterns of job and buying power, with both their associated strains and promise, along with woman's traditional burdens of household and lower status and her childbearing potential, brings a not surprising prospect of poorer health for women. It also, however, offers clues to changing those prospects.

changing the future

Viewing the fabric of modern women's lives, woven as it is into the social, economic, and technological changes occurring in American living, makes clear that improvements in health services alone will do little to alter the prospects for women's health. At best, the health care system may detect and treat women on an equal basis with men, as they acquire heart or liver disease or cancer, thereby allowing women to enter old age with as much disability as men, prolonging life that is accompanied by debility. Changes in policy that affect the financing and delivery of services could indeed, and should, give women more options as to where to obtain health services and from whom. Changes could provide easier access to ambulatory and in-home care as well as safer and less costly forms of treatment. Policy improvement could offer full maternity and preconception benefits, now grossly underfunded. Such changes will improve the short-term prospects for the health of low-income women especially.

But they will do virtually nothing that can effectively prevent the onset of those chronic conditions that are the greatest and growing threat to women's health—to which poorer women are even more vulnerable than the more affluent. Nor will the prevalent emphasis on reproduction-related health problems of women help solve their larger problem of chronic illness.

The real health policy issues—those that most affect the health of women and of all Americans—extend far beyond health services policy. They include economics and employment, environment and energy, agriculture and food, and substance abuse control. For it is these that make the difference in shaping the options and the opportunities available to women throughout their lives. They lay out the array of the possible from which women may only then choose how they will live. These policies—whether or not part of woman's consciousness—determine how likely will be their chances for job and adequate earnings; how clean their air, water, and food; how safe their workplace, house, and travel; how sedentary their employment or modes of transportation; how easy for them to buy health-limiting products instead of health-promoting ones.

In other words, these policies are the shapers of the environments in which women live, strongly affecting the stresses with which women must deal, strongly influencing the patterns of living, the life-style they have.

For example, economic policies that allow widespread unemployment affect women more than men in several ways. Not only do women workers bear a higher share of job loss, but their deteriorating income begins at a lower base income, threatening food and shelter. Under these circumstances, chronic illness is known to increase. Furthermore, pregnant women, employed or not, are at greater risk of complications in their newborn children when they are part of an unemployed household.

In the special case of employment policy related to health services, women are especially affected. If the frequently discussed and needed shifts in health care occur, providing more services in ambulatory centers than in hospitals, the burden of job loss would fall on women since they form the largest components of hospital personnel, especially at the lower paid rungs. The shift to ambulatory care will indeed benefit both women patients and, eventually, health workers, because of the smaller, safer, more personable working conditions inherent in noninstitutional care. Nevertheless, the burden of change—income loss, uncertainty, and the risks to health associated with them—will be borne unfairly by women workers unless compensating transition policies are included. These might provide phased job retraining and relocation of workers at ambulatory centers, early retirement benefits for some, and adequate income

maintenance for those adversely affected.

So, clearly, policies affecting adult education, job training, public service employment, and unemployment insurance, among others, are of special importance to women and their health. This is even more true for women in farm and domestic work, two occupations not at all protected by unemployment insurance and minimally by Social Security retirement benefits or health insurance programs.

So seemingly remote an issue as energy policy is also very directly related to the problems of women's health. For example, policy aimed at using alternative sources of energy rather than current dependence on nonrenewable fossil fuels would mean new health-promoting options for women. It would include using people-power, women-power, that is, the ever-renewable source of energy based in people's ability to learn and do; it would mean more labor-intensive (not energy-intensive) jobs and small-scale technology. And these most easily could be developed on a community-specific basis, providing as well for currently unmet needs. This might include services for health, recreation, nontraditional education, home assistance, housing repair, child care, and transportation. It could link distant schools, colleges, and industries to houses and neighborhoods through communications media, developing modern "cottage industries" and localized training and education.

These new directions would not only create jobs and meet community needs, but would offer more personalized worksites, safer working conditions, and consume less energy by reducing the need for constructing and operating large buildings. It would save transportation costs and fuel and also lower the air pollution resulting from vehicle traffic. And while clearing the air, it would diminish the need to use (and the hazards of) cars, thereby allowing more walking and time for exercise. The advantages of home and community-based work and education are especially great for women with young children and elders, most of whom are women.

Another area that at first glance may seem removed from women's health issues is the policy link between energy and agriculture. The most energy-intensive and, therefore, costly and inflationary agricultural and food products are beef and its feed grains, tobacco, and processed sugar goods. These are also among the high health risk consumer products for Americans, being implicated in chronic heart and lung diseases, high blood pressure, stroke, cancer, diabetes, stomach ulcers, acute respiratory problems, some maternity-related disorders, and dental caries. There is also sound economic evidence to show that a wide array of farm, economic, and tax policies favor the production, processing, and consumption of these risky products compared with the more health-promoting components of the national food supply, such as wheat, dairy, soy and peanut products, potatoes, and fresh fruits and vegetables. According to recommendations developed by over a dozen panels of experts from several countries including the United States, the food supply of Americans is the most risky for health of any of the advanced industrial nations.

This means, in short, that public farm-food policy is providing an array of consumer options for Americans in which the health-limiting types are easier to choose—because of availability, cost, convenience, promotion, attractiveness, and so on—than the more health-promoting types, and the former bring far higher profits than the latter. Given women's increasing buying power, as well as their increasing dual-role strains, it is predictable that they will be consuming more of the health-limiting products and so become increasingly exposed to the health risks associated with them.

If, indeed, policy affecting women's and all Americans' health encompasses a spectrum from economics to agriculture, as well as health services, how would women induce the policy changes necessary to improve their prospects for health? How might they gain support for such health-making policies as the development of sources of renewable energy and other useful-job-creating thrusts; for adequate retraining and income maintenance during periods of transition in people's lives; for full use of environmental and occupational health and safety measures, and development of a health-promoting national farm-food supply?

The task is formidable and the stakes are high, in health and well-being, as well as dollars. It is not the work of individuals struggling alone. It requires organized strategies. It is not an effort obviously for the women's movement alone, but one requiring alliances with all groups who seek health-generating, health-making changes in American life.

Opposition to such changes is strong. It is found in the lobbies financed by industries whose economic interests are involved, often including those in health services. These lobbies have grown rapidly in recent years. Industry influence has expanded further through election campaigns seen in the unprecedented proliferation of new political action committees.

At the same time, there may be readiness among segments of the public to respond to clear, understandable, consistent leadership. Women voters for instance, as well as blacks, the poor, and elders, believe they have little influence and that the major party leaders do not act in their interests. In opinion polls, the public has favored health improvement policies concerning food, smoking, safety, and economic security.

Furthermore, the health-making policies mentioned here have been, and are increasingly being, implemented in other affluent nations. There, not only are the chances for life in infants and elders better, but the rates of chronic disease in the middle years of life are lower, especially among women. Such policies are then possible to undertake and do show potential for improved prospects for health.

legislation and organization

In the 1970s, national legislation provided legal tools to allow consumers, employees, and citizens to monitor, question, and to some extent alter the direction of public policy decisions. This includes such health-important areas as pollution control, occupational safety and health, consumer product safety, and, to a lesser extent, drug and medical device effectiveness and safety. Beyond these, the National Health Planning and Development Act of 1974, which was slowly implemented, requires a 60 percent consumer majority on the policy boards of the over 200 health systems agencies (HSA's), which now cover the entire American population. These consumer members are to reflect in general the population of the area in age, race, income, language, and rural-urban residence. Women, however, have not been, nor were they required through the implementing regulations to be, proportionately represented among either consumer or health care provider members of these boards.

The statutory purpose of the HSA's is to develop plans that will both improve the health of, and health services for, the community population. The scope of their work is, therefore, very broad, encompassing environmental and workplace issues, vehicle and product safety, nutrition, smoking and, of course, personal health services. In reality, to the end of the 1970s, the overwhelming focus of HSA's has been on personal health services, and more specifically on cost-containment issues centering on reducing the supply of unneeded hospital beds. In one exceptional and much publicized case, an HSA did seriously address the wider areas of health promotion in its plans. Having thus threatened a number of vested interests, this brought a flurry of legislative amendments in Congress proposing to restrict both the scope and authority of the HSA's.

As this experience illustrates, while it is necessary to have legal and administrative channels to bring about policy changes, they do not in themselves assure that the health-promoting intent of policy is carried out. Active participation is needed at the local level, on HSA boards, and in other health-affecting programs, in workplace organizations, such as unions and professional groups, and in electoral processes, promoted and all backed by women's and other groups who can be mutually supportive.

Among the local, health-making changes that such groups might influence are, for example, full access to Food Stamp and the Women's, Infants and Children (WIC) supplemental food programs; provision of more healthful food options in eating places, markets, cafeterias, and vending machines; segregated smoking areas; development of child care arrangements; affirmative-action hiring, training, and promotion programs. Educational, consciousness-raising efforts can be directed not only at women, or the general public, but may be more effective by targeting local opinion leaders, including journalists and broadcasters. Local television will and must allow time for messages that provide alternative views of events. Talk shows and newspaper stories are often not difficult to arrange.

Such activity, of course, requires organization and, therefore, funds, however small. It also requires a degree of consensus on the priority of issues, backed by a strategy that can encompass the spectrum of problems most important for women's health.

Even so, local endeavors in communities, worksites, schools, health facilities, public agencies, and governments are not enough. Increasingly, the shape of local policies, both governmental and within private organizations and businesses, flows from national policy. Too often local efforts can be cut off by national changes in legislation or regulation, just as the potential of the HSA's may in the 1980s be measureably stifled by Congressional amendments.

This means, then, that local efforts must be linked to national organizations, which can monitor and attempt to influence policy at that level. Furthermore, a national unit can more efficiently provide essential resources that cannot be easily duplicated in every local group. This includes leadership training, materials development, consultation on legal, communications, and technical issues, provision of expert witnesses for public hearings, coordination with other groups' efforts and not least, analysis and interpretation of the vast amounts of publicly available data that goes unused, even though it can document both current problems and the soundness of a variety of solutions. Accurate and usable "translations" of these data would go far toward getting the health message across to

women, to the mass media, the general public, and policymakers. It is an essential part of the constant task to goad government to act in the public interest, which includes its health interests.

With so broad and complex a set of problems as are involved in improving the health prospects for women, and all Americans, it is only women acting together, organized, who can hope to acquire the essential information and other resources to pursue the necessarily sustained effort and do so with timely and realistic tactics. National and local links are required as well as alliances with other groups who share some of the same concerns. The breadth of health issues is such that many alliances are possible. The seriousness of the issues, the scope of their impact on today's and future generations, if not the likelihood of success, make the venture worthwhile.

If organizations do their job in influencing policy decisions—and if women entering policy positions do theirs—so that more healthful options become available to women, then women as individuals will have a less weighty burden. When the individual woman eventually faces her choices in clinic, on campus, at the personnel office or marketplace, she will not be required, as so often now, to engage in a fruitless struggle to create a more healthful option than is available to her; to pay an excessively high personal cost in time, energy, anxiety, money, or dignity. She will, rather, have a choice to make among more, healthful options, finally *enabling* her to "take responsibility for her own health."

Gori, G. Dietary and nutritional implications in the multifactorial etiology of certain prevalent human cancers. *Cancer,* May 1979, *43,* 2151-61, Suppl.

Haynes, S. et al. The relationship of psychosocial factors to coronary heart disease in the Framingham study. *Am J Epi,* Pt. 1, 1978, *107,* 362-400.

Milio, N. A women's view of women at work: A different view? An analytic summary of the literature in

Symposium on Occupational Safety and Health 1979. Washington, DC: National Institutes of Occupational Health and Safety, 1979.

Milio, N. Health policy and women's health. *Health Care Management Rev.*, April 1977.

Milio, N. *Promoting health through public policy.* Philadelphia: Davis, 1981.

Mushkin S., & Wagner, D. Expected mortality as a criterion in health policy evaluation, rep. no. 12. Washington, D.C.: Georgetown Univ. Public Services Lab., 1978.

Schottenfeld, D. Alcohol as a co-factor in the etiology of cancer. *Cancer*, May 1979, 43, 1962-66, Suppl.